DR. ATKINS'
HEALTH
REVOLUTION

DR. ATKINS' HEALTH REVOLUTION

How Complementary Medicine Can Extend Your Life

. . .

ROBERT C. ATKINS, M.D.

HOUGHTON MIFFLIN COMPANY · BOSTON · 1988

Library of Congress Cataloging-in-Publication Data

Atkins, Robert C.

Dr. Atkins' health revolution : how complementary medicine can
extend your life / Robert C. Atkins.

p.   cm.

Bibliography: p.

Includes index.

ISBN 0-395-46780-2

1. Low-carbohydrate diet.   2. Diet therapy — Case studies.
I. Title.

RM237.73.A83   1988   88-12827

615.8'54 — dc19   CIP

Printed in the United States of America

P 10 9 8 7 6 5 4 3 2 1

Dedicated to the memory of
CARLTON FREDERICKS, PH.D.,
who was my mentor and the mentor of many
of the great minds
in Complementary Medicine

Contents

Preface

Although this is a book that very plainly explains highly effective nutritional and other treatments for a number of serious illnesses, it should not be used as a manual for *self*-diagnosis and *self*-treatment. Such treatment is always potentially hazardous, even when the elements of the treatment are as safe as the nutrients prescribed by a complementary doctor.

Therefore, the author and the publisher cannot take responsibility for changes in your medical and nutritional program that have not also been approved by your personal physician.

It is almost certainly in your best interest to find a responsible and caring physician who will work with you and guide the course of your treatment.

I urge you to find a doctor who is sympathetic to the idea of using good nutrition and the techniques of Complementary Medicine before drug therapy. Allow the physician to know your medical status thoroughly, and give him or her the responsibility to make the medical decisions appropriate to your condition.

Robert C. Atkins, M.D.

BOOK ONE

. . .

THE
PHILOSOPHY

• • •

INTRODUCTION

To those of you who don't know me, and to those who think they do but really don't, allow me to introduce myself.

I am not a writer who happens to be a doctor; rather, I am a practicing physician, happily burdened with the responsibilities of providing a unique kind of patient care and of running an extremely large, hectic outpatient center devoted to a new type of medical practice. I am a writer only during those all-too-few remaining moments of spare time that any sensible person would devote to his family and to relaxation.

I would not be sacrificing my cherished personal time to write this book if I had not learned from my day-to-day experiences in medical care of a need — and of a solution to that need — of such far-reaching significance that it had to be made known to the public.

The need is to replace the present system of medicine, which has begun to petrify around its own mistakes. The solution is a new medicine, which is best described by the name Complementary Medicine.

I write, therefore, as a physician. This book is a statement of the philosophy that accompanies me on my daily rounds, as I share in the medical and health decisions of my patients, who truly represent a cross section of patienthood. I apply the same philosophy in dealing with other physicians — those I work with, those I would like to work with, and those I could never work with.

My Philosophy

This book describes the rationale underlying the medical system I see evolving around me. It explains why, when Joe Smith asks me, "What can you give me for my headache?" I say, "Instructions on how to make sure you never get another one." And why, when Lester Lesnorsdorfel asks me, "What's my diagnosis, Doc?" I say, "You're a Lester Lesnorsdorfel, and there's no one else like you. I can describe the ways you are not in perfect harmony, but I don't want to give you a diagnosis that puts you in a pigeonhole. I'm sure you don't want to be a pigeon."

This book also represents my responses to the questions of medical colleagues who have joined me to work in the Atkins Center for Complementary Medicine in New York City. In speaking with them, I've sometimes been forced to convince academically trained doctors that there is something more to medicine than what we've all been taught.

And this book represents an important way station in an ongoing odyssey that has taken me from the middle of the pack to a place where a wondrous, yet-to-be-defined system of healing is gradually being put into practice.

My Odyssey

My adventures began in 1963 when I discovered, for myself, the health benefits that accompanied the weight loss on a low-carbohydrate diet. I realized then that the sacred theory that weight changes could all be explained by calories had an obvious refutation, which was already neatly described in the scientific literature. Yet none of it was accepted because it ran counter to the existing dogma.

This taught me Personal Lesson Number One: *Medical dogma is not necessarily overcome by scientific observations.*

In 1972 I did for the first time what I am doing now. I stole time from my career as a practicing physician to write a book about what I had been doing successfully, because no one else was doing it and the story needed to be told. Thus was born *Dr. Atkins' Diet Revo-*

lution, the book for which I am best known, for it attained a total printing of 10 million copies in all of the world's major languages.

Since that book had been based on my experiences with the ten thousand patients I had treated between 1965 and 1972, its scientific observations were destined to stand the test of time, and I have never seen a single one of them scientifically refuted. But that did not stop the American Medical Association (AMA) from issuing a scathing indictment of my book, armed with innuendo and a recitation of "facts" that simply didn't apply. As disheartening as this was, it taught me several of my most important lessons.

More Lessons I Have Learned

From the AMA experience, I learned Personal Lesson Number Two: *Medicine, as an organization, acts more out of economic motives than scientific ones.*

Lesson Number Three: *Medicine often denies truths learned only from empirical observations.*

Lesson Number Four: *That which is true is not necessarily that which is accepted.*

Thus dislodged from my orthodox moorings, I began to seek my own personal truth as a physician, all the while conducting an extremely busy private practice. Through some process of natural selection, most of the patients who came to me in the seventies had disorders of carbohydrate metabolism. There were thousands who were simply obese, but there were even more who had diabetes, hypoglycemia, cardiovascular disorders, or hypertension — all conditions for which a low-carbohydrate diet is a perfect match. As I studied these patients' glucose and insulin responses to their dietary sugar, I began to see our culture-wide overconsumption of sugar (and other refined carbohydrates) as the cause, hyperinsulinism as the mediator, and obesity, diabetes, atherosclerosis, and hypertension as the consequences of a new twentieth-century epidemic that provided the lion's share of our medical problems. As I wrote this message in my 1977 book, *Dr. Atkins' Superenergy Diet*, I was learning Personal Lesson Number Five: *Virtually every patient can be benefited, and many can be treated fully, by arranging the diet to stabilize blood sugar.*

And Personal Lesson Number Six: *Understanding causation of disease can be more valuable than knowing the diagnosis.*

At the time my second book was published, my quest for an ever-expanding understanding of medicine was still proceeding. I began to see more patients with other illnesses and began to learn more and more nutritionally based techniques of treatment, a nutrition pharmacology, if you will. And I particularly noted that my patients benefited as much from their withdrawal from conventional medications as from the nutritional supplements they were given.

My book *Dr. Atkins' Nutrition Breakthrough* represented my learning two more important lessons.

Personal Lesson Number Seven: *Nutrients, which are enabling agents, provide a better therapy than do drugs, which are blocking agents.*

Personal Lesson Number Eight: *Working with nature is better medicine than opposing it. The body is capable of healing itself, if presented with the proper substances.*

Since You Heard from Me Last

My regular readers may have broken contact with me at that point and assumed that I was continuing my development as a medical nutritionist. This would have been a reasonable development.

But in fact, the quest has taken a somewhat different turn. I began to explore chelation therapy, herbal medicine, acupuncture, homeopathy, biologic medicine, immunology, bioenergetics, musculoskeletal techniques — a diverse mixture of healing arts, not necessarily nutritional, but with a single common denominator: All were *safer* modalities than those in common medical usage.

At the same time, I made a commitment to expand my practice from a one-man operation to a large medical center that would embrace valid practitioners of naturopathy, chiropractic, oriental medicine, and neurolinguistics, as well as physicians trained in immunology, biochemistry, and most of the medical specialities. I rejoiced in my patients' successes as I saw these component healing specialties work together with a beneficial synergy. I became absolutely certain that a greater and greater proportion of my patients were getting better and better with the combined approaches. As this exhilarating experience took place, I learned many more of my personal lessons.

The single most important lesson I learned, Personal Lesson Number Nine, is this: *Any valid healing art used on behalf of an individual can have an additive benefit when combined with other valid healing arts.* The corollary to this lesson is: *The greater the number of valid systems used, the greater is the probability of success.*

The New Medicine

This lesson, the lesson of Complementary Medicine, was a personal breakthrough for me. It led to a still-ongoing search through dozens of candidates within the scope of alternative medicine. As I found treatments that worked, they took their place alongside the orthodox medical-nutritional combination that was my basic therapy. The more alternative treatments I and my team of doctors had to draw on, the more were the successes of our patients. Not only did the majority of our patients get better, but those with seemingly incurable conditions such as cancer, crippling arthritis, and multiple sclerosis began to get better, too.

I can never go back to practicing orthodox medicine. I know it is too limited; there are too many areas it cannot enter. There are too many people it cannot help. *Orthodox medicine is not to be discarded; it is simply to be added to.* Once a physician knows what the additions can do, his ethics will not allow him to withhold them.

The War

Why do I talk here about withholding valid treatments? In case you haven't noticed, there's a war going on. It's a bitter ideological struggle, and at present one of the adversaries, orthodox medicine, clearly has the upper hand. The other healers, many of whom hardly notice they are involved in no-holds-barred combat, are threatened with loss of their practice, or even their license to practice, whenever they discover the validity of a healing system beyond the pale of medical orthodoxy and use it in an attempt to help their patients.

Before I tell you more about the remarkable discoveries that have been part of my odyssey, I would like to tell you about this struggle — who the participants are, how it came about, how it has extended to the present day, and what you and I can do about it.

The Three Types of Medicine

Let's start out by defining our terms. Throughout this book, I shall be referring to three types of medicine — orthodox, alternative, and complementary.

Orthodox medicine refers to the existing type of medicine taught in medical schools, practiced in all hospitals, and approved by the AMA, by the government, and by the third-party (insurance) carriers. You may also see it referred to as allopathic medicine, traditional medicine,* academic or school medicine, conventional medicine, establishment medicine, scientific medicine, or the dominant medicine.

Very few people ask me to define orthodox medicine. The reason for this is probably that it is the medicine we are all familiar with. Many people, on the other hand, ask me: What is alternative medicine? They are not familiar with that term. The definition I use is very simple — *whatever medicine is not orthodox medicine is alternative medicine.* Please bear in mind that my definition makes these two medicines mutually exclusive. That serves to keep the concepts straight, but it does not really conform to reality. In point of fact, there is a little bit of alternativist in most every orthodox physician and a little bit of orthodoxy in most alternativists.

What then is Complementary Medicine? It is the synthesis of these two medicines, put together in such a way as to integrate the best of both. Complementary Medicine must be the survivor of the struggle between orthodox and alternative medicine if we are to make any progress in our pursuit of good health.

There is another term that needs defining because it is in such

---

*Not so in China. There, the traditional medicine is in the same category as Western alternative medicine, since Western medicine is quite foreign to the oriental tradition.

common use, and that is *holistic medicine*. In usage, it is almost synonymous with the term *alternative medicine*. It means treating the whole person and/or treating each person as a whole, indivisible entity. That concept is used strongly in alternative medicine and will be emphasized as a major tenet of my proposed Complementary Medicine. But holism, by definition, is an opposing concept to specialization. The reawakening of interest in the orthodox medical specialty of family practice is a good example of holistic medicine within orthodox medicine. This enlightened countermovement provides one reason the term is not useful for describing the sharp demarcation between the two schools of thought.

Now, About That War

My interaction with thousands of patients and acquaintances has taught me that many of you are completely unaware of the warfare currently being waged, especially in the United States, between medical orthodoxy and every form of alternative medicine, and that only a handful of those who know of the struggle fully comprehend just how far-reaching it has become.

You may not even notice the war because it is as one-sided as a conflict between the Soviet Union and the Principality of Liechtenstein. This frightening analogy gives a pretty true picture of the superiority in size and strength that orthodox medicine currently enjoys over the alternative healing arts. And, since one of the techniques of this sort of cold war is control of the media and public awareness, you may only learn about it under headlines such as "Medical Society Polices Incompetents — War Against Quackery Deemed Success." What that news item signifies, more often than not, is that some outstanding physician who was so far ahead of the rest of the profession that they could not understand his accomplishments has had his license to practice medicine revoked or suspended by the local medical society.

How We All Hate Quackery!

Fighting evil is a noble ideal, and nothing could sound more noble than a war against quackery. What could be a loftier goal than to purge the profession of charlatans, those fraudulent pretenders to medical knowledge who bilk unsuspecting patients of their life savings, all the while costing them their health and denying them a chance for effective treatment? Certainly, I can think of none — except perhaps to purge the profession of those who use the campaign against quackery to persecute supercompetent, innovative physicians whose very success threatens the livelihood of the mediocre.

The War Against Quackery is a carefully orchestrated, heavily endowed campaign sponsored by extremists holding positions of power in the orthodox hierarchy. They work through organizations with names such as National Council Against Health Fraud, American Council on Science and Health, and the Quackery Action Council. They even have nonprofit status, which gives their adherents, often the officers and stockholders of major pharmaceutical firms, a chance to pay less in taxes than do hardworking stiffs like you and me.

They have raised enough funds to issue a steady stream of press conferences and press releases, which reach the magazines, wire services, networks, and physicians' journals monthly. They have succeeded in getting the federal Food and Drug Administration (FDA) and the advertising council of the pharmaceutical industry to issue joint communications warning about "quackery." It shouldn't take a mental giant to see that as a federal conflict of interest of heroic proportions, and a potential embarrassment to any administration.

They even came close to achieving the passage of legislation sponsored by Congressman Claude Pepper of Florida — House bills 6049, 6050, and 6051 — that would have allowed "quacks" to be driven out of practice without due process of law because of extraordinary powers given to the FDA, the U.S. Postal Service, and the Federal Trade Commission. Fortunately, an avalanche of protest mail by a belatedly awakened but outraged public led to the withdrawal of the infamous Pepper bills.

The Extremists' Objectives

The salient fact is this: This multimillion-dollar campaign against quackery was never meant to root out incompetent doctors; *it was, and is, designed specifically to destroy alternative medicine.* The profession has always done a creditable job of removing the isolated incompetents and can always do so without a need to deny due process of law. No need to raise funds for that, you can be sure. The millions were raised and spent because orthodox medicine sees alternative, *drugless* medicine as a real threat to its economic power.

And right they are! If I, by using nutrition and a nontoxic, biologic medicine, have been able to cut down my drug prescribing by 90 percent and can get obviously far better results than I ever got practicing "by the book," then why couldn't every doctor, once similarly enlightened? When this comes to pass, as it inevitably must if there is any validity to the adage "Truth will out," then the majority of the drug houses will not survive.

In case I haven't yet convinced you that the antiquackery war is, in reality, an anti–alternative medicine campaign, then let me show you that it is by calling your attention to the very definition used by the FDA, the Pharmaceutical Ad Council, and Congressman Pepper. Quackery in these writings is defined as using "unproven techniques."

When you realize that *most* of medicine and certainly its entire vanguard, or cutting edge, is not yet proven, then you will see that all of alternative medicine, whose fundamental precept it is to be at the cutting edge, must be, by *their* definition, classified as quackery.

Authority Without Checks and Balances

What you must first understand is that much of what orthodoxy characterizes as unproven is very well established by means of numerous carefully conducted case studies and the results tabulated on the basis of those studies. The "unproven" label fits only to the extent that the proof is not in the form of the double-blind studies that are standard in developing new drugs. (I'll explain double-blind proof in chapter 3.)

Second, you should realize that whenever you hear orthodox spokesmen explaining their viewpoint, they're doing so from a position of unique strength. They, after all, never have to answer to anyone. If they wish to belittle and break their rivals, they can do so without fear of retaliation, because there is no establishment in medicine apart from the American Medical Association.

The health field is the only field where inequity, conflict of interest, and gross public deception can remain unchecked. After all, the people in the FDA and in all the branches of government that deal with health come from the same orthodox school of thought as the heads of the AMA.

And the well-worn phrase "Tell me what to do, I'm not a doctor" represents the attitude of the public as well as the federal government. The orthodox establishment is happy to oblige. Not even the news media feel they have the ability to sit in judgment on medicine. The result is that all those forces in society that mold opinion and criticize incompetence have relinquished responsibility in the huge area of health.

One of the reasons I have written this book is to blow the whistle on this situation and prevent the orthodox extremists from using the word *quackery* as a vehicle for persecution.

More About Warfare

There is more to the life-and-death struggle over which kind of health care you may receive than an antiquackery campaign. There is always a subtle, and sometimes not-so-subtle, pressure on physicians to conform to "accepted" practices. Loss of referrals, loss of hospital privileges, or just plain social ostracism constitute threat enough to cause almost all doctors to fear being branded as engaging in alternative practices.

To give one example: There is an effective, nontoxic nutritional treatment for the nearly untreatable neurologic condition called multiple sclerosis (MS). It is the calcium salt of the neurotransmitter colamine phosphate, called calcium-EAP. I have treated over one hundred MS patients with it. Because most of my patients live a good distance from Manhattan, where my office is located, and because this nutrient must be given by injection three times a week, it is usually necessary to ask the patient's family physician to administer the calcium-EAP. This is a two-minute task for which the doctor would be paid. I kept a fairly accurate tabulation of the doctors' responses. Of the first sixty doctors who were asked by the patients, fifty-one refused to do so. This survey may give you some picture of the degree to which conformity to the party line takes precedence over the physician's innate humanitarian instincts.

From a self-preservation standpoint, these seemingly uncaring physicians are absolutely correct. The penalties imposed on a doctor who dares to follow his own drummer can indeed be horrific. In the past decade there have been over one hundred alternatively oriented physicians who have been stripped, permanently or temporarily, by state and local medical boards, of their right to practice their profession. These boards, composed entirely of orthodox physicians, declared the doctors "incompetent"; but any quick study of the doctors' accomplishments would put the lie to that notion. These "war victims," many of whom were leaders of alternative movements, were prosecuted (or persecuted) because they dared to practice alternative medicine. I have known many of these physicians, doctors like Alan Nittler, Michael Gerber, Robert Vance, James Privitera, Emanuel Revici, and a host of others, and can vouch for their broad knowledge, expertise, and devotion to their patients.

Dr. Halstead's Story

Let me provide a single example, the case of Bruce Halstead, M.D. Dr. Halstead is a physician-scientist of great repute; he has written more than 160 medical papers and several books, mostly describing the scientific basis underlying such medically unpopular subjects as chelation therapy or nontoxic cancer management. He was not only given a five-year jail sentence, but was stripped of the right to practice medicine, to write or lecture on medical subjects, to use his earned M.D. degree after his name, or even to publicly acknowledge that he had once had a medical education! He was even forbidden to operate his nonmedical, nonprofit oceanographic research foundation. For Dr. Halstead had been duly convicted of a crime that in the mind of California Superior Court Judge Marvin D. Rowen obviously deserved such penalties. The crime? Dr. Halstead prescribed and sold to several of his cancer patients some herbal remedies whose effectiveness in supporting the immune system he had learned of during a recent trip to Japan.

Although none of the patients was damaged in any way by the herbs, and none issued any complaint, and although Dr. Halstead specifically instructed the patients that the herbs were for immune support, not anticancer therapy, he did violate a rather onerous California law that forbids a doctor to treat a cancer patient with anything other than chemotherapy, radiation, or surgery.

I trust that some of you will be alert enough to recognize that the punishment is a little too severe for the "crime," which might raise in your mind the question: Who's out to get whom? Or the more sophisticated query: Who's protecting whom?

What About the Patients?

Don't think doctors are the only war casualties; the patients are very real sufferers, too. Thanks to the efforts of third-party carriers, the medical insurance companies most of us rely on to help us cover our medical expenses, alternative medical approaches are not usually reimbursable. All the carriers have review boards, composed exclusively of orthodoxists, who use the ploy of declaring the most reliable techniques of alternative practitioners to be "experimental" or "not usual and customary," and therefore not reimbursable. This can place patients on the horns of a dilemma. I have treated dozens of cancer patients, to give one type of example, who had to choose between receiving chemotherapy, which admittedly had no chance to cure them and which promised to cause distressing and demoralizing symptoms from the first day of administration — but for which they would receive full reimbursement — or being treated according to a nontoxic alternative program with a track record of great success, but for which medical coverage would be rejected by those "all-heart" insurance carriers because the treatment was not "usual or customary."

Now that you know of the great medical cold war, it is time that you learned how it all came about.

1
...

MEDICINE'S
DUAL TRADITIONS

I once did a series of TV talk show debates that pitted me against some rather dyed-in-the-wool orthodox physicians. Most of them took the position that I was the upstart and they represented traditional medicine. My answer was that they really weren't displaying much knowledge of the history of medicine.

The real tradition of medicine, which goes back to pre-Hippocratic times, has emerged from two opposing schools of thought — rationalism and empiricism — which, over the centuries, have vied for dominance as the historical pendulum has favored first one, then the other.

Today's orthodox medicine has risen from rationalism; and today's alternative medicine, from empiricism.

What Is the Main Difference Between Rationalism and Empiricism?

Some of you may not be philosophically oriented, but let me pose this question: Which is a more appropriate source of truth and knowledge — reason or experience? Or, to stick to our subject: Which is a better way to acquire expertise in matters of health and medicine — through reason or through experience?

If your answer was "Reason," you are a rationalist; if your answer was "Experience," then you are an empiricist. Now, if you are a little uncomfortable choosing just one, and you really want to answer "Both," then you are in a good position to go to where I've already been — to Complementary Medicine, a rational empiricism, or an empiric rationalism.

When we attempt to distinguish the two poles of medical thought, this simple reason-versus-experience dichotomy takes on far more specific characteristics.

Empiricism

The empiricist can look at the human body as a system of subsystems, but in reality he sees it as integrated into a whole. Early empiricists saw the human system as a unit interacting with its environment. To the empirical physician, symptoms were the result of the body's reaction to some aspect of environmental stress, such as food, pollutants, climate, medicine, and the like. The approach was to base treatment upon *all* of the patient's symptoms. Often, some of the symptoms characterized the individual and were not necessarily common to other persons suffering from the given "disease." Therefore, the empiricist did not categorize but saw each individual as a unique case relating to his environment in his own unique way.

I am sure that you can see the weakness in such a system if you wanted to develop a science or do something beyond merely helping the patient. How do you explain the illness? How do you repeat a successful treatment? The empiricist's failure to provide a rational basis for understanding his methods meant that his method was not suitable for the development of a body of scientific knowledge, and the empirical approach would later prove to be a misfit in cultures that prized scientific achievements.

Rationalism

On the other side of the medical street were the rationalists, who looked for "greater precision." They perceived the experiential approach as too imprecise, for it did not explicitly delineate the relationship between environmental influences and the patient's signs and symptoms. Their reasoning led to a search for common denominators and to basing medical treatment on the symptoms that were found to be identical in all patients having the same disease.

The rationalist orientation, from the beginning, was anti disease. This disease opposition opened the door to heroics — strong measures designed to kill or destroy the enemy. The balance of forces within the body itself became secondary, in the rationalist philosophy, to a direct attack upon the specific disease. Major interventions such as bloodletting made sense in the rationalist approach, for they reasoned that with the letting of blood the disease also came out. They focused so much on eradicating the disease that the unwanted but unavoidable result was the weakening of the body. The hope was that as the body became an inhospitable host, the enemy within must leave or die. This certainly was a radical, or heroic, approach. The continuity of rationalist thought has made this initial orientation a tradition around which all future orthodox postulates and actions have evolved. The perfect modern example is the debilitating chemotherapy routinely administered to cancer victims.

Over time, these philosophical differences grew wider. The empiricist saw the healing force as being within the body, and the physician's role was to be teacher, assistant, mediator. The rationalist saw the disease as the primary concern and assumed that he possessed the ability to affect the healing inasmuch as nature had "gone wrong."

What Medical History Teaches Us

Against this backdrop, let's take a quick peek at the history of medicine to see how we got here.

If you ask your doctor of traditional medicine the question "From whom does your medical tradition originate?" chances are his answer will be "From Hippocrates, of course." And why not? It is the oath of this great healer and teacher that all physicians take as they complete their medical training, and it is by his ethical precepts that they govern their professional lives. Hippocratic teachings remained influential for about two millennia.

So, Was Hippocrates a Rationalist or an Empiricist?

Hippocrates was a Greek physician who lived some four centuries before Christ, and his tradition clearly is empirical. He taught physicians to work with nature, emphasizing that nature is the best healer. His treatments were experiential, not deductive. And his most significant dictum may be read as a stern warning against rationalist medicine's penchant for intervention: *"Primum, non nocere"* — "First, do no harm." As we go along, you will see that this is the dictum I feel most strongly about, and the one around which any proposal for a new medicine must be built.

The immediate counterbalance to Hippocrates was Aristotle, who lived a century later and who developed the philosophy of rationalism. But it took several centuries until a rationalist physician, Galen (129–c. 199 A.D.), came along to create a rationalist medicine. For the next fourteen hundred years, much more of medicine was patterned after the Galenic model than the Hippocratic model. Looking back upon it with our contemporary hindsight, we are, of course, struck by how hard it would be to achieve a workable medicine by making deductions based on a science that was grossly inaccurate by today's standards. It is clear that most of the usable medical teachings of the post-Roman years had to derive from empirical observations, if not from empiricist teachings.

Paracelsus

Empiricism was swept back into dominance with the posthumous publication of the work of a sixteenth-century German mathematician-theologian-physician. Paracelsus (1493–1541) voiced the principles of empiricism in large part as we know them today. As I read some of his writings, I cannot help imagining him dressed in a white coat and sneakers and transplanted to a holistic clinic in California. He would be ready to start work tomorrow. His main contribution: In medicine, experience, not theory, contains the answers.

The Scientific Era Begins

The pendulum swung again with the influence of philosopher René Descartes (1596–1650) and the founder of modern physics, Sir Isaac Newton (1642–1727). Both used their own scientific inclinations to demand that we, as thinking beings, begin to analyze the world about us. The search in physics was to discover the *mechanisms* by which things worked. The goal in medicine was to use this mechanistic approach to understand the human body and its diseases. The physician's treatment would be to oppose that which he understood as the mechanism of the disease.

The wide usage today of the terms *Cartesian logic* or *Newtonian science* testifies to the vast influence these two thinkers had upon the development of modern scientific medicine.

With the development of physics and chemistry, and with the discovery by William Harvey (1578–1657) of the fact that our blood circulates, meaningful explanations of the mechanics and physiology of the body were sought and were forthcoming. (Incidentally, imagine how successful the rationalist deductions must have been in the days before they even knew that blood circulated!)

Cartesian thought ushered in a shift in the prevailing philosophy of knowledge. The key scientific process became one of *analysis* — scrutinize the parts to learn about the whole. The main philosophic understanding was that the whole was the sum of its parts. Medically, this led us to study our bodies in terms of organs, then of tissues, then of cells and of biochemical processes. It led us away from the consideration of the forces that integrate us in a single entity; it moved us from the empirical principle of holism to the mechanistic principle of analysis.

Theory Affects Treatment: "Opposites" Versus "Similars"

As would be expected, the two approaches used different methods of treatment. Beginning in the eighteenth century (but not "scientifically proven" until the late nineteenth century), the European rationalist saw disease as a product of pathogenic, or disease-causing, microorganisms. They focused on developing substances that killed the organism in vitro (in an artificial environment — a culture dish or test tube, for example — outside the human body) and then applied them in vivo (into the living organism). Here we see the origin of what was to become the cornerstone of modern medicine — testing the effect of disease and drugs on animals and extrapolating the findings to humans. The therapeutics tested, and used, were based on the principle of destruction of disease. Often this meant doing the opposite of what was required to keep the body healthy.

This brings up what may be the most significant difference in treatment approaches — the use of "similars" versus the use of "opposites." Most treatment in medicine today is so centered around the *opposition* to symptoms that we absolutely take it for granted that that must be the only way it was ever done. Blood pressure too high? Lower it. Have diarrhea? Stop it. Runny nose? Dry it up. Headache? Kill the pain. Vomiting? Take an anti-emetic. Skin rash? Suppress it.

But on the other hand, must we lose sight of the fact that symptoms generally represent the response of the body to something that has gone wrong? When we suggest a gentle enema to "clean out" someone with diarrhea or an emetic to encourage vomiting in a food-poisoned individual, we are going *with* the symptoms and treating according to the principle of similars.

Rationalist medicine was, and is, based almost exclusively on the principle of opposites. Most empiricists, in the tradition of Hippocrates and Paracelsus, treated by the principle of similars.

Since I employ both similars and opposites in my contemporary practice, I view the ideological struggle with much curiosity. I believe the real problem was not so much the *direction* of the therapy as the *intensity* of it. The doctor who opposed illness, upon finding that his treatment was not getting the job done, would be tempted to oppose the illness even more and thus treat with dosages that would overwhelm both the disease and the patient. The similarist, by contrast, would always find it inappropriate to do more than gently stimulate the patient's healing responses, and was thus less likely to upset the balance of nature.

Hahnemann and Homeopathy: The Ultimate Empiricism

It was less than two centuries ago, in Germany, that a scientific-minded empiricist named Samuel Hahnemann (1755–1843) developed the principle of similars, along with some rather astounding dosage concepts that have yet to be fully explained, into the science, or art, of homeopathy. Hahnemann's medicine was the best-developed example of the empiricist approach and at the same time was its last gasp, prior to its utter dominance by today's orthodox medicine.

Even though homeopathic medicine is not one of my special skills, I have seen it work and I hold it in great esteem. It is not to dwell on homeopathy but rather on the broader principle of empirical medicine that we must look at Hahnemann's contribution in greater detail.

Hahnemann wrote about similars in this manner:

> Each individual case of disease is most surely, radically, rapidly, and permanently annihilated and removed only by a medicine capable of producing [in the human system] in the most similar and complete manner the totality of [the disease] symptoms, which at the same time are stronger than the disease.[1]

The homeopathic system of treatment thus introduces into the patient minute quantities of a remedy that in large doses would produce the symptoms being treated. Hahnemann himself painstakingly determined the effect of hundreds of herbal medications by giving them to the well and noticing the symptoms produced. This method led to the use of these substances on sick people who had such symptoms.

The most empirical aspect of Hahnemann's teachings was the constant search to find the perfect "constitutional remedy," that is, the substance which induced a correction in an individual because of his uniquely individual characteristics, not because of his membership in a disease category.

The Infinitesimal Dose

Most startling was the Hahnemannian model's concept of dosage. In the homeopathic system, the more dilute dosages are considered the strongest. In fact, most homeopathic remedies have been diluted through a process of trituration to the point that they do not contain a single molecule of the substance indicated on the label! Allopathic doctors (here the term *allo-* refers to the orthodox concept of opposites), because they were unable to find a suitable rational explanation, tended to dismiss homeopathy as "quackery."

A typical homeopathic ploy to convince doubters is to offer the skeptic a 6oX homeopathic dilution of ipecac, which does not contain a single molecule of this emetic. If the skeptic is disdainful enough to take the bait, and the dilution, he will invariably barf up his latest meal.

Yes, there should be a rational explanation for the empirically observed effects of homeopathic dilutions. To me, it bespeaks a bioenergetic system in which an energy pattern, a sort of echo, exists where the molecular substance previously existed.

The Great Affront

The important lesson is that homeopathy, which defies rational explanation, and works only because it seems to work, is a total affront to a mind that lives solely by its deductive powers. A rationalist may be annoyed with empiricism, but he will absolutely detest homeopathy.

Can it be surprising, then, that such differences of thought become irreconcilable? Ideas become hardened positions and hardened positions become battlegrounds. So, too, it was between the rationalists, whose traditions led to medical orthodoxy, and the empiricists, whose traditions set the stage for alternative medicine. Positions thus established, any member of either camp who questioned its respective tradition "betrayed" the cause. These traditions were entrenched by the time medicine came to America.

Heroics on America's Shores

It should come as no surprise that by the early nineteenth century there were two dominant medical philosophies in the United States vying for supremacy. They were allopathy, the rationalist orthodoxy, and homeopathy, the empirical tradition (along with other alternative therapies, such as Indian medicine and botanical medicine).

As you might expect, the American schism was not very different from the centuries-old European rationalist-empiricist struggle. Generally, rationalists studied in European medical schools or were trained by physicians who had. The empirical homeopaths and naturopaths were not typically affiliated with the urban hospitals that were then in their infancy; they were practitioners without much formal medical training of the kind we know today. But they served a large segment of the population. It was they who employed the more conservative treatments — herbals, botanicals, mild doses of medications.

The allopathic doctors learned a rationalist medicine whose traditions they acquired in Europe and successfully transplanted into an American academic hierarchy. This rationalist medicine was extremely "heroic" and interventive; it employed bloodletting and combinations of strong medicines designed to oppose the disease processes. The early American orthodox position is best exemplified by Dr. Benjamin Rush, professor of medicine at the University of Pennsylvania from 1769 until 1813.

Rush's medicine involved the use of extremely large doses of powerful mineral substances, such as calomel (mercury) plus emetics, cathartics, blisters, cold baths, and bloodletting. In his writings, he echoed the principles of heroics, intervention, and opposition to disease. "The physician must be bold and dictate . . . the use of powerful and painful remedies in violent disease," he stated.[2]

Case in Point: George Washington

American presidents get the best care that the rationalist medicine of the day can offer. Let's go back to the deathbed of George Washington in 1799 to see our medical tradition in action. The description is given by Dr. Wooster Beach, writing in 1832:

> Think of a man being, within the brief space of little more than twelve hours, deprived of 80 or 90 ounces of blood; afterward swallowing two *moderate* American doses of calomel, which were accompanied by an injection; then five grains of calomel and five or six grains of emetic tartar; vapours of water and vinegar frequently inhaled; blisters applied to his extremities; a cataplasm of bran and vinegar applied to his throat, upon which a blister had already been fixed. Is it surprising that when thus treated, the afflicted general, after various ineffectual struggles for utterance, at length articulated a desire that he might be allowed to die without interruption![3]

I Said This Was a Rational Medicine

So let's look at the rationale behind the most widely used drug of nineteenth-century America, a harsh purgative, the mercurial compound called calomel. According to the Massachusetts Medical Society journal of 1836, mercury worked as an *alterative*, transforming the patient's disease into a "mercurial disease."[4] Mercurialism was known to be self-healing. This meant, to the rationalist mentality of that day, that the original disease would be healed by the backlash of the self-correcting mercurialism.

If there are AMA types out there who are still proud of the "traditions" from which they sprang, let them become more familiar with nineteenth-century American medicine.

Nonetheless, the tradition continued and, armed with only a little knowledge about disease compared to what physicians know today, American orthodoxy was already embarked on an anti-disease crusade, convinced that it knew more about curing the body than did nature itself. They viewed the struggle as man versus nature, not, as empirical medicine did, as man in harmony with nature.

Fear Entrenches the Tradition of Heroics

The conflict between orthodoxy and the alternative healers grew worse as homeopaths made major inroads into orthodoxy's power base by treating an increasing percentage of the nation's patients. Their economic success brought about open conflict between the two camps. Orthodoxy not only resented the flimsy, almost nonexistent educational background of alternative therapists, but now saw the homeopaths as a threat to their own interests. It was at this point in 1849 that orthodoxy established the American Medical Association, expressly for the purpose of combating the effectiveness of what they did not hesitate to call the "enemy."[5]

Thus the AMA began its glorious tradition, spanning nearly 140 years, of unbroken commitment to the same noble ideals — economic self-interest and the squelching of all intellectual opposition.

How the AMA Destroyed Homeopathy

Not only did the newly formed AMA bar homeopathic doctors from its ranks, it prohibited its own membership from using any homeopathic techniques. It even barred physicians who *referred* patients to homeopaths or who worked at hospitals where homeopaths were allowed to practice. With these strong measures, the AMA won the day, and within sixty years there was near-total uniformity to American medicine, with hardly a dissenting voice to be heard.

The AMA's inevitable supremacy was aided by the Civil War, which in turn provided the impetus for a burgeoning new industry: pharmaceuticals. The Civil War, like all wars, required medical heroics. Allopathic physicians performed the amputations and operations, and the drug industry supplied the bandages, splints, sulfur, antiseptics, morphine, and so forth. The heroic tradition of orthodoxy was allowed free rein.

The war propelled the pharmaceutical industry beyond its infancy. Companies like Squibb and Sharpe & Dohme provided medicine and medical supplies for the Civil War troops. After the war they developed the sales concept of "proprietary" medicines, for sale directly to the general public. These were patent medicines but with a new twist: their ingredients were identified on the labels, thus circumventing laws that restricted the sale of nondisclosed medicines. Its name, or advertisements in medical journals, indicated the specific disease the medicine was to cure. Late nineteenth-century physicians bought this concept hook, line, and sinker. This centralized compounding of medicines spared them the intellectual effort needed to learn how to use their own techniques of curing their patients. As physicians abandoned prescription-writing in favor of these compounded nostrums, a significant new industry emerged. By 1916 there were over thirty-nine thousand different patented medicines.[6] But all of this came about due to a sales promotion campaign that is carried out even more vigorously today than it was then.

Pharmaceutical Seduction

Between 1870 and 1880 orthodox medical spokesmen attacked the value of these drugs and these firms, according to the medical science and ethics of that era, which had taught that the physician should *himself* know the therapies he would use on his patients. But the doctors' attacks grew weaker and weaker as the fledgling drug industry grew economically stronger and concentrated on winning over the orthodox medical establishment. The industry began producing literature to educate the practicing doctor to new diseases and methods of cure using the compounded formulas they had patented. They developed the idea of the industry sending out "detail men," salespersons trained to educate doctors, give free samples, and provide literature. This strategy is still in widespread use today, but in the 1880s it was of an even greater impact. In many parts of the country, because of poor or nonexistent roads, physicians simply did not travel. There were few conventions and no refresher courses in those days. For many, the drug salesmen became the key method of "staying up" with medical research. Some of the pharmaceutical houses even supplied pharmacists with the financing, pamphlets, and supplies to begin their businesses. With the drug industry supporting both pharmacists and physicians, it had no competition except with itself, and medicine gradually evolved a drug-industry-oriented treatment philosophy. The tail (physician-approved drug suppliers) was now wagging the dog (the medical profession). Now traditional medicine was ready for seduction.

Whose Journal Is It Anyway?

The pharmaceutical companies realized how much orthodox physicians depended on their medical journals, so they began buying them. For example, Parke-Davis between 1877 and 1883 bought several successful medical journals, each headed by orthodox physicians, professors at prestigious medical schools. The cream of orthodoxy was now being salaried by the pharmaceutical industry.

The drug industry's companion technique was advertising. Of

the 250 medical journals in existence in 1906, all but one were supported by advertising from the drug industry.

All this, and more, goes on today. The pharmaceutical industry's efforts to seduce physicians through detail persons, free seminars, drug-testing research, journal ownership, and advertising should be well known to you all. A recounting of this should raise no eyebrows. But in the nineteenth century, generations before the terms *public relations* or *marketing strategy* were even introduced, it was an exceedingly precocious and effective technique. It seduced an entire profession. Physicians had once been open to any therapeutic system that appealed to a rationalist's intellect. Now they assumed that the only answer was pharmaceutical.

The irony of it all was that for the first time, there was a plausible scientific background to support a rationalist medicine.

The Role of Pathologists and the Bacteriology Breakthrough

Most of the great physicians and medical educators of the nineteenth century were also pathologists. By studying the preserved organs of individuals dying with a variety of diseases, they became the quintessential carriers of a rationalist medicine. They defined disease, thus creating categories called diagnoses in which patients could be neatly pigeonholed. As their microscopes were switched to higher magnifications, they were able to engage in the Cartesian analysis of organs, then of tissue, and finally, of cells. Their very discipline was a movement away from holism. And they found interrelationships between various organs, thus providing a narrative to explain the causation of disease. The greater the knowledge of pathology, the more powerful was the intellectual satisfaction of a nonempirical medicine.

At the same time, the discoveries of Robert Koch, Louis Pasteur, and other bacteriologists seemed clearly to demonstrate that most illness was caused by microorganisms. This provided the greatest impetus of all for a rationalist medicine. *Diseases had individuality; individuals did not, they had the diseases.* More often than not, victims of the same microorganism-caused illness had certain common denominators. One case of cholera or of yellow fever was very like another. No room here for Hahnemann's quest for a constitutional remedy.

This does not mean that allopathy was getting the better results. In 1878 the Mississippi Valley was ravaged by a yellow fever epidemic. The death rate was over 20 percent; in Memphis, there were 5,000 deaths out of 18,590 reported cases. But of those treated by homeopathic physicians (in New Orleans), the death rate was only 5.6 percent (110 out of 1,945 cases).[7]

Until the basic sciences could provide specific therapies for the allopaths, the experience-based practitioners of homeopathy were still beating them at their own game.

The Age of Specific Therapies

A few decades after the first era of great bacteriological discovery came the era of "magic bullets." The German bacteriologist Paul Ehrlich (1854–1915) first discovered strong chemical substances such as arsenicals, which provided a disease-eradicating type of treatment for syphilis, then a number-one killer disease. Other "bullets" followed, and for the first time, medicine could work with drugs designed to wipe out a disease.

These brilliant discoveries, mostly made in the late nineteenth and early twentieth centuries, are the greatest triumphs in the entire two-thousand-year history of rationalist medicine, and the medical establishment has been living on the goodwill earned by them ever since. It is, after all, very difficult to convince the average person that drug treatment is not the solution to most medical problems when, within the memory of living people, a score of major illnesses were eradicated by drugs.

For almost a century now, medicine has been pursuing a path based on a magic bullet philosophy.* *For every disease, there must be a specific cure that will stamp out the disease.* There are two major problems with that philosophy. First, it is rarely applicable anymore — the applicability being limited to conditions for which

---

* Dr. René Dubos, who was one of my teachers at Cornell Medical College, named this the doctrine of specific etiology (*etiology* is a medical word meaning *cause*). The doctrine holds that illness can be broken down into specific diseases, each one of which has a unique primary cause.

microorganisms *are* the primary cause. Medicine's magic bullets have mostly wiped out some illnesses, such as tuberculosis, syphilis, and leprosy, and its magic preventatives (immunology procedures, which we are not discussing here) have done the same for smallpox, polio, diphtheria, and the like. But we still have disease. Many of today's diseases — hypertension, heart disease, diabetes, arthritis, and perhaps cancer — are caused by our lifestyle, and magic bullets don't correct them.

Ehrlich's Wisdom

Second, magic bullets are not without effect on their host, the very person we are trying to save. Paul Ehrlich himself recognized this fact better than did most of the enthusiasts who followed his lead. This is Ehrlich's caveat, made in a 1906 address:

> It must be regarded as in the highest degree probable that substances of this kind, magic substances, foreign to the body, will be attracted also by the organs, and that, since we shall be dealing with a range of different substances, all with pronounced activities, these are not unlikely to injure the organism as a whole, or some part of it.[8]

The magic bullet philosophy made progress by fits and starts but achieved full fruition half a century later, when World War II ushered in the era of antibiotics. This provided orthodox medicine with its greatest support in its conviction that man was indeed a greater healer than nature.

Osler Ushers in Contemporary Medicine

The twentieth century began with two noteworthy influences that further shaped orthodox medicine into what it is today, and neither left any place for the empirical tradition. The first was the teachings of Sir William Osler (1849–1919), the chief physician at Johns Hopkins School of Medicine. Osler emphasized the scientific method in medicine and taught us to accept research that could be replicated. Out of this developed the need to do controlled experiments and eventually the double-blind study, which became one of the main sacraments of medicine's orthodox "religion."

Flexner Changes the Face of Medical Education

The second influence was a specific document usually referred to as the Flexner Report of 1910. At the time, American medical education was in total disarray, some schools representing the highest level of rationalist academic tradition, but others providing, for profit, the flimsiest of learning opportunities. Abraham Flexner (1866–1959) was commissioned to set America's medical teaching house in order, which he did with *Medical Education in the United States and Canada* — the Flexner Report. As a result, the majority of small medical schools went out of business and those that survived adopted a rather uniform curriculum. That curriculum had no courses in nutrition, and the only instruction directed toward therapeutics was a rather lengthy course in pharmacology. Thus a doctor's only knowledge of how to treat patients came from what he knew about drugs; he was not given the wherewithal to use anything else.

Thus set in motion, twentieth-century medicine witnessed the total domination of an orthodoxy that was at first symbiotic with, and then eventually controlled by, a philosophy consistent with the financial interests of an ever-expanding pharmaceutics industry. Voices that questioned this conflict of interest were gradually stilled, and the lay press, overwhelmed by the accumulation of scientific knowledge it could little understand, adopted a you-teach-us-and-we'll-print-it posture. Stripped of public and official support, the empirical medicines withered to the point of near extinction, when they were not simply openly suppressed.

As was intended, we were left with the concept that all healing is mediated through the hospital-based hierarchy. And it's to that that we products of the twentieth century simply give the name Medicine.

And so, ladies and gentlemen, now you know how it came about that of the two valid traditions of medicine, you have been exposed to only one. Unless you are (a) European or oriental, (b) very, very old, or (c) very, very contemporary, you will have had no exposure to an empirical system of healing.

But What of Empiricism?

Somehow, empirical medicine managed to survive.* In many cases, it survived on non-American soil. Homeopathy did very well in its native soil of Germany, where it has also enjoyed a successful admixture with botanical medicine and an acupuncture-based system of bioenergetics. In England, thanks to the support of Prince Charles and Princess Diana, it serves as the cornerstone of a flourishing mix of alternative medicines. Traditional oriental medicine is pure empiricism — it is an extremely successful blend of acupuncture theory and gentle herbal combinations.

In America, the struggles have all been bitter. The manipulation technique of chiropractic has survived an ugly all-out effort of the AMA to destroy it and is now flourishing. Osteopathy, on the other hand, has followed the if-you-can't-lick-'em-join-'em strategy and is now virtually indistinguishable from medical orthodoxy. Naturopathy has become an interesting pastiche of American folk medicine traditions, herbalism, homeopathy, and nutrition, and is gaining some acceptance, with naturopathic graduates being allowed to practice in some states.

How Alternativism Originates Today

The American medical hierarchy has become so hidebound that new areas for medical alternativism are created every few years from it own ranks. All that seems to be necessary for an approach to be categorized as alternativism is that the concept be innovative and empirical (i.e., its success is demonstrated through experience). It thus runs afoul of a strong "If it hasn't been proven, it can't be any good" bias. Areas of medical treatment that have fallen under the shadow of this peculiar sort of intellectual bigotry include chelation therapy, clinical ecology, candidology (the science

---

*Although empiricism survived the assaults directed against its right to exist, it lost the propaganda word game. In defining the medical use of the word *empiricism*, the *Oxford English Dictionary* begins with, "Practice founded upon experiment and observation," but concludes with the damning words "ignorant and unscientific practice; quackery." How far this is from John Stuart Mill, writing in 1846, whose subtle and original observation was that "an empirical law then, is an observed uniformity, presumed to be resolvable into simpler laws, but not yet resolved into them."

of diagnosing and treating systemic yeast infections), heavy metal toxicology, and most appalling of all — nutrition.

Nutrition Is Not Rational?

No, Virginia, nutrition is not a part of present-day orthodox medicine. That is, if we can go by a statement made by a highly regarded (by orthodox activists), oft-quoted leader of orthodox medicine named Victor Herbert, M.D. His words: "A quack is any doctor who prescribes vitamins."

To be perfectly fair, there is a nutrition of sorts taught and accepted by orthodox medicine, but it does not include nutritional pharmacology. The science of using nutrients as safe alternatives to drugs is a rejected rationalist science, relegated to the dump heap (as viewed by orthodoxy) of alternative medicine. In their view, it is okay to use vitamin therapy to correct a deficiency state; it is not okay to use vitamin C to enhance the immune system, magnesium to lower the blood pressure, tryptophan to treat insomnia, vitamin E as an anticoagulant, or primrose oil to prevent premenstrual syndrome.

The Alternative Team Line-up

Nutrition together with some of the empirical treatment systems mentioned above (and some not yet mentioned) forms the backbone of the alternative medicine team — a team that can provide some pretty stiff competition for the drug-oriented approach practiced in academic and hospital circles.

If you can see that there really are two kinds of medicine to choose from, that there is a two-party system, the ins and the outs, then you're ready to go on to the next step. Let's scrutinize them both and see how they stack up.

2

...

COMPARING
THE TRADITIONS

This book is about several old medicines and one proposed new one. It is about physicians, people who have devoted their lives to helping others achieve well-being. In analyzing these various medical systems, I have been emphasizing their differences, but I wish now to emphasize the commonality of purpose of all physicians. All share a desire to use the best of their abilities to help you and others achieve or restore the best possible state of health. In many cases, all physicians, regardless of their orientation, might handle similar problems in identical ways. All might lance a boil, keep open an obstructed airway, reduce a high fever, or administer drugs for intractable pain. But, as we shall see, in many other areas, the differences can be profound.

Comparing Modern-day Orthodoxy with Alternative Medicine

I hope I have succeeded in demonstrating that history can trace two basic types of medical approach. I would now like to bring them up to the present time and offer them for comparison.

Since my thesis is that today's orthodox medicine derives from the rationalist tradition, and the alternative medicines (all that is not orthodox) spring, by and large, from the philosophy of empiricism, let's see what that distinction means in contemporary terms.

Orthodox, rationalist medicine is a medicine of reason, of logic, and of science. It deals in what is known, what can be understood, and what can be proven. Alternative, empirical medicine is a medicine of experience. It deals in what works, what has worked, what seems to work, and what promises to work.

Now, What Does That Mean to Us?

It means that orthodoxy will never fall for some harebrained system of gobbledygook or endorse a half-baked therapy based on wishful thinking; but it also means that it will reject any system it cannot explain or understand, such as homeopathy or acupuncture. Alternative medicine's contrasting attitude is rather direct: "Show us that it works, that patients benefit from it, and we will use it."

Let's see what these differences mean in practice.

Orthodoxy Is Anti Disease, Alternativism Is Pro Health

Anti disease or pro health. This is probably the most important distinction of all, and its implications are manifold. Contemporary orthodoxy is preoccupied with identifying and combating disease and gives short shrift to the gradations of health shown by the patient. The prevailing attitude seems to be: "If it ain't broke, don't fix it." But the real difficulty of the orthodox stance comes from the fact that most agents that fight disease also fight health. Consider cancer chemotherapy. And then go on and find out about some of the side effects of the drugs used to treat arthritis, or heart rhythm disorders. You'll see some of the obvious risks that go with disease-opposition.

The alternativist can identify health (*it is balance, and disease is merely the absence of balance*) and will work to restore it. He combats disease not by opposing it but by replacing it with an improved state of health. This means improving the immune system, reducing stress, optimizing physical exercise and nutrition, helping the patient achieve spiritual harmony, improving bowel function, removing toxic environmental elements, and more. In fact, most of this book will deal with the way my patients have used a health-enhancing system to overcome their illness. I think the case histories in this book will convince the most hardened skeptic that it is possible to cure illness and enhance health simultaneously.

Therapies or Tonics?

Oftentimes some of the best treatment systems in empirical medicine are derisively criticized by orthodoxy with the phrase "That's just a tonic."* The implication of that statement is that substances which exert a general health benefit but don't treat a disease simply aren't much good. The U.S. government (FDA) seems to agree. In the 1950s the FDA approved a drug called Spartase, a nutritional compound consisting of aspartates. Tests showed it made patients feel better and overcome "that tired feeling." A few years later the FDA removed Spartase from the market, not because of some risky side effects but simply because the drug did not treat a disease.

Empiricists, by contrast with the FDA, like therapies that have a beneficial effect on everyone. Empiricists would gladly use them on patients who have no disease, patients who want to feel better or improve their already "acceptable" level of health. As you will learn from our case histories, many of our patients' health problems were solved by the combined usage of nutritional and other substances that had no direct antidisease effect, but which were in some way restorative to balance or were health-promoting simply because they are good for nearly everyone. Orthodox medicine works in quite a different way.

Blockers Versus Enablers

The distinction between the two camps on the antidisease or prohealth issue extends to the substances used in treatment. Should we treat with agents that *prevent an undesired reaction* from taking place or with agents that *allow for a desired action* to occur? In the former case, we will use blocking agents; in the latter, enabling agents.

Most pharmaceutical substances are blocking agents. There are surprisingly few exceptions to that axiom. They act with selective toxicity. A good drug will distort the biochemical processes of a specific enzyme system and prevent a specific biochemical reaction from taking place. The result is that the imbalance caused by the

---

*The term *tonic* refers to substances that have a general effect of promoting well-being but are not appropriate as disease therapy.

illness is replaced with a drug-induced imbalance. In other words, *drugs work by substituting one imbalance for another*. It is vital to remember, then, that drugs cannot be of benefit except when there is disease.

Perhaps this helps to explain why a pharmaceutically seduced profession has evolved to the point that it only works by opposing illness.

The other approach, that of providing the body what it requires to enable it to perform its functions of rectifying itself, means, in essence, providing nutrients. One can, quite fairly, define nutrients as "those substances which enable all the body's biochemical processes to take place." Needless to say, those enabling agents work just as well in the absence of illness, and when given in optimal combination (whatever that is) can lead to optimal health.

Although the principle of enablers is, by and large, an alternative approach, it is certainly one that would be recognized by scientific rationalists. In fact, it was two-time Nobel laureate (chemistry in 1954, peace in 1962) Dr. Linus Pauling who first set forth the principle of orthomolecular medicine, which means treating by regulating the concentrations of substances normally present in the body. This credo of enabling-agent therapeutics, one of the basic tenets of nutritional pharmacology, is rejected by orthodox medicine, even though it is derived more from rationalism than empiricism.

Heroics Versus Nonintervention

One of the glories of orthodox medicine is its ability to take bold strokes to overcome catastrophic disease. We all applaud the TV medical hero who can, with his deft neurosurgical skills, remove a life-threatening brain tumor or who can stop a nearly fatal heart rhythm with the intravenous use of potentially dangerous drugs. And we know that in our real-life hospitals, doctors in a similar fashion save lives every day. Contemporary American medicine has evolved very nicely from the tradition of medical heroics laid down by Dr. Benjamin Rush.

The question is: When are heroics appropriate, and when inappropriate? Heroics, or interventive medicine, *is* the preferred treatment in times of crisis; there are times when only bold measures will get the job done. But just how well do heroics apply in chronic degenerative diseases that take a lifetime to develop?

An obvious case in point is the widespread use of heart bypass surgery for symptom-free patients in whom modern medical technology was able to diagnose "blockages" in coronary blood vessels due to a process called atherosclerosis. That process had gone on for decades and continued unabated *after* the surgery. More than a decade after the first rush of heart bypasses, it has become apparent that those who underwent the heroic treatment have fared no better than a matched group who did not. More significantly, nonorthodox medicine has, all along, offered a variety of effective treatments for the underlying condition of atherosclerosis that by all experiential criteria work better than any orthodox therapy. We shall be dealing with them at great length.

Crisis Medicine Versus Maladaption Management

By now you may have guessed I am not totally enamored of all the directions medicine has taken, but you can rest assured that if I were in a state of medical emergency, I would want to be in a well-equipped, specialist-staffed orthodox hospital. For nowhere in our history has crisis medicine been developed to the level of effectiveness that now exists in our best hospitals.

The question is this: Do we have to wait until the patient reaches a crisis state before we can use our efforts to benefit that person?

There are many reasons why orthodox medicine is good at being a crisis medicine. The same reasons also explain why orthodox medicine employs emergency-room techniques when it is not appropriate to do so.

American medical education is hospital-based. This means that medical students, interns, and residents, by and large, come into contact with patients (each one, incidentally, not as an individual but as a case history, an example of a specific disease) only when their illness reaches a state severe enough to require hospitalization. This means seeing the asthmatic during an attack, the epileptic immediately after a seizure, the arthritic during a flare-up, or the heart patient in acute pulmonary edema (heart failure). Doctors-in-training learn to treat these illnesses in their most vulnerable state. Here intervention and heroics are the appropriate therapy. Then, thanks to the successful emergency heroics the doctors employed, the patient goes home, where he leads 99 percent of his life as a patient. Hospital-trained doctors are not taught much about that 99 percent of the case. *The tendency is to employ a maintenance dose of crisis medicine.* In using these techniques in a crisis, orthodox medicine is at its strongest; in trying to force these techniques to adapt to the management of chronic illness, it is at its weakest.

Why Not Head It Off at the Pass?

Allow me to take sides on this one. Alternative medicine does it better because alternative medicine works from a more correct understanding of chronic illness, according to the theory of clinical ecologist William Philpott, M.D. Chronic illnesses, even the kinds that eventuate in medical crisis, start off on a small scale as maladaptive reactions. The diabetic in acidosis was at an earlier time either a hypoglycemic eating an incorrect diet or a person forming antibodies to his own insulin. The arthritic or asthmatic was making a poor adjustment to dietary factors of chemicals in his environment. In any case, the appropriate treatment is to recognize the illness when it is the pre-illness — the maladaptive state — and then avoid what can be avoided, or desensitize the allergic manifestations, or provide the nutritional enablers to strengthen the healthy immune response.

Only rarely would an illness so treated in its incipient state reach the stage where crisis management was necessary.

Cure Versus Prevention

Both camps agree that it is better to prevent illness than to seek a cure for it once it is established. Orthodox medicine does indeed offer a bona fide specialty called preventive medicine, as taught in all post-Flexner medical school curricula. But it is much more a science of large-scale prevention in *populations*, not *individuals*. This is where epidemiology, hygiene, infectious disease transmission, and the like, are studied. American alternativists take it one step further — preventive medicine is the name they give their own specialty of nutrition-based medicine. Two leading alternative societies are (or were) named accordingly: the International Academy of Preventive Medicine (IAPM) and the American Academy of Medical Preventics (AAMP).*

The question here is worthy of lengthy debate: Who does prevention better and is better equipped to handle preventive aspects of our health?

For all the reasons cited above — the emphasis on heroics, the need to oppose a disease, a crisis-based education — I have found the orthodox specialty of preventive medicine to be woefully incomplete and constituting a far too small segment of the total medicine. Modern orthodoxy is a drug-based medicine, and there are very few, if any, drugs that do a good job of prevention. Many that were proposed as preventives have, after scientific scrutiny, failed to prevent illness. Drugs to prevent complications of diabetes, of hypertension, or of lipid disorders have been shown to produce more harm than good (but not until billions of dollars of profit accrued to the drug industry).

Meanwhile, present-day alternative medicine is trying so hard to emphasize prevention that its practitioners often must appear in front of state license review committees to explain *why they are treating patients in the absence of a proven disease.* This should tell you something about the alternativist orientation as well as something about the attitude toward prevention held by the orthodox physicians who sit on these boards.

If you want my personal opinion, I believe that disease starts with imbalances, and if you can identify those imbalances, keep the person away from what harms him, and give him what seems to be good for him, then you can and will prevent lots of illnesses.

A Mechanistic or an Integrated Philosophy?

In our historical discussion, I made the point that Newton and Descartes ushered in an era in which, as science developed, medicine was able to study more and more fundamental subdivisions of the body. As each level was studied — the organs, then the tis-

---

* Until its name change in 1986, to the American College of Advancement in Medicine.

sues, then the individual cells, then the biochemical units — a more and more "scientific" understanding of the body and of medicine was achieved. Medicine thus became imbued with a mechanistic philosophy.

Orthodox medicine today follows the same mechanistic approach — analysis of parts of the whole. As more and more of its membership specializes, fewer and fewer remain to integrate the patient's entire picture so that it can be seen as a whole. And even then, they never go as far as does empirical medicine in seeking, the way Hahnemann recommended, the factors that make each individual unique.

I believe the above distinction is a fair statement of one major difference between the two kinds of medicine. This does not mean I prefer one to the other. A good physician must be aware of the workings of both the parts and the whole.

But neither does this mean I approve of patient management by specialists. There is too much of medicine to be known for any one mortal (assuming, in contrast to some doctors' prevailing opinions, that doctors are mortals) to know. And a doctor who wishes to practice Complementary Medicine must know four times again as much, or so it seems to me. But the managing physician *must* be able to see the patient as an individual and must be able to integrate all the fragments of specialized information about him into a comprehensive, understandable picture. I never said it was easy!

People with a Diagnosis or Individuals?

The main pitfall of failing to remember that individuals are individuals is that they get categorized and become group members. Thus, if Sadie Smith gets rheumatoid arthritis, the question arises, Will she be treated as (a) Sadie Smith or (b) a case of rheumatoid arthritis? The implications for treatment are colossal.

According to orthodox medicine, all members of a disease group should be treated according to the same protocol, or standard program of treatment, unless there is some clear, complicating obstacle that prevents a particular patient from receiving that treatment. Thus, if there were a study of the fictional drug "Antiarthrheum" which reported that 57 percent of the patients showed more relief on it than on placebo (an inactive substance used as a control in an experiment) and 15 percent showed more relief than on three other anti-arthritic drugs tested comparatively, then Sadie — and any other rheumatoid arthritis patient the doctor had — would be prescribed Antiarthrheum.

The alternativist approach would be to find out whether Sadie showed a reaction to nightshade foods or to wheat gluten, or to whatever her food-intolerance test indicated, as well as learning whether she was low in copper, manganese, or other minerals, or whether she would respond to vitamin C or several members of the B complex of vitamins. The alternativist (or complementarist, as we shall soon find out) wants to know much more about Sadie than about rheumatoid arthritis.

As we will be discussing shortly, assigning individuals to diagnostic categories can be useful in evaluating a therapy or a medical approach. But as a system for treating patients, it can lead to protocol-following and away from personalized therapy. A 57 percent success rate, or whatever the impersonalized protocol achieves, is not satisfactory for the 43 percent who don't benefit. With an individualized empirical system, almost 100 percent can benefit, even though no two of them will be treated exactly the same way.

The Role of the Physician

I don't think there is much argument from either camp as to what the role of the physician *should* be. One of the great teachers during my residency at Columbia University was Dr. David Seegal, who drummed into us this axiom: "A doctor's duty is to *convince*." It is no coincidence that Dr. Seegal held a unique academic position; he was director of a hospital service devoted to chronic diseases (the kind that most of us have and will continue to have). He recognized two important points. First, that in the care of chronic illness, the patients need convincing. They need to be convinced that their less-than-perfect habits contribute most to the chronicity of their illness. Second, the role of the physician should be that of an effective teacher.

We all know examples of another type of doctor. The one who says: "I am the doctor, you are only a patient. I know what's good for you." Such an authoritarian doctor can get his instructions followed explicitly; but he encourages passivity and blind faith on the patient's part. He's at the furthest extreme from the doctor who sees the doctor-patient relationship as a teacher-pupil relationship and encourages his patients' participation in decision-making and in carrying out their own health programs. And it's that sort of patient participation that results in the patient's thinking about his whole health situation and planning for the future well-being of his body.

Let me give you an example, close to home. I have a business adviser, who is not my patient; he has confidence in his orthodox physician. His eating habits are acceptable except that he drinks a pint of sugar-sweetened cola beverage with each of his meals. When I urge him to give up the sugar, citing studies that indicate it can lead to heart disease, diabetes, hypertension, mental illness, and a litany of other problems, he answers me, "My doctor gave me a thorough checkup and found nothing wrong. Since I feel fine, why should I change what I'm doing?"

A patient who had learned to participate in planning his own health probably wouldn't have said that. He'd have realized that accepting this free-of-disease-for-the-moment conclusion can leave in place some pretty treacherous lifestyle patterns. I urge my patients to strive for perfection in their lifestyle no matter how good the routine lab tests happen to be.

Is It Religious Fervor That Produces Medical Rigidity?

But let's get back to our authoritarian doctor, or rather to the whole authoritarian habit of mind that is found within modern establishment medicine. Orthodox medicine has entrenched itself within a formalized structure that is surprisingly codified. Centered around the teaching hospital, this structure includes ritual, pomp and ceremony, a hierarchy, a belief system, and a profound faith in those beliefs. It is very like a religion.

I have a clear recollection of attending the Saturday morning medical conferences at Columbia Presbyterian Hospital during my residency training. The professor introduced the assistant professors, who in turn presented cases or told of their research accomplishments. All did so skillfully but always after engaging in a ritual of self-effacement clearly showing their humility in front of the greater god, medical science itself. I was so caught up in the emotion of being a small part of that hallowed teaching institution that a voice within me solemnly proclaimed: "I do not need a religion; medicine can serve as my church."

I do not know how many doctors have adopted medicine as their religion, but I suspect they do so in large numbers. Medicine has such an appeal.

But as a religion it promotes a blind emotional attachment to its tenets and, consequently, a blind antipathy to what it perceives as heresy. As in a strong church, anything that is not orthodox is heretical.

Not unlike other religions, medical orthodoxy believes in proselytizing the uncommitted. In this endeavor it has succeeded, and most of the general public has been converted to its beliefs.

But don't think that alternativists do not have a strong sense of faith. Because they do; it is probably greater than that of the orthodoxists. But in this instance the locus of the faith has shifted from the hospital to the patient's bedside. The alternative physicians I have met tell me that they feel God's presence as they do their work. In my own case, my sense of religion increased manifoldly when I "converted" to nonorthodoxy — and in a very pointed way. I no longer felt "Medicine is my God"; I felt "God is my Medicine."

Medicine-worship

Even when medicine is not a religion substitute, it is an object of adoration for its orthodox membership. This is the trait I find most frustrating in my day-to-day dealings with other doctors or insurance review boards, protecting my practice and trying to disseminate my findings.

Most doctors indulge in medicine-worship to the extent that they cannot be reasoned with. To them the entire scope of knowledge about health begins and ends with what appears in medical journals and texts. Would you like to know how many times in my career I've had to deal with this response: "If it were any good, don't you think we'd all be doing it?" It's well over a thousand times.

If you have ever debated theology with a religious fanatic of a different faith, and watched him reason from his preconceived dogmatic tenets, then you have had a similar experience.

Self-worship Leads to Arrogance

There is a difference. In the theology of medicine, the devotee-physician is not merely a humble believer but is himself a sort of demigod. This, I believe, is the source of a trait many of you must have encountered — arrogance. Arrogance results when one is given the belief that he is one of a chosen few, without being given the humility to handle it.

How many of you remember the joke that takes place in the cafeteria of heaven? There, a self-possessed figure dressed in a green surgical scrub suit and face mask persisted in going to the head of the line, demanding and expecting special service.

"Who's that?" a newcomer asked.

"Oh, that's God. He's always trying to play Doctor."

Apparently, someone else has also noticed the role that many physicians choose to play. I'm sure you've heard the expression "The doctor gave him only six months to live." Well, the doctor didn't do the giving. He merely asserted his perception, based on what he knew of the facts and what he didn't know of other healing arts. After all, the orthodox physician's dedication to science combined with his ignorance of alternatives is a powerful mixture and often places him in the position of having to tell some patients: "There's nothing medical science can do for you; get your affairs in order." The empiricist healer would rarely do that, for he knows, as I do, that the demoralizing effect of such a prognosis will usually make it a self-fulfilling prophecy. *I offer this critique as a person who does not believe in incurable diseases, even though I do believe there are incurable people.*

By contrast, I must say I have met very few arrogant alternativists. Most do share the feeling that they have been chosen, but chosen to be God's servants, not his junior partners. I can only attribute that distinction to the fact that the alternativists have been cast adrift from the mother church and have had to maintain their faith in the humbling context of going it alone.

Winning Through Intimidation

How has a strong central church traditionally kept its followers in line? How does it control heretical notions? By intimidation. By instilling the fear of hellfire and brimstone. So it is with the powerful orthodoxy of medicine.

When institutions believe that "ours is the only way," and when they are confronted with potential nonbelievers, a most commonly used technique is to intimidate to insure conformity. I have had countless patients who meekly acceded to questionable surgery, invasive diagnostic testing, or powerful chemotherapy in situations in which far safer alternatives were available to them, although they had not been so informed. When I queried why they had taken such risks with their own health, their answers were always along the same theme: "They made me feel I had no options, had no time to waste." All had been intimidated by the hospital-based hierarchy.

Who Does the Healing?

All this follows from the premise of mainstream medicine, which reads: "Put yourself in the doctor's hands. He provides the treatment; your role is to comply."

Contrast this with the basic premise of the alternative side: "Take charge of your own health. You will do your own healing. The doctor can teach you how." When I or my confreres intervene, it is as a teacher, or sometimes as a stern taskmaster, but always with the understanding that we will not be doing something for the patient; we can merely show him what he can do for himself. If and when we do intimidate, it is for the purpose of motivating the patient to take charge of his own fate and not passively accept the treatment given him.

Even the diagnostic approaches favored by the two schools reflect this difference. A recent example is a patient who saw me and an orthodox cardiologist for a workup just a few days apart. He

was complaining of chest pain, typical of coronary artery insufficiency. The cardiologist started off by ordering an angiocardiogram; he was obviously looking to see if his surgical colleague could
help the patient. I started off by ordering tests for glucose tolerance, blood lipids, and food intolerance; I was looking to see if the
patient, by following the appropriate diet, could help himself.

The Cause of Disease: External or Internal?

There is another distinction that needs to be made, although it
does not strictly follow the rationalist-empiricist boundary line.

How do the medical philosophies in question view the origin of
most illness? Are the causes found outside the body or within?

One of orthodox medicine's more recent traditions is that it is
still emerging from the age of infectious disease and is still very
much in the era of antibiotics. It continues to view its role as that
of protecting the patient from sources of illness foreign to the body.
In this role, the doctor can do things for the patient that the patient
cannot do for himself. He can still maintain his "doctor knows best"
posture.

As most infectious diseases have faded from the picture and chronic
degenerative diseases have taken center stage, it is becoming increasingly recognized that most illness does represent an internal
imbalance.

The difference is that orthodox medicine is just awakening to
that point whereas alternative medicine (or the proposed new
Complementary Medicine) has always recognized it. Alternativists/
empiricists have always acted from the assumption that the body
heals itself by balancing itself from within.

A Pediatric Illustration

Let me show you how this distinction works in real life. If you
know many children, chances are you know one who is plagued
with chronic ear infections, or recurrent otitis, a most common and
distressing pediatric problem. If the family uses an orthodox pedia-
trician, chances are the treatment will be a course of antibiotics.
This will seem to work, but the problem will come back again and
again, until a chronic disease affecting the child's entire health pat-

tern develops (usually a systemic yeast infection caused by the use of the antibiotics).

The modern-day complementarist will start by making internal corrections. He will prescribe vitamin C, bioflavonoids, zinc, pantothenic acid, and beta carotene; he will remove sugar from the diet and test for food intolerances and for the allergy that is the probable contributing cause of the otitis.

With the pre-eminence of chronic illnesses caused by our interaction with our environment — and, in my view, most specifically an overly refined diet — *the doctors best equipped to handle patients are those who are most determined to convince a patient to change his diet and his lifestyle.* The doctor who absolves the patient from his responsibilities will be less and less successful.

The Establishment Versus the Anti-Establishment

There is a major difference between the two poles of the medical continuum that did not exist through the centuries, but that holds true now, and provides a major distinction for our comparative analysis. Having held sway for the last century and having aligned itself quite successfully with every source of economic backing with which it has come in contact, medical orthodoxy is totally entrenched within that widespread power network called the establishment. I need not remind you that there is virtually no connection between that establishment and the entire slate of medical alternatives.

The entire superstructure embraced under the general term *health care* is based on the establishment's medical system. Look how far-reaching that is. It means that the government and its agencies and legislative acts; the private sector, with its concentration of wealth, including but not limited to the pharmaceutical, direct health care, and food industries; plus the philanthropic foundations, the media, the insurance carriers, the hospital system, the licensing boards, even our own education programs — are all integrated to protect the ins and keep the outs out.

What Does the Establishment Connection Mean to You?

There are countless advantages to being a patient in harmony with the entrenched establishment. Over the years, a well-intentioned

bipartisan government effort has provided you with a federal sub-
sidy system, including Medicare and Medicaid; has provided billions for medical research; has set up the National Institutes of
Health; and has supported impressive nonprofit teaching hospitals.
At the same time, numerous philanthropic contributors, in the form
of foundations, have supported hospitals, research, some medical
care financing, and mixed in with their propaganda, a little public
education. The private sector also harbors our widespread medical
insurance system, which is capable, when it chooses, of paying most
of your medical bills (with your money, of course).

With the support of the establishment, Big Brother can take care
of you when you get sick. It has all been provided for you in all the
ways that are already quite familiar to you. You know where your
doctor's office is, where the emergency care centers are, where the
nearest and best hospitals are, where the pharmacy is, and some of
you even know how to find someone who will make a house call.
Best of all, you know how to fill out your medical insurance forms
so that none of it will cost you much more than the premiums you
(or your employer) pay anyway. That is the security blanket called
contemporary American health care and you've already been told
and retold that it "just doesn't get any better than this." If you buy
that package, you know what you're getting. It's the path that most
everyone takes; it is better known as the path of least resistance.
You may live and die within that system, and you will not have
made any waves.

But suppose something I have said or will say catches your attention, and you say: "That's for me! I'm going with Complementary
Medicine."

Now you have just stripped yourself of most of your support system. You'll be on your previous doctor's "bad" list, and so you'll
wonder what will happen to you if, God forbid, there is an emergency. You'll be afraid of hospitals, knowing they will surely take
you off the new diet and nutrition program you're beginning to
depend on. Your insurance carrier will, more often than not, give
you various types of "hard times" in getting your reimbursement.
Your friends and some of your family will try to talk you out of your
folly and bring you back into the fold, where all the normal people
are. You're even likely to hear, or read, that your new alternativist

doctor is a quack. And the greatest affront of all is that your new doctor is going to expect you to do your own getting well; he isn't even going to do it *for* you.

What it all comes down to is that you've lost your security blanket.

So Why Do It?

Only because it might just be the difference between staying sick and getting healthy. To learn more about that, you'll just have to read on.

Establishment connections provide some insight into more distinctions between orthodoxy and the "pretenders to the throne." The fact that there are large sums of money pouring into our health care system from a lot of sources other than patients' fee payments is having an effect on orthodoxy, but not on alternativism, which is spared the responsibility of dealing with money from these sources.

The great hospitals depend in large part on charitable donations from community-minded individuals and corporations. A lot of the clout within the hospital political hierarchy is awarded to the doctors who secure the greatest contributions of this kind. To reach these benefactors, one must appeal to their own psychology, and that means appealing to the corporate mentality. Remember that almost all *individuals* who support medical projects are, in reality, individuals with *corporate* connections.

Time after time, I have seen these wealthy benefactors go to alternative physicians, have splendid results, and vow that they owe their lives to those doctors. And yet when it comes time to give their philanthropic financial support, they donate to the local hospital or to a foundation named after the disease it seems to perpetuate. Why?

I believe this kind of behavior indicates the stranglehold that establishment membership has on the psyche of its members. The patient-benefactor wants to be accepted by his peers and wants it known that he is doing the "correct" thing.

The upshot is that the doctor is a better fund raiser if he joins the war and opposes the empirical opposition.

The Self-serving Benefactors of Research

The question of research grants is more clear-cut. Here the drug industry itself is often the "benefactor," paying specifically to have research done on exactly the pharmaceuticals it intends to promote. When the government pays for the research, that mechanism is one step less direct. Government research grants are authorized by scientists, all of whom have a track record of supporting and engaging in pharmaceutical-sponsored research. They merely act in a manner consistent with their past affiliations, and the federally funded research grants continue to operate in support of a drug-oriented medical system.

All this means that despite a rather impressive list of clinical studies published in Europe, an anticancer protocol of antioxidant vitamins, including vitamins C, E, beta carotene, and selenium, along with, perhaps, some enzymes and other biologicals, does not get studied at all, while chemotherapy combinations are studied by the thousands under the government's aegis.

It also means, thanks to the stonewalling role of the media (another corporate establishment constituent), that you or your doctor don't even know that such unorthodox studies are being conducted, and reported upon. Research on promising biologic approaches should obviously be done, but through the passive resistance technique known as calculated ignorance, no one in authority admits to being aware that there is work that bears replicating. To give a specific example, I find it hard to believe that officials of the National Cancer Institute, whose entire careers are devoted to knowing about cancer research, would be *unaware* of conferences in Switzerland and Germany where high-quality research papers about successful nontoxic, biologic treatments are being presented. It is much more plausible to presume that they are aware of what's going on and *choose* to pretend that it does not exist. If you need to know the reason, it's this: The entire concept of a biologic, nontoxic cancer therapy would signal the beginning of the end of the highly profitable chemotherapy industry, an industry that is deeply entrenched in establishment economics. Acknowledging the biologic conferences would be an extreme anti-establishment act. These people are salaried, you know.

The Prepaid Versus Fee-for-Service Dilemma

There is another distinction, based on economics, looming on the health care horizon. A growing percentage of Americans, because of the burgeoning phenomenon of health maintenance organizations (HMOs), are being covered by a system of prepayment for medical fees. The economic thrust is the opposite of our traditional fee-for-service system. As honest as we all try to be, economics forces errors.

In fee-for-service economics, the more interventive the doctor is, the more money he makes. An extra electrocardiogram, endoscopic procedure, medicine check, cancer screen, and the like all enhance the doctor's income. In a prepayment program, the doctor receives a capitation fee for every patient enrolled, and it is the doctor who in effect pays for the procedures, inasmuch as they are expenses deducted from his already pledged income. Here the tendency is to do as little as possible.

I don't know which situation is worse. One friend of mine, a very successful London general practitioner, informed me that his patients are treated only for their immediate complaint and never even have their blood pressure taken. The capitation fee in Britain's National Health Service prepayment system is so low, "we can't afford to do otherwise," he confided.

On the other hand, I know of several American neurologists who order CT scans (computerized tomography, also called CAT scans) routinely on every patient complaining of headache.

If the prospect of a minimalization of medical care disturbs you, then the prospect of HMO membership may give you pause. If you opt for nonorthodox medicine, you are very unlikely to be a part of HMO economics. At this writing, I know of no HMOs that admit alternative-thinking physicians.

I have gone to great lengths to help make you aware of the two options we all have in developing our own health care strategy. You'd think I could not have left very much out. But I have saved for last what is the most important distinction of all and the most passionately guarded issue: the issue of proof.

3
...
THE ISSUE OF PROOF

No matter what the historical pathways tracing the traditions of the dominant medicine and its alternatives, the main issue that separates them today is the issue of proof.

From the first time that Alexander von Humboldt, circa 1830, issued his criteria for proof, the mainstream of rationalist medicine grasped it to its bosom and adopted it as its credo. "Our medicine is based on science; now, with these principles it can itself become a science."

One of the first and certainly one of the most significant applications of the need for proof was uttered by Robert Koch, who proposed four criteria that must be met in order to *prove* that a given bacterial agent caused a given disease. Koch's Postulates, as they were called, provided the guidelines for the golden age of bacteriologic discovery that included the achievements of Louis Pasteur and others.

And on American shores, the influence of Sir William Osler was significant. Mainstream American medicine was to be built only upon provable discoveries from his time forward.

But Proof Is an Issue

It took me twenty-five years as a physician to discover that proof not only is an issue, it is *the* issue. Let me show you why.

Suppose someone very dear to you is suffering from an illness known to be incurable by all techniques of modern medical science. And suppose you learn of a new technique that is being used to treat that very illness with great success in some remote part of the globe. That technique is, of course, too new to be proven. The patient thus will be confronted with a dilemma: Should I resign myself to the fate that medical science has outlined for me, or should I deal in the unproven and perhaps be cured?

I'm sure you recognize that whenever such an option enters a person's life, the impact is, indeed, gravely important. But you might be surprised to learn that dilemmas of this sort, perhaps on a somewhat lesser scale, are anything but rare.

Let me offer my own experience as a physician. Now that I have treated thirty-five thousand patients in my private practice or at the Atkins Center, I can state that virtually all of them have been treated, at least in part, with unproven therapies or techniques. What follows is, of course, my personal evaluation, but I estimate that had I used only the proven techniques, a full 90 percent of them would not have done so well, and many who now lead normal, healthy lives would have been dead.

So let us take a closer look at this matter of proof and try to decide whether it is our friend or foe.

Must Our Medicine Be Proven?

I have listed over a dozen distinctions between orthodox medicine and the medicines emerging from the empiricist tradition, but all pale by comparison to the significance of this distinction. One could well call the two competing medicines proven medicine and yet-to-be-proven medicine.

Rationalist medicine entered the modern era and became the dominant medicine when it began to live by its demand for proof. Before that, it was a tradition of opinions, a hodgepodge of therapies without standards and without any certainty that they even worked; it was an unscientific "science." There it would still be today had not its farsighted leaders insisted that a rational system of proving its precepts be meticulously adhered to. The century-old tradition of proof is the force that provided the impetus for medicine to emerge from its own dark ages to the awesome system it is today.

When empirical medicines attempted to abide by the same standards of provability, they found that, for a variety of reasons I hope to offer shortly, they simply could not provide what was accepted as proof. Because of this, they lost ground and almost perished from world view.

The Requisites of Proof

At first the criteria for proving the worth of medical therapies were not overly burdensome. After all, the world's medical knowledge to that point had been accumulated by virtue of subjective observations on the part of some pretty astute clinicians. (Not the least of which was the impressive body of clinical observations made by the leading empiricist, Samuel Hahnemann.)

There were test-tube (or culture plate) proofs, referred to as in vitro techniques; there were animal experiments, and finally, human experiments, the in vivo techniques. Clinical observations were still done by the age-old system of tabulating results and comparing them.

Comparing with What?

Initially the standards of comparison were simply against what was expected from previous understanding of the illness. When Paul Ehrlich tested his arsenical compounds against the relentlessly progressive illness syphilis and was able to observe some patients improve, his peers accepted that he had "proven" his magic bullets to be effective. But the scientific vanguard of medicine soon recognized that there were loopholes: What about illnesses with unpredictable outcomes? What about those which waxed and waned? When patients get better after a proposed in vivo therapy, that doesn't *prove* anything. It might have happened anyway.

Their answer, in the interest of keeping medicine scientific, was the idea of "controlled" studies. Some patients, called the control groups, would not receive the proposed treatment under study, just so they could be observed and compared with the group that was treated. Then the experimenters discovered, as empiricists had long known, that the act of being treated had a healing effect of its own. So they began to insist that the control group also receive treatment, but in the form of placebos, inert substances whose only purpose was to "fool" the patient into thinking he had received the active test substance.

This sufficed for a decade or so, until the scientists discovered, again as empiricists had long known, that the doctor was much more effective when he believed in his therapy than when he did not. At this point the placebo-controlled study was no longer considered good research and no longer of much value toward the accumulation of "proof." The new requisite for proof henceforward was the "double-blind" study. Not only could the *patient* not know whether he or she was receiving the active therapy, neither could the treating *physician*. Who got what was not known until after the study was completed, when a secret code was cracked by someone not heretofore connected with the study. It was a security system the CIA would be proud of.

Medical Traditions and the Double Blind

Since much of our previous discussion has centered around the traditions from which modern-day medicine has emerged, let's pick up the threads of that discussion and see how traditions have affected today's medical research.

One of medicine's nobler traditions has been the replacement of opinion with science and its insistence on the scientific method. One of medicine's more ignoble traditions, I'm sure most fair-minded people would agree, is the squelching of opposing medical thought, the original purpose behind the founding of the AMA.

It soon became apparent to the ignobles, the economic protectors of medicine, that they could use the techniques of the nobles, the scientific protectors of medicine, to permanently suppress, and perhaps destroy, all economic threats to the "trade union."

This Is How It Works

The double blind is an excellent test for evaluating pharmaceuticals and single variables. I agree that, when it is applicable, it should be used. The problem is that, as the protocols get stricter and stricter in their exclusion of subjectivity, the area of applicability becomes narrower and narrower. The real blind spot in the double blind is that the leadership in medicine continues to insist upon it as the *only* acceptable proof even though its applicability is so limited.

The problem is that for many good therapies, a double-blind protocol *cannot even be devised*.

For example, if the medication to be tested has a taste or smell that cannot be disguised, or produces an immediate reaction like a flush, a tingling, fever, nausea, or diarrhea, the test will not be considered properly "blinded," and thus acceptable as proof, until a suitable inactive substance, for use as the placebo, can be found to cause exactly the same combination of sensations.

Further, the tests are usually, in comparison to the lifetime that chronic degenerative conditions last, too brief and unable to pick up delayed risks or benefits. That's why many drugs enter commerce highly touted because of their "proven" efficacy, achieve widespread usage, and then after being prescribed for a few decades fall into disrepute when their long-range drawbacks are discovered. Examples of this are the oral antidiabetic agents, several anticholesterol compounds, many anti-arthritics, and most of the diuretics.

Is the Double Blind Suitable for Drugless Medicine?

So far, we have discussed problems with testing drugs. But what about nondrug medicine? What about all the empiricist techniques I have been mentioning and will be telling you about in the chapters to come? Here the double blind is about as inappropriate as an evening gown at a mud-wrestling match.

How can one even devise a double-blind experiment to test a diet? Or chiropractic manipulation? Or acupuncture done the classical oriental way? Or homeopathy, where a hundred different patients would require a hundred *different* treatments? Or a nutritional balance system, in which the therapist must use the results to govern his treatment schedule?

The truth is that any therapy that requires an interaction between healer and "healee," as is essential to all empirical approaches, cannot employ any sort of doctor-blinded technique in its self-evaluation. I assume that all of you can easily grasp this point. I think it is a very straightforward point. Now, if this point is so easy to grasp, why do you think that the leadership of medicine can't grasp it? Is it that they are not as bright as you, or is it that they, very purposefully, refuse to?

J'accuse

I accuse the political leadership of orthodox medicine of fostering the worship of the double-blind requisite for proof as a specific technique for suppressing the alternative/empirical healing systems. And I also accuse the mainstream of practicing physicians of being so wrapped up in their fear of nonconformity that they fail to see that they have been systematically brainwashed.

My Evidence

One of the dominant medicine's most effective techniques is what I refer to as a white paper. This is an editorial analysis of an alternative medical approach published in a prestigious medical journal for the purpose of dissuading the journal's readers from looking further into the matter. The white paper is usually written by a "blue-ribbon panel" drawn from the membership of the specialty society being economically threatened by the innovative technique; occasionally, it is written by a blue-ribbon individual.

I have seen white papers published against orthomolecular (nutritional) psychiatry, clinical ecology, neutralizing dose allergy treatments, numerous alternative cancer treatments, the diagnosis and treatment of chronic systemic yeast infections, mercury amalgam toxicity, chelation therapy, nutritional arthritis treatments, and on and on. My first experience with a white paper was the one directed against the Atkins Diet in 1973, the rebuttals for which appear in the Bantam paperback editions of *Dr. Atkins' Diet Revolution* and *Dr. Atkins' Superenergy Diet.*

All White Papers Do the Same Thing

All use a common ploy; all attack the innovative technique on the basis that it is *unproven.* Most of them specifically decry the fact that there are no double-blind studies in support of the technique being "hatcheted." Sometimes the double blind's essentiality can be inferred from statements such as "There is no evidence for . . ." or "No good evidence exists that . . ." written without reference to the fact that considerable evidence other than double-blind studies exists in favor of the victimized technique.

I use the terms I do because all white papers have another common denominator. They present only the "contra" side of the issue. In the business and political world, one-sided editorials are expected and can be taken for what they are. But you must understand that the contemporary physician plays by a more genteel rule book. In his professional reading he has come to expect balanced "review articles" on all medical subjects, rather painstakingly delineating the pros and cons of each unsettled subject. His mind is not geared to assimilate a hatchet job. Thus, he is left with the assumption that what he has read represents the whole story on the subject; he does not even recognize that he has been presented with only what the leadership wants him to know.

Other Problems with the Double Blind

In addition to the fact that the double-blind technique was devised for pharmaceutical testing and is not suitable for testing empirical healing systems, there are other obvious problems with it.

First, it demands a fixed protocol; there is no room for flexibility. Granted, in certain instances in which medicine is still an art, such as psychoanalysis and rehabilitation (physiatry), practitioners are spared the responsibility of doing double-blind research. But what medical leadership won't realize is that all of medicine requires flexibility in case management. Even medical problems for which the double-blind study is the holy scripture — such as the treatment of headache, arthritis, colitis, hypertension, and the like — really demand flexibility of treatment and interaction with an aware and concerned physician.

Then There Is the Matter of Money

I hope you realize that medical research costs money and has to be subsidized. Where is that money going to come from? First of all,

I must tell you that no doctor practicing alternative or Complementary Medicine in America makes enough money to do much more than cover expenses. Even entire groups of doctors in alternative societies can raise just enough funds to hold annual meetings. Remember, for them, there is none of the pharmaceutical research money their orthodox counterparts can call upon, almost at will.

In medical school we were taught to remain academically disciplined, and were told that even doctors in private practice could do some very valuable clinical research. To which I now say, "Bleep bleep." That was true in the days when tabular results were accepted, but medicine apparently no longer accepts tabular results as proof. More about this subject momentarily.

Doctors in fee-for-service private practice cannot do research that demands a control group unless they are subsidized. And alternative-thinking doctors have never been subsidized and there are no prospects that they will be.

This does not keep mainstream medicine from applying the Catch-22 screws to the innovator by smugly and patronizingly asserting: "You can be sure that nothing would make us happier than if your claims were true. Show us your proof and we'll be all too glad to accept them." All the while they know that proof is the most difficult achievement in all of medicine.

It is easier to cure a hundred incurables than it is to prove that the treatment works.

And There Is the Matter of Ethics

Now let's look at this probability. Clinicians, doctors in the front line treating sick people, do make wonderful discoveries. It happens all the time. Confronted with a difficult case, or treating a patient they care very much about, they often try new therapies. Many times, these new treatments work far beyond their expectations. Enthused, the doctor tries the same treatment on other patients with similar problems, and lo and behold, the treatment works again. This happens thousands of times in a decade. Yet only a handful of these discoveries make it into mainstream medicine. Why?

Because the profession insists: "Doctor, prove it." Now, by the time the innovative doctor realizes that he has something that needs to be proven, he already *knows* that it works. Withholding such treatment from a patient who needs it is unethical and immoral. His usual course of action is to continue to use the treatment and leave the proof to someone else. This is the course of action I instinctively took when I discovered the therapeutic advantages of a low-carbohydrate reducing diet. The immorality of my allowing an overweight patient to eat an English muffin is not earth-shattering, but if I were withholding an effective treatment from an otherwise terminally ill cancer patient, the moral question would be a heavy one indeed.

Who Accepts Unproven Therapies?

We have been very diligently analyzing the differences between the two medicines and have stressed the importance of the issue of proof. I now intend to show you that this is the most important distinction of all.

The distinction is this: Orthodox medicine rejects the unproven; alternative medicines accept and utilize unproven therapies.

What Does This Mean to You?

This means that if you opt for mainstream medicine, you will not be treated with any procedures that have not been adequately tested, or are not in widespread use. But it also means that you will not have an opportunity to be treated with anything at the frontier of the healing arts, nothing based on ideas which are truly innovative. In rejecting the unproven, mainstream medicine has consistently shut out medical innovation.

If you have a condition for which conventional medicine has devised an effective treatment, then perhaps an orthodox approach will prove satisfactory. But if you have a condition for which the track record of orthodoxy leaves something to be desired, then, of course, a decision to remain with the dominant medicine forces you to accept those shortcomings.

If you have such an illness, your only chance to get well may be to move to the nonorthodox side of the schism. That area, the area at the cutting edge, is the exclusive property of alternative medicine.

Now, those of you who follow the press releases about all the new developments at this medical center or that, should say, "Dr. Atkins, here's where we part company. I know there are loads of major breakthroughs in medical science taking place this very week."

Of course, there are developments that are hyped as breakthroughs, but by and large they are nothing more than variations on old themes. A new chemotherapy combination, a new antihypertensive or antidiabetes medication — these are not breakthroughs and they are not new medical concepts. When the advance is something truly different, it faces the kind of skepticism we have been describing, and here the demand for proof is raised.

"But what about the very high-tech use of interleukin-2 in cancer patients I've recently read about? That's a different mainstream approach — immunology, not chemotherapy. What about that?" you ask. Let me point out that German complementarists have been using a biologic medicine that stimulates the same system as does interleukin, only they've been doing it for twenty years and can do it without the toxic reactions interleukin causes. I believe that the cutting edge of Complementary Medicine consistently stays ten to twenty years ahead of the mainstream, simply because it takes that amount of time to progress from discovery to proof.

Remember, *the demand for double-blind testing is not universal in scientific medicine.* It is, in fact, peculiar to the medicine of America and countries that follow America's lead. Where the traditions are different, alternative medicines may still flourish. For example, if you, or better yet, your doctor, were to spend the first week in November of every year in Baden-Baden, the famous West German spa city, he could attend, along with more than two thousand other doctors, the annual meeting of over a dozen nonorthodox medical societies. Here during Medical Week, many of the subdivisions of Complementary Medicine meet in scientific session so that members may present papers for review by their peers. Here is a prototype for medicine of the future, an empirical medicine studied by scientific techniques. It will serve the future *because* it does not require the double blind for proof. Thus unencumbered, it can provide a more sophisticated healing system.

In demanding double-blind proof, medicine cuts itself off from its own avant-garde. Time after time, I have seen superior orthodox physicians alienated from the mainstream of medicine simply because the advances they proposed were too far ahead of the existing paradigms. Many of these breakthrough-oriented individuals found comfort and acceptance working with other doctors of innovative medicine — the complementarists.

That is why it is nonorthodox medicine and not mainstream medicine that can properly stake claim to the vast territory between discovery and proof.

How Can a Science Develop Without Proof?

I hope you have been asking that, because that's the right question.

I have been describing the scenario whereby the innovative doctor tries a treatment on a patient and it works. The patient gets well. Now, all properly skeptical people will say, "People with just about any illness can get better on their own; how can you say with a single case that your treatment did it?"

My answer is: Sometimes you can't, but many times you can. Cause and effect is not such a difficult concept to prove. All it takes is replication, and it happens in medicine every day. All doctors use it, even if they are dyed-in-the-wool, card-carrying AMA members.

Let Me Show You How It Works

Most nonorthodox physicians today believe in the existence of a condition called nightshade-induced arthritis, even though the mainstream rheumatology party line denies its existence. In this condition, the ingestion of a toxic natural substance called solanin will cause a prompt flare-up of an inflammatory (rheumatoid) type of arthritis. Solanin is a substance contained in a diverse, widely consumed food group called the nightshade family. Nightshades include potatoes, tomatoes, green and red peppers, paprika, eggplant, and even tobacco.

Since I am not encumbered by orthodox dogma, I suspected that the arthritis of one of my patients, Mrs. Helen Corwin,* might be in part due to her daily nightshade ingestion. I put her on a no-nightshade version of the sugarless Meat and Millet Diet (see Appendix B) and she promptly responded by having days in which she was free of arthritic complaints. Occasionally, however, she would have a three-to-five-day flare-up of symptoms. It turned out that these occurred whenever she broke the no-nightshade dictum, but it took us a while to catch on to the cause-and-effect relationship because we had eliminated so many possible culprits and had given some pretty valuable nutritional supplements. When Helen and I realized the probable role the nightshades were playing, she avoided them like the plague. Over the next year, Helen had only four moderate, and brief, flare-ups of her joint discomfort. She followed up each recurrence with some personal sleuthing and was able to uncover the fact that in each instance she, while eating out or at dinner parties, had been given either meat loaf with a potato stuffing, a hidden tomato-based salad dressing, or a garnish containing green pepper. In each case the flare-up followed the hidden transgression by about one day. I trust there is no well-intentioned doctor anywhere, not even the chief propagandist for the Arthritis Foundation, who wouldn't concur in advising Helen to stay away from the nightshades, thus tacitly admitting the presence of at least one case of nightshade-induced arthritis.

Helen demonstrates the point I want to make. *Important medical knowledge can be gained from a single case history.*

Now, if one case could prove the existence of nightshade arthritis, imagine what ten cases could do. Now imagine a hundred cases and then a thousand. One could write a helluva paper on the subject, and without doing a controlled or double-blind study.

Case History: Rejected Concept or Accepted?

This is the point of distinction between our two medical systems. Orthodoxy rejects the case history as a step toward proof; the em-

---

*Mrs. Corwin and all the other patients whose medical histories are discussed in this book are real people, and the course of treatment for each case is described exactly as it took place. However, in all cases the patient's identity has been concealed, and the name has been changed.

pirical medical approaches depend on it. Of course, it's not so cut and dried as that. Orthodoxists have two names for case histories. If the case history is about something they like, such as a new application of a popular drug, it is called "preliminary evidence." When it supports something they don't like, such as chelation therapy or a biological nontoxic cancer success, it is called "anecdotal evidence." (The printed word does not do justice to the loathing and derision that an orthodox physician can give to the pronunciation of "anecdotal evidence.")

Yet, if a doctor learns from his clinical experience, most of that learning is from repeated examples of "anecdotal evidence." Nevertheless, would you believe that there are some doctors who don't trust their own personal experience and believe *only* what they read in medical journals? Well, from my dealings with mainstreamers, and mind you this is not a scientific survey, I would estimate that slightly more than half of them are like that. Many times, we have had inquiries about this innovative treatment or that, and they always ask: "Do you have any literature?" When I answer, "There is no literature; it's all happening right now," they then take a "not interested" posture.

Anecdotal Evidence: You Be the Judge

In many ways, this book is a testimonial to anecdotal evidence. I shall present you with the case histories of a number of people who have been patients at the Atkins Center. You will learn of their experiences with chronic illnesses both before and after they were exposed to Complementary Medicine. As you read them, I want you to be the judge as to whether there is something to be learned from individual case histories.

In all fairness, I must point out to you that the orthodox resistance to anecdotal evidence is not altogether inappropriate. There are laws of probability, and a single case rarely overturns them. The case history of a person who wins $10 million in the state lottery certainly does not prove that lotteries are a good investment. But a second case, or a tenth case, or a hundredth case of a cure effected by the application of a particular therapy can become very convincing. The key here is replication; the more times an experience can be repeated, the more it can be shown that the experience represents a significant variation from what would otherwise be expected according to the rules of probability.

Replication Is Needed to Rule Out Coincidence

But replication can be achieved in a single individual. This is a basic everyday observation. Most shellfish-allergic people, for example, make their own diagnosis, not through sophisticated allergy testing, but by tracking down the cause-and-effect relationship of their own symptoms after eating shellfish. By having the experience repeated often enough, they can make the diagnosis.

Good Clinicians Are Good Observers

Throughout medicine's history, new knowledge was developed and propagated through the simple, direct expedient of an astute physician, at the bedside, making his observations and drawing his conclusions. Those who remained empirical and relied on their experience rather than imposing their logical expectations were seldom wrong.

It was only in the twentieth century that doctors turned their backs on this system of learning.

I agree with the idea that medical practices should, wherever possible, be proven. I do, however, wish to redefine what constitutes proof. *Medicine is not an absolute science; therefore, medicine should not require absolute proof.* A biologic science is not an exact science, and the patient who is sick *now* must be treated *now*. How can he wait years or even decades for "proof"?

My suggestion for medical proof is the tabular study. A tabular study is a group of case histories, all similar yet all, because of individual uniqueness, a little different from one another. The results, after a given treatment, are evaluated and tabulated according to the degree of improvement or worsening, or to some numerical readout on a test, or to length of illness, or to whatever is measurable and significant. To constitute proof, it is essential that this compilation of results be compared with something that represents how it would turn out if the condition remained untreated or were treated in some heretofore acceptable way.

Standards for Comparison

The major problem involves what should be the comparison standard. Orthodoxy now insists that the comparison (control) group *must* be run concurrently with the treated group, and without a hint that there are many differences in the treatment the groups are receiving. Nonorthodox disciplines, citing the problems with simultaneous controls we have discussed (cost, ethics, and inflexibility of protocol), contend that the best we can do in most cases is to compare our tabular results against "historical controls." This means using what is known about the illness, usually learned by analyzing previously reported medical studies, as the standard for comparison. Thus, to evaluate a new treatment for pancreatic cancer, for example, one would use survival statistics from previously published studies in lieu of a simultaneous control group. This works quite well because the historical studies for this affliction show a nearly uniform fatal outcome. But there is a real problem in studying asthma, arthritis, colitis, or the like this way, because these illnesses vary so in their severity. How can one be sure that the group offered for comparison had problems as great as those of the patients in the tabular study group?

Lack of Comparability Can Be a Weakness

There is no question that this lack of accurate comparison standards was the weakness that pulled the tabular study from its onetime status as the gold standard of proof down to the level of unacceptability. But in pursuing "pure science," medicine has sacrificed too much in the way of applicability. I maintain that the tabular study, which served medicine well for most of the past century, still provides appropriate proof and should be accepted as such. More important, I maintain that those who judge medical systems should recognize that the revered double-blind study cannot be used for judging complex or flexible therapies.

I hope that this rather detailed comparison of the two existing medicines has provided you some insight into the dilemmas facing you or anyone concerned with securing the best in health care. When you are basically healthy, you can thrive in either situation. But when you or your loved ones face a serious illness, requiring good medicine *and* a good support system, you will find yourself, in today's society, between a rock and a hard place.

I have promised you a solution because I am working with a system that seems to answer some of the difficult problems. Now I would like to show you how it works.

4
...

COMPLEMENTARY MEDICINE
The Health Revolution

You have now read about the strengths and weaknesses of our science-based mainstream medicine and of the strengths and weaknesses of the experiential alternatives. You know of the antipathy between the two camps and you know why that forces you, in matters of health, to make a choice between the two.

How My Own Brand of Complementary Medicine Was Born

I have gotten through life, when confronted with a dilemma, by making it a rule never to grasp either horn but to alter the dilemma itself, so that the choice is different and is easier to make. As an independent medical practitioner, I found this relatively easy to accomplish in my own practice.

I simply decided to put all the medical disciplines I knew on the table and then select from them all. Where some systems were weak, others might be strong. As simple as this was, it was a breakthrough. It seems most everyone was concentrating on a single approach; some doctors were orthodox, some were homeopaths, others were herbalists or acupuncturists, chiropractors or nutritionists. If there is a validity to each discipline, then why not use them all? All healing arts, if they are valid in the first place, can and should complement one another.

And so when I first heard the term *Complementary Medicine*, my reaction was: "That's it! That's really what my practice is all about." It is Complementary Medicine, then, that I propose to you.

Complementary Medicine: Altering the Dilemma

The solution to everyone's dilemma is not to choose orthodox medicine or alternative medicine, but to choose both. Let me give you an example. It is my practice to discourage patients from using pharmaceuticals if similar benefits can be obtained by other means. Thus, when the first suggestions of using aspirin as an anticlotting agent came forth a few years ago, I took a firmly negative stance. Aspirin is a drug, all right, and its side effects — including gastric bleeding — are by no means negligible. If we need an anticlotting agent, I said, then let's use a natural one like vitamin E.

Then in January 1988, the *New England Journal of Medicine* released the results of its five-year controlled study on the effects of aspirin on the incidence of coronary heart disease in twenty-two thousand physicians. Eleven thousand physicians had taken one aspirin every second day for the period of the study and had suffered almost 50 percent fewer heart attacks than their eleven thousand colleagues who took no regular dose.

Two days after the study came out, I was on the air doing my talk show on WOR radio, and I reversed my position publicly. The fact is that the benefit-to-risk ratio had altered dramatically. One aspirin every two days is an impressively low dosage that most people can handle without difficulty, and the statistical benefits shown by the study were not to be shrugged off. I've swallowed an aspirin every other day since then myself. (Incidentally, I still remain bitterly opposed to aspirin in the management of arthritis, headache, and any other condition for which the dosage would be significant.)

From that example you can see that I'm not firmly committed to one school of medical thought over another; what I remain firmly committed to is the welfare of my patients, and that, I think, is the basis of Complementary Medicine.

I have known thousands of my fellow physicians over my thirty-five years in medicine. The overwhelming majority of them are caring, compassionate, and patient-oriented. I find it hard to believe that they would not accept the basic premise of Complementary Medicine if only they knew that it was a possibility whose time has come and that they would not be penalized for accepting it.

The Idea Whose Time Has Come

We have reached the stage at which rationalism can finally give scientific support to empiricism at the same time that empiricism teaches rationalism to respect the wholeness of the individual. Complementary Medicine, then, is a contemporary rational empiricism. Or, it is a contemporary empirical rationalism. Now is the time to declare its birth. This is the first point in recorded history at which a rationalist medicine has sufficient scientific backing to be correct. Previously, its science was wrong. Just how successful could a system based on logic be when its basic science dictated that there were four elements — earth, air, fire, and water? But now that the underlying science can be believed, now that we understand the function of T- and B-lymphocytes, of prostaglandins, free radicals, antioxidants, and the like, we can make deductions based on some bona fide knowledge and come up with therapies that work.

But why not tie this vast body of scientific information to the one tradition that has worked through the centuries when the other has not? Why not combine it with the principles of empirical medicine, the discipline whose success derived from the fact that it is based on results?

With Complementary Medicine, you get to utilize our scientific breakthroughs *and* work with *vis medicatrix naturae,* the healing power of nature. The doctor can know his patient as one with many component parts *and* a single unifying vital energy. We can see him as a person in a specific disease category *and* as a unique individual.

The time for Complementary Medicine is now; it could not have worked much sooner than this. This is the first point in time when *both* its subsystems have come of age. The funds of rational and of empirical knowledge have become so vast that the only logical step is the wedding of the two.

It is beginning to take place, anyway. The empirical nutritional use of marine lipids (fatty acids found in fish oils) is being studied, and accepted, in orthodox peer-review journals. Immunology, a health-enhancing approach, is gradually supplanting the toxic, opposition-oriented chemotherapy in cancer management. Acupuncture is being studied scientifically, and showing results in comparative studies. And quite recently the prestigious journal *Lancet* published controlled studies proving the benefit of homeopathy. All that is needed is the will to make it happen on a grand scale. I fervently hope that this book will make some contribution to that end.

BOOK TWO

. . .

THE ILLNESS

∎ ∎ ∎
INTRODUCTION

I t just so happens that, as a physician, I am a pragmatist, and this is how I became one. Once I was cut adrift from orthodoxy by the AMA attack on what I felt was proven — the benefits of low-carbohydrate dieting for overweight people — I felt compelled to plot a little revenge. My motto became "The best revenge is success." To me this meant a successful form of medicine, and that success had to be measured by the "bottom line." In a word, I became obsessed with getting better results than my detractors.

This obsession with getting results led me to the result-oriented side of medicine — to empiricism. And the obsession with doing it better led me to search along the edge of discovery, in the areas of unproven innovation that the medical mainstream hasn't been ready to accept.

I didn't realize it at the time, but what I was learning was setting the stage for a new system of medicine — an innovative, multifaceted, empirical, nature-allied, health-enhancing, individualized, yet unproven system that deserved the name Complementary Medicine.

I used it in my practice and watched it expand, month by month. And as it expanded, my patients' results, that bottom line I was seeking, got better and better. By the time my hypertensives threw away their medicine, my angina-invalided heart patients went back to water-skiing, and my multiple sclerosis patients gave up their wheelchairs, I knew the system was far better than that which I, and all doctors, had been taught. And when some of my terminal cancer patients began to get well, I knew the system belonged in the public's hands, where the institutions of medicine could develop it further.

Those of you who are how-to oriented and who have indulged me in my philosophizing are about to get your reward. I would like to show you how the Atkins Center brand of Complementary Medicine has worked in a variety of types of patients. Perhaps, from the case histories of the individuals we have treated, you may receive some insight as to how a similar problem you or a loved one may have might be approached.

I trust it is explicitly clear that *these are medical reports, not medical advice*. I haven't treated any two patients exactly alike yet, so don't expect that sort of activity to start now.

PART I

. . .

Diet-Related Disorders

5

· · ·

TO KNOW THE CAUSE . . .

Before I discuss the diseases in this section of the book, there's one more point that's so well worth making that I've given it this little section to itself.

I want to talk about the tremendously useful habit Complementary Medicine has of looking for the *cause* of an illness.

This is important, because when complementarists find the cause, they treat the cause. Orthodox medicine, on the other hand, tends to treat the symptom, and once it has made the symptom go away, it tells the patient that his or her condition is cured or at least controlled. Actually, in most cases, the *disease* hasn't been treated at all. Its symptoms have been masked or obliterated, but in due time the disease may well assert itself in another direction.

The most devastating example of this process is found in cancer, where a concentration on the symptom to the exclusion of the cause leads oncologists to an obsession with the tumor. The tumor is indeed the flashpoint of the disease, but it is not the disease itself; and though the orthodox physician may burn, cut, or poison it out of existence, all too often he finds the cancer is still present and has metastasized elsewhere. Thus we see that the cause of the cancer is more important than the visible tumor — necessary though it may be to remove it — and the cause is often found to be a disorder of the immune system, which the physician must therefore strengthen. When orthodoxy fails to look to that cause, it too often embarks on a destructive course of chemotherapy that can cripple the patient's chance of survival.

Indifference to causation, however, troubles orthodoxy at all levels and discourages thought even among general practitioners. Sad to say, the orthodox physician frequently doesn't feel compelled to discover the cause of an illness, because once he can name it — once he has a diagnosis — his troubles are over. All he has to do is recommend the prescribed remedy of the moment. That's why internists in hospitals are often called diagnosticians — naming the disease is the most important thing they ever get to do, since the treatment has already been prescribed. Is this good medicine? You'd better bet not, but it's safe medicine — for the practitioner. He who stays firmly within its bounds will never lose a malpractice suit. He won't have a very good success rate with his patients either, but he may not know it, since he'll have more or less the same success rate as all the other orthodox physicians he sees around him. And if he isn't searching out the ultimate causation of his patients' problems — whether it be in the food they eat, or the environmental conditions around them, or the nutrients they're not getting — *it will be for the very good reason that he doesn't even know he should.*

This is where Complementary Medicine takes a different path, as the next eighteen chapters will show you. It's because we find the *cause* of the patients' diabetes or fatigue or headache that we treat them with a success unknown to the academic medical world.

I might add — not in an attempt to conciliate the outraged guardians of orthodoxy, but simply as a matter of fact — that physicians are a varied bunch, and orthodox medicine *does* include many people of creative vision and enlarged curiosity who go deeper than a superficial diagnosis and who insist on pecking away at the irksome question of causation. Such physicians are harbingers of hope, but to the extent they practice medicine this way, they're actually practicing Complementary Medicine. Whether they know it or not.

6

. . .

DIABETES
The Basic Epidemic

It would be hard to scrutinize the weaknesses of orthodox medicine and point out the need for a new medicine without using as a prime example the major disorders of blood sugar, diabetes and hypoglycemia. These two illnesses are not opposites but rather distinct facets of a single category of illnesses which has no special name other than blood sugar disorders. (The term *glycopathy*, which applies, certainly is not in widespread use.)

More than any other category of illness, the glycopathies are *the* major illnesses of the twentieth century. It is fair to say this, because there is increasing evidence (which we'll discuss in the cardiovascular section of the book) that atherosclerosis largely overlaps the blood sugar disorders and shares many of the same metabolic disturbances.*

If that's the case, then *diet* becomes, clearly and obviously, both the cause and the cure of this century's major cause of death. And none of orthodoxy's characteristic responses, from aloof disdain based on sheer ignorance to vindictive persecution based on fear, will succeed in concealing that fact forever.

These Are Diseases of Modern Times

What is thought of as the classic blood sugar disorder is, of course, diabetes. *Classic* is an interesting word in this context, since dia-

---
*This thesis was elaborated upon in a two-volume book edited by Howard M. Katzen and Richard J. Mahler called *Diabetes, Obesity and Vascular Disease*. In it, the numerous metabolic interconnections are outlined for the medical scientist.

betes really became widely known only in the last century, and then it was anything but common. Before that century, one can search the rough medical case histories of the past and come up with only a thin stream of cases that resemble diabetes. Why? Very simply because diabetes is the direct result of sugar consumption, and refined sugar didn't become important until the nineteenth century, when Napoleon built sugar factories in Europe.

In 1815 the average Englishman consumed 7½ pounds of sugar a year. In 1976 the average American consumed 120 pounds. I'll tell you now that before you finish this book I intend to convince you that if there were such a thing as a national act of health suicide, that's what it would be like.

What Sort of Disease Is This?

The short definition of diabetes is that it is the improper relation between blood sugar and insulin in the body. The ultimate results of this misrelation can be fatal if not attended to. Typically the disease produces complications in small blood vessels (arterioles) in areas such as the eyes and the kidneys and also adversely affects the overall cardiovascular system and can result in coronary heart disease and other cardiovascular complications.

Hypoglycemia Begins It

Diabetes in an individual usually progresses for several decades before it becomes so overt that a patient is defined as diabetic — I am talking here about the more common form of the disease, adult-onset, or Type II, diabetes. What has happened before that is that the patient has generally been hypoglycemic. Let me explain how this works.

Hypoglycemia (which is simply a Greek word for low blood sugar) is a condition so common that a large minority, if not an actual majority, of Americans suffer from it. I have found in my practice that whatever illness patients come in to be treated for — from headache to heart disease — 40 percent of them will be significantly hypoglycemic (at least according to the criteria I accept as most useful).

Low blood sugar is something of a misnomer, however, since the condition is actually a response to an *excessive* amount of sugar in the blood. What happens is that when a person consumes large quantities of sugar, the body releases large quantities of insulin to control it. Insulin — a hormone secreted in the pancreas — transports glucose (the body's form of sugar) from the blood to body cells, where the glucose is converted into glycogen, which serves as a stored carbohydrate, or, when there is an excess, into a fat called triglyceride.

Now, the insulin is simply doing its job, but if you regularly consume large amounts of sugar (and refined carbohydrates, which soon break down into sugar), your body eventually begins to over-react, and instead of producing just the amount of insulin it needs to handle the really formidable task you've set for it, produces even more. This excess insulin drives the blood sugar level below its starting point. Thus, as a consequence of consuming large amounts of sugar, you end up with less blood sugar than you had to begin with and you feel exhausted. Usually you respond to this by eating even more, and the body responds by secreting even more insulin, and so on.

The Diabetic and Insulin

The most hurtful consequence of an excessive consumption of sugar and refined carbohydrates is, therefore, the high level of insulin that is secreted. The still-common layman's notion is that diabetes is caused by a shortage of insulin. In Type II (adult-onset) diabetes, that is generally the opposite of the actual situation. Of course, Type I diabetes, a somewhat less common form of the disease that characteristically begins in children and young adults, *is* insulin-dependent. In Type I, the pancreas's ability to produce insulin is indeed lost.

Type II diabetics have usually been hypoglycemic and have been producing large quantities of insulin to deal with their blood sugar for many years before the diabetes is diagnosed. And insulin — which among other things contributes to obesity (you'll remember that excess glucose is converted into triglyceride fat) — is responsible for much harm to the body. Indeed, there is now evidence implicating it as a major cause of atherosclerosis.[1] That's where the linkage between blood sugar disorders and cardiovascular illnesses is found. I will be explaining that a few chapters farther on.

The Breakdown Occurs

After several decades of hyperinsulinism, the diabetic's body becomes unable to cope. In some cases, the pancreas is exhausted and can no longer produce the amount of insulin needed. In others, the insulin is produced in ever-larger quantities, but the insulin receptors in the body have become defective and only a small quantity of insulin can get through and process the glucose in the blood. At this point, the diabetic may begin to "spill sugar" into his urine. The disease has reached the stage at which it is commonly diagnosed, although a physician studying the tolerance of glucose could have diagnosed the inevitable onset twenty years before.

Why Does It Happen?

At the risk of being repetitive, I'll now pose two questions to you, both of which have the same answer. First question: Why have blood sugar disorders been so widespread over the last three generations? Second question: Why is orthodox medicine so ill equipped to handle these conditions?

Answer for both questions: *Because these are predominantly diet-related disorders (DRD).*

Before I Prove My Point

Let me first define *diet-related disorders*. This is a very useful term that all too few people use. It means, simply, those illnesses or conditions which are in some significant degree caused by or corrected by dietary or nutritional factors.

The more we learn about nutrition techniques, the more DRD patients we recognize. Every condition I have written about in this book falls into this category. A more useful question might be: What conditions are *not* diet-related? The best answer might be to look at the illness line-up in well-nourished primitive cultures. It is totally different from ours. The most plausible explanation is that their diet is so different from ours.

The bottom line is that 95 percent of the patients we see at the Atkins Center have DRD. And in the vast majority of cases the most active stimulator of their disorder is sugar.

The Case Against Sugar

The definitive essay on the subject is Surgeon-Captain T. L. Cleave's book *The Saccharine Disease.*[2] Cleave shows example after example of societies in which the addition of sugar to the diet was the obvious starting point for the development of diabetes and of atherosclerosis in the epidemic proportions typical of a Western nation. Two striking examples in Cleave's global studies were in Iceland beginning in 1920 and among the nomadic Yemenite Jews. Before sugar was introduced into their cultures, there was absolutely no diabetes or atherosclerosis. Two decades after their diets became similar to ours, because sugar was added, they began to develop nearly as high an incidence of these illnesses as we have.

Another of Cleave's great contributions was the discovery of the Law of Twenty Years. In every culture he studied, it took exactly twenty years after the dietary change for the first cases of diabetes and atherosclerosis to appear. In American terms, this means that the increase in consumption of sugar and of highly refined flour between 1895 and 1910 could easily be invoked to explain the beginning of the heart attack era and the increase in diabetes prevalence noted between 1915 and 1930. This increase has continued — in the years between 1935 and 1968 the prevalence increased by 600 percent.

Animal Studies Abound

In 1972 A. M. Cohen, who was Israel's leading scientist in this field, published a landmark paper on the causation of diabetes in the prestigious American journal *Metabolism*. In his paper, titled "Genetics and Diet as Factors in the Development of Diabetes Mellitus: An Experimental Model," he described how he and his associates were able to create an entire strain of diabetic rats by feeding them sugar and selectively breeding the most sugar-sus-ceptible rats. The process took just six generations! (Could it be that we, like Cohen's rats, are in the process of being genetically mutated by the effects of what is now the fourth generation of in-ordinate sugar consumption?) This work was confirmed with strik-ing similarity by two scientists from the University of Ulm in West Germany, H. Laube and R. Pfieffer, who were contributing editors to the book *Diabetes, Obesity and Vascular Disease.*[3]

Now, I won't bog you down with all the evidence implicating sugar as a contributing cause of diabetes — along with hereditary predisposition — as laid out in Dr. Cohen's rat model. That would be a book in itself. But it seems to be proven that sugar raises insulin and triglyceride levels and has been used to create diabe-tes. Insulin and triglycerides, in turn, have been shown to help cause atherosclerosis. I hope you can see the connection.

The Case Against All Refined Carbohydrates

I believe the case against sugar is well proven.[4] There is a second dietary factor, refined carbohydrates (such as white flour, corn-starch, rice flour, etc.), which might also be tarred with the same brush. Here the epidemiologic evidence is almost as impressive, but the support from animal studies is lacking. Sophisticated nutri-tionists (that is, those who don't get paychecks from cereal makers) are quick to point out that all overly refined carbohydrates share the same glaring defect — they have to be metabolized (or pro-cessed) by the body, yet the micronutrients (vitamins and min-erals) that were a part of them as they grew in nature, and which enabled them to be metabolized by those who consumed them, have been removed. This means that the person who eats them must draw upon his own store of the nutrients involved in carbo-hydrate metabolism, thus using them up. In this way, refined car-bohydrates are, in regard to the essential B-complex vitamins, an-tinutrients.*

---

*That the AMA and the orthodox medical community refuse to accept the idea that refined sugar is an antinutrient is amply documented. In fact, one of their major disagreements with me, cited by the AMA's panel of "experts" in their critique of my first book, was that they took exception to my referring to sugar as an antinutrient.

My Second Point

Since it is not oriented toward handling nutritional problems, orthodoxy is poorly equipped to handle patients with these problems.

I don't have to remind you that nutrition is virtually not taught in medical school. I went to Cornell Medical College, one of the best, and I can vouch for the fact that I knew *nothing* useful about nutrition until eight years *after* I was graduated — and everything I learned was apart from my formal medical education. And worse yet, when it is taught, it is taught with a strong bias against clinical nutrition. You know, the teaching that runs: "Choose from the four basic food groups and you won't have to take those dangerous vitamins."

How can doctors with this kind of background manage patients with a major diet-related disorder? The answer is: Not as well as they should.

The facts seems to bear this out. At the Atkins Center we have treated more than six thousand patients in various stages of diabetes. Most of these had been under the care of other doctors, and many of the physicians were among the finest in their communities; yet we were able to improve the clinical evaluations of over 90 percent of them. All we did was apply nutritional knowledge to a condition that is largely the result of bad nutrition.

Before I introduce you, by way of case histories, to some of the patients we've treated at the Atkins Center, let me digress slightly. It will be a somewhat personal digression but, I trust, a useful one. The reason I'm putting it here is that, in most of the case histories, I'll be saying things like, "We put her on our standard low-carbohydrate diet," or, "He began by going on the Meat and Millet Diet." To me this seems to be as good a place as any to tell you what those diets are and how I got into nutrition medicine.

The Making of a Nutritionist

I was trained as a cardiologist and gave nutrition as little thought as any other cardiologist does (and, even today, that's not much).

It took something weighty and personal to make me think about the significance of what I stuck in my mouth each day. You guessed it — I'm probably the only gourmand ever to become a diet doctor, and by the early 1960s I was pretty heavy. I simply had to do something to curb my out-of-sight appetite, so I tried a typical low-calorie diet and found out, for the first time, how much fun starvation is. In case you don't know, draw a circle. That's how much.

That experience showed me that what most dietitians were offering wasn't for me, and so, while everyone else was figuring out how to be austere, I tried to find another way. I came up with the idea of a qualitative rather than quantitative diet, and at about that time an article in the *Journal of the American Medical Association* gave me the idea that such a diet might be low in carbohydrates and high in almost everything else. I tried it and was amazed to find it worked in spite of the fact that I was eating all day long.

Next I tried it out on some patients who were available to me through an industrial medical position I held. They lost weight, and when I asked them about the diet, the universal response was: "I'm never hungry."

The Eyes Begin to Open

I had to realize I was on to something, and as I refined the diet further, I tried to make it even more enjoyable. It took a while before I saw it had health advantages far beyond the mere loss of weight. Even in 1972, when I wrote *Dr. Atkins' Diet Revolution* and it became a national best seller, I was only beginning to understand the full potential of nutrition medicine. It takes a long time for a fully orthodox physician to discover heresy.

The Atkins Diet

The diet that I offered then and, with some slight revisions, put my overweight patients on today is a low-carbohydrate diet. The basic thrust of the diet is that it forbids *all* refined carbohydrates — not simply that nutritional horror sugar, but flour, cornstarch, white rice, potato starch, bread, crackers, and pasta. But it also restricts unrefined carbohydrate foods if their carbohydrate content is too high. In this category are many vegetables and most fruit, milk, yogurt, and a wide variety of nuts, grains, and legumes.

The diet stabilizes blood sugar, decreases insulin response, and is the most direct technique for inducing stored fat to serve as fuel. Most characteristically, it also does what diets are not expected to do: It decreases hunger dramatically.

The Atkins Diet is, after all, the most luxurious of all reducing diets. Meat, fish, fowl, and eggs are unrestricted, and many other foods are permitted in part. (The complete diet is found at the back of the book in Appendix A.)

The other reason for the lack of hunger experienced on the diet is, of course, the collapse of the hypoglycemic cycle. Without sugars and refined carbohydrates, the body simply doesn't fall to that low blood sugar level that causes exhaustion and a massive attack of hunger.

The Meat and Millet Diet

The low-carbohydrate diet is a weight-loss diet. For people who are at their ideal body weight or below it, I developed a second diet, to which I finally gave the name the Meat and Millet Diet. It is less stringent than the low-carbohydrate diet in that it allows you to eat some carbohydrates, but they will be starches instead of sugars, and they will be whole foods rather than partitioned ones. The no-sugars rule may mean that popular items such as milk and yogurt (lactose) and fruit and juice (glucose, fructose) will be curtailed or even eliminated. But your insulin levels will be regulated; this is the cornerstone of an effective diet plan.

Back to Diabetes

Now that we have set a nutritional standard, let's see how it works for individuals. I have chosen several case histories, the first of which is an example of so-called insulin-dependent, or juvenile, diabetes.

Thomas Kastor

Tom Kastor is twenty years old, an age at which one could develop either juvenile or adult-onset diabetes. Tom's troubles all began when he noticed he was losing weight without trying to, he was extremely thirsty, and he developed an increase in urinary output. He was in law school and was under a lot of stress studying for exams, doing everything he could to stay awake. The symptoms continued for several months, until Tom developed a throat infection and ended up in the hospital. There, his sugar levels were astronomical (over 500 milligrams percent*) and he was diagnosed as a Type I (insulin-dependent) diabetic. He was discharged on a daily dose of 47 units of the long-acting insulin NPH, plus nystatin, an antifungal, because the throat infection was diagnosed as thrush (the *Candida albicans* infection).

I met with Tom in August 1985, after he had had extensive testing at the Atkins Center. His blood sugar, glycohemoglobin, and serum insulin readings reflected moderately good recent control of his diabetes with the insulin regimen.

"Can you help me?" he asked. "I'm really devastated about having to take insulin the rest of my life."

I'm afraid I answered his question with a question: "You were studying for exams when this illness began, weren't you? What did you take to keep awake?"

"Coffee, all night, with milk and sugar. And Coke. I don't think I've ever drunk so much Coca-Cola in my life."

Then I answered: "You might be surprised. There are several hopeful signs. First of all, you haven't had your diabetes very long; I've seen some dramatic turnarounds in early cases. Second, your sugar decompensated in connection with a throat infection. Without that infection it might not be as bad as it seemed to be at first. Most of all, all that sugar you consumed! I've seen enough cases of diabetes precipitated by sugar — maybe that applies to you. You're young, but you might not be a juvenile diabetic. Yours could just as easily be an acute instance of an adult diabetic pattern triggered by a combination of diet, stress, and infection."

---

*All blood sugar readings are presented in milligrams percent, meaning the number of milligrams of glucose in 100 cubic centimeters of blood. The normal range is 70–100 milligrams percent.

I EXPLAINED TO TOM WHAT OUR PLAN OF ATTACK WOULD BE

First of all, there would be a strict diet and a new system for dosing the insulin. Then, he would need nutritional support for diabetes — the minerals chromium, zinc, magnesium, and manganese. Chromium is especially important, since it has been shown to increase glucose tolerance. I also wanted his treatment to take into account the possibility that any acute Type I diabetes might be an autoimmune disorder. Recent studies have shown that antibodies against islet cells (the ones that produce insulin) are detected in as many as 70 percent of Type I diabetics if they are studied at the time of diagnosis. These antibodies are rarely seen in normal subjects.[5]

The increasingly popular suggestion that immune suppressants such as cyclosporin be used in Type I diabetes is evidence that mainstream medicine is not only convinced that autoimmunity plays a role but is taking interventive action in support of that belief. I certainly believe all newly discovered diabetes should be treated with this awareness. Accordingly, I prescribed generous quantities of primrose oil and EPA (eicosapentaenoic acid, a fatty acid present in fish oils), to provide the sort of prostaglandins that protect the immune system.

Tom was placed on a low-carbohydrate diet. Carbohydrates release more glucose into the blood than other foods and so require more insulin. Therefore, I wanted to take advantage of the fact that the lowest carbohydrate intake requires the least insulin. The end of the re-education process came when I explained to Tom our system of providing insulin.

We try to mimic the physiological pattern of insulin administration. A healthy individual normally maintains an extremely low insulin level all through the day except just after a meal. The insulin increases abruptly with eating and then goes back to a low baseline level. In contrast, individuals on NPH or other long-lasting insulin have high levels of insulin twenty-four hours a day. The net result is that a much higher total insulin dosage will be required. At the center, we use regular insulin thirty minutes before meals, with the dose being determined by a blood sugar test the patient performs just before he gives himself the insulin. In this way the patient who is eating three times a day takes the insulin three times a day with just the right timing and a dosage proportionate to the blood sugar. Most insulin-dependent diabetics, unlike Tom, are too thin to thrive on a low-carbohydrate diet. Here we eliminate foods containing simple carbohydrates, such as fruit, milk, and sweets, for they will have more of an adverse effect on blood glucose than will complex carbohydrates. Using the technique of revamping the diet-insulin relationship we have been able to reduce our patients' total insulin requirements to 50 to 60 percent of what they were previously.

In Tom's case, he was told to follow this procedure and to test his blood sugar four times a day. He was to take one unit of insulin for every 10 points that his blood sugar registered over 140 milligrams percent.* Tom was an excellent patient in this respect and complied by performing four blood tests every day for four months. Within a few weeks' time, his blood sugar went below 140, which meant no more insulin was needed, and then down to a normal level (90–100). He did not deviate from the prescribed diet.

He continued to do well through October 1985, but in January 1986 his blood sugar began to increase to 150, with an average reading of 140, readings typical of a non-insulin-dependent diabetic. What had changed and caused this increase? Simply that Tom had gone off his diet and had put on some extra weight.

It is most important that a newly detected diabetic of any type be treated with the idea that this is a potentially reversible condition. If Tom had stayed with the doctors who limited their treatment to merely instituting an insulin program, it is certain he would still be on insulin. Although Tom is not cured, there is a strong possibility that the diagnosis of insulin dependency by his physicians was a misdiagnosis.

The Two Kinds of Diabetes

I have alluded to the fact that there are two kinds of diabetes. They are so different in their causation that they are probably two different diseases. And each of these has so many subdivisions that a

---

*This dose was specifically designed for Tom; for other patients, who are probably on less insulin to begin with, the dosage scale is usually somewhat less.

"splitter" (the opposite of a "lumper") could have a field day in defining all the distinctions.

Juvenile diabetes, the type called Type I or IDDM (insulin-dependent diabetes mellitus), usually strikes children and adolescents as a rather acute illness. In addition to the rapid onset of symptoms (dehydration and unexplained weight loss, increased thirst and urinary output), the diagnosis is easily made by the high sugar levels in blood and urine, combined with the low or absent levels of insulin.

But, as I pointed out at the beginning of the chapter, the common form of diabetes is associated with a *greater* than normal amount of insulin, at least in the early stages. The sugar disorder is not a defect in the pancreas, as in the juvenile type, but in the insulin receptors. In juvenile diabetes (Type I), insulin must be provided; in diet-related diabetes (Type II), insulin levels should be suppressed.

Tom was an interesting example of one of the few times that the differential diagnosis between the two types of diabetes could be legitimately confused. Even now that Tom is surely a Type II diabetic, the question remains: Did we simply manage an acute Type II better, or did we, with our attention to his immune system, "cure" a Type I pancreatic failure diabetic?

The next case is more illustrative of 95 percent of all diabetics we see — patients in whom the pancreas still produces insulin.

Marian Peck

Marian's story is a typical example of mature-onset diabetes, a diet-related disorder that was mistreated. When Marian complained to her physician about her fatigue and low energy she was told she had a diabetic tendency and was placed on the American Diabetes Association diet. The diet was higher in calories and contained many more carbohydrates than Marian was used to eating. Within two weeks of following the diet, she felt worse. She had no energy at all and she felt quite fatigued.

> *"I had been on the Atkins Diet years ago, lost a good amount of weight, and felt really well, so I decided to make an appointment."*

Marian visited the center on March 11, 1986, and a series of tests and exams were done. She had no energy at all, she had polyuria (excessive urinary output), polydipsia (excessive thirst), and anxiety attacks. Marian's blood test showed a blood glucose level of 296. The battery of tests confirmed diabetes and candidiasis (a yeast infection). I immediately placed her on our carbohydrate-deprivation diet for a period of two weeks. The diet was supplemented with our Basic Formula (see Appendix C); B-complex vitamins; zinc, manganese, chromium, and magnesium; the amino acids taurine, ornithine, and glutathione; and EPA; plus a regimen of homeopathy and caprylic acid directed against the *Candida albicans* (see chapter 8).

Marian began the program and by her March 18 visit, her glucose was down to 211 and she was feeling less tremulous, her vision was clearer, and her urinary frequency had decreased.

By March 25, Marian was having energy bursts and her headaches were gone.

> *"I improved on the low-carbohydrate diet almost immediately. The change was like night and day. It's truly unbelievable. I find myself feeling stronger and I can focus better. I cherish my life more and I know I'm on the right track. I'm so grateful to you and the staff."*

In the course of the next few months, Marian's glucose reached a nearly normal 124. Her blood pressure incidentally fell from an initial level of 160/92 to 140/80. All her symptoms were improved. What is most astounding in Marian's case is that her previous physician felt he was doing something for her but in reality was treating himself. At no time did he use a low-carbohydrate diet, which has been written about in medical journals since 1790. Yet I have seen patient after patient on the diet make incredible strides toward health. In particular, the low-carbohydrate diet works well with sugar metabolism disorders; yet other physicians are still pushing the American Diabetes Association diet.

> *"The ADA's 1800-calorie diabetes diet contained a higher amount of carbohydrates than I ever ate. I was given no*

rules about complex carbohydrates as opposed to refined carbohydrates. The diet you prescribed for me changed gradually and I was slowly adding back whole grains and some fruit — the difference in both the diets and how I now feel is unreal. I feel well."

The kind of diabetes that Marian has is the most common kind, and it seems to be on the increase. The American Diabetes Association, which monitors these things, denies that it is increasing but does admit that there are 6 million diabetics in America, which translates into over 2 percent of the population.

I often wonder whether the ADA is taking the diabetes epidemic a little too personally, as if its members were the ones who were responsible. The reason I suggest this is that we surely would have had a greater increase in numbers of diabetics if the ADA had not changed the criteria for diagnosing diabetes.

What the ADA Did

It simply created a new category of patient. It took all the low-grade or borderline diabetics out of the diabetes group and reclassified them, calling their condition "impaired carbohydrate tolerance." But this category is very prevalent and adds as many as 6 million more people, depending on who does the estimating. At the Atkins Center 21 percent of our patients fall into this "gray area."

This quick work with the bureaucratic redefining pen insures that we won't have to worry about diabetes becoming an epidemic. When the ADA found it couldn't lower the river, it raised the bridge.

The Diabetes-Hyperinsulinism-Obesity-Heart Connection

It is quite important that you understand that:

- The majority of adult-onset diabetics (80 percent) are or have been overweight.
- At least half of the grossly obese are diabetic.

- Virtually all obese people and most adult-onset diabetics have hyperinsulinism.
- Hyperinsulinism, diabetes, and obesity are all risk factors for heart disease.

From this you can see just how pivotal is the problem of hyperinsulinism (excessive insulin response to carbohydrate feeding).

The final point I want to make is the absolutely critical point that *this hyperinsulin response can be bypassed by avoiding the foods that evoke it*. This is the major reason for the effectiveness of a low-carbohydrate or a sugarless diet in all of the above conditions. This is the reason all the adult-onset diabetics at our center are given such a diet. That's why Marian was given the Atkins Diet on her first visit and why her blood sugar improved to the extent it did. And it is why over 90 percent of the six thousand diabetics treated at the center show measurable improvement when they follow their prescribed diet.

The Glycemic Index

A food's ability to provoke the insulin response is proportionate to its glycemic index, which has been calculated for a variety of foods. The index is a measure of the degree of blood glucose elevation that follows the ingestion of the specific food being indexed. The findings roughly parallel the simplified "pecking order" that we use at the center (from worst to least): (1) sugars; (2) fruits; (3) lactose (milk); (4) starchy vegetables; (5) low-carbohydrate vegetables; (6) nuts and seeds; (7) proteins; and (8) fats. According to glycemic index work, certain vegetables and grains belong in the "premium" class and are more glycemic than most fruits (examples: carrots, parsnips, potatoes, white rice, corn flakes). By the same token, there are some surprisingly low glycemic index fruits, such as cherries, grapefruit, peaches, and plums.

Carbohydrate Restriction: Nobody Does It Better

Applying a system of carbohydrate restriction in treating the obese diabetic simply requires a good understanding of the illness and of the underlying scientific studies, as established by orthodox, academic medicine. It could be utilized with equal aplomb by an orthodox, an alternative, or a complementary physician. All that is required is a modicum of common sense and a willingness to stand apart from the pack. Apparently this is not often found. Most of the diabetics we treated were following a doctor's instructions and yet still required medications and/or were not in good control of their sugar levels. We simply applied what is generally known about nutrition and were consistently able to demonstrate improvements.

Why Is This Approach Being Ignored?

Simply because it calls for a knowledge of nutrition, and it doesn't call for writing a drug prescription. Also, no one in the hierarchy of medical opinion-molding has written it up in a medical journal, and most doctors suffer from what they proudly call "medical conservatism." The real name for it is "fear of the new." But how can their position be considered conservative, since it leads to the widespread prescribing of a class of drugs *proven* to do more harm than good?

Proven to Do Harm?

Yes, I'm referring to the oral antidiabetic medications, which are still being prescribed a thousand times more often than is the appropriate low-carbohydrate diet. If you find my allegation hard to swallow, simply do this: Get hold of the *Physicians' Desk Reference* and look up any of the oral antidiabetic medications (Orinase, Tolinase, Diabinese, whatever) or get the package insert. You will see in block capital letters the statement WARNING: INCREASED RISK OF CARDIOVASCULAR MORTALITY.

Now let's think this one through. Stable diabetics don't get into trouble from sugar elevation because they don't tend to go into acidosis (a metabolic imbalance caused by lack of alkali) — but if they did, it would be appropriate to give them insulin. The purpose of controlling the blood sugar, then, is to prevent the complications of diabetes. Almost all these complications are cardiovascular. Of what benefit, then, would a drug that *increases* that risk be?

The basis of the need for that all-too-significant disclaimer* was a vast, multicenter study on these medications (some fifteen years after they were in widespread use) called the University Group Diabetes Program (UGDP).[6] The test was long-term and was conducted on 823 patients with the revered double-blind design. When the code was broken, it was clear that those who were treated with the placebo, and who had to do a little more conscientious dieting when they spilled sugar, were more fortunate than the group treated with the drugs, who were lulled into a false sense of security by the fact that their blood and urine sugars were so "good." Results: a cardiovascular mortality (death rate) approximately two-and-one-half times that of patients treated with diet alone.

Now, if orthodox medicine were as dedicated to the scientific method as it claims to be, that study would have sounded the death knell for this class of drug. But instead the doctors quarreled over the findings, called the study "controversial," and continued their prescribing practices. To this date, over 2 million American diabetics are treated with these drugs. (Needless to say, my six thousand diabetic patients have not been among them.)

The UGDP sequence of events shows clearly that, if respect for scientifically performed studies is a characteristic of establishment medicine, then respect for the prescription pad is an even stronger one.

The Other Side of the Diabetes Coin

The irony of the whole matter is that we have achieved our success only in relative terms — relative to the nearly universal mismanagement our patients received before they came to the Atkins Center. Because I must, in all candor, confess that we have as yet come up with very little that fundamentally reverses the underlying diabetes. All the low-carbohydrate diet does is *bypass* the problem.

---

*This is not an isolated instance. Almost any prescription drug comes with a published litany of its officially recorded side effects. I strongly suggest that you develop the habit of reading the package inserts before you agree to a pharmaceutical intervention. This may keep you from doing something just as foolish as taking oral antidiabetics.

Specifically, the low-carbohydrate diet provides a better technique for managing that 80 percent majority of adult-onset diabetics who are (or were) overweight and who are still in a hyperinsulin stage; and although it contributes somewhat less to diabetics who are slim or low in insulin, it makes management with insulin much easier. In fact, Dr. Richard K. Bernstein, the Westchester, New York, diabetologist and author of the book *Diabetes*, finds that an ultra-low-carbohydrate intake (approximately 35 grams daily) is the best diet prescription to match with his painstaking system of achieving very tight glucose control with regular insulin.

For the slim diabetics, who rarely experience hyperinsulinism, we offer a diet low in sugar and high glycemic index foods; they are counseled to avoid caffeine and alcohol and to add the nutrients I'm about to discuss. But the improvement these patients achieve is limited, especially if they were already following a careful diet.

Before I tell you about some of the nutrients we use in dealing with diabetes, let me give you one more case history, that of a patient whose diabetes was not in any sense a new development.

Marilyn Greenspan

Marilyn Greenspan's case is a good example of how the simple adherence to a single principle (i.e., insulin is good for diabetics) can lead to gross mismanagement in diabetes, and it also shows that such adherence is evidently the policy of the biggest institutions. Marilyn Greenspan had been my patient in 1973, when she was simply overweight, with a prediabetic tendency. At that time I taught her that she must stay away from carbohydrates on a lifetime basis, but after she left my care she eventually gave up on the diet.

Instead, she kept gaining weight, until she was diagnosed as fully diabetic in 1980. Her treatment by her regular physician was more of the same wonderful diet that gave her the diabetes in the first place, plus oral medication. In 1984 that was changed to insulin, but the sugar level in her blood wouldn't drop.

Finally she hit upon the definitive solution. She would check into Boston's prestigious Joslin Clinic/Diabetes Center and do whatever they outlined for her.

"I thought they were the Bible."

To most American physicians the Joslin Clinic is the gold standard in terms of diabetes treatment. Joslin's approach is to achieve "tight control" of the blood glucose. Within a week, Marilyn's insulin dose was upped from 50 to 150 units (remember, a typical daily insulin dose is 25 units, and remember, too, that obese diabetics have excessive insulin levels to begin with). All this accomplished was to allow her to gain twenty more pounds and become hypertensive, for which she was given hydrochlorothiazide (a diuretic known to all the world as the blood pressure medicine that aggravates diabetes).

Then Marilyn Greenspan remembered that she had lost thirty pounds with me, and, unconcerned about her diabetes, decided to come to me to lose weight. Before seeing me, she had seen other physicians, who restricted her carbohydrates but kept her on insulin. After two months there had been some insulin reactions (induced hypoglycemia) but no weight loss.

Finally, we met again on June 15, 1987. I reviewed her lab tests and told her that we found evidence of excess insulin at every turn. Her insulin levels were ten times the normal value and her triglycerides (blood fat produced by insulin) were astronomical — 545 milligrams percent. I knew that Marilyn shouldn't be getting *any* insulin, but I compromised on a schedule of one unit of regular insulin for every 10 points the sugar registered over 200 points. And, of course, she was told to eat no carbohydrates. At the Joslin Clinic, she had been allowed three to five slices of bread a day, three fruits, and even some ice cream on occasion.

This treatment program meant an immediate drop to 12 units of insulin, a 93 percent decrease, overnight. Almost immediately the diet began to make itself felt. "My sugar dropped like crazy," Marilyn recalls. Her weight fell, too — from 198 pounds in May to 172 pounds in December 1987. Two other problems Marilyn had been experiencing improved dramatically. She found that the considerable afternoon fatigue she had gotten used to went away — a typical result on a low-carbohydrate diet — and the hot flushes and night sweats she had had became rare occurrences. And when she did have them, she looked back over the previous day and almost invariably discovered she had cheated on the diet. But now, when she doesn't cheat, she is able to go for days *without insulin*. The hypothesis that obese, high-insulin diabetics should not get insulin is intriguingly supported by this case.

These Are the Things That Help

Having given you a broad picture of our treatment as it applies to individual patients, I'd now like to focus on particular elements of our treatment protocol. First and foremost, there is a massive body of evidence based on dozens of scientific papers over the last twenty years that the trace mineral chromium is the key element in a complex molecule called glucose tolerance factor (GTF).[7] The administration of trivalent chromium, usually from a yeast source, in many studies has been shown to increase glucose tolerance. Here is an example of a nutrient that satisfies every criterion that orthodoxy requires, but is rarely offered to diabetic patients. Why not? Can it be that its use is not pushed by any drug industry detail men and that it is purchasable not in drugstores but only in health food stores? I see no reason not to administer chromium *routinely* to every diabetic or prediabetic patient, or even to those predisposed to heart disease. Even if the beneficial results are obscured by all the other useful aspects of the treatment program, as is the case in our center, there is every reason to use chromium for whatever help it can provide. There is no downside risk at the dosages used in nutritional medicine.

After Chromium Comes Zinc

Zinc is a mineral that plays so many roles in the body that many of them are yet to be discovered. I am struck with the pivotal role zinc plays in supporting the immune system and the distinct possibility that diabetes may be, in many instances, an immune disorder.

I also see roles for magnesium (especially in preventing vascular complications) as well as manganese. I try to give more than adequate amounts of all three of these nutrients plus chromium to any patient with a blood sugar disorder. I will usually be guided by the mineral levels in blood, hair, and urine specimens, and will emphasize those which seem the most deficient.

The Essential Fatty Acids

Essential fatty acids are so called because they must be supplied by the diet, since the body cannot manufacture them. Researchers at the University of Rotterdam conducted a five-year study of one of the essential fatty acids, linoleic acid, and showed that the diabetic complications to the heart, kidneys, and eyes could be significantly reduced with regular doses.[8] Work in progress under the aegis of David F. Horrobin suggests that an even better effect can be achieved by gamma-linolenic acid (GLA).* At any rate, fatty acids serving as precursors for beneficial prostaglandins (I include EPA, in the form of salmon oil, here) hold great promise for helping ease the course of diabetes; their use must be considered in all diabetics. It may be exactly what Tom Kastor benefited from most.

Helpful Nutrients — Is There a Breakthrough on the Horizon?

In working with nontoxic nutritional substances, Complementary Medicine is using some agents that just *might* bear results. The most promising of these is pyridoxine alpha-ketoglutarate (PAK), which we began working with in 1988. Studies done in Italy showed that this compound of two nutrients significantly reduced the sugar elevations in diabetics of both Type I and Type II.[9]

Similarly, Japanese researchers demonstrated improvement in diabetic parameters using Coenzyme Q_{10} (the first study actually used Q_7).[10] We were particularly excited about the idea of using the unsung B vitamin biotin in milligram doses, rather than the

*One such study, by G. A. Jamal, was reported in *Lancet* in 1986. The study involved twenty-two subjects with diabetic neuropathy. After six months of daily primrose oil (the major dietary source of GLA) totaling 4 grams (8 capsules) all tests were *improved* in the treated group and *worsened* in the placebo-controlled group.

*micro*gram doses we usually administer, and, after studying a report in the *Annals of the New York Academy of Science* showing a significant improvement in glucose readings, we incorporated megabiotin therapy into our routine.[11]

We have developed a supplement for diabetics, our DM formula (see Appendix C) used in conjunction with PAK, GLA, and EPA. Our initial impression is that this nutrient combination offers tangible benefits to our diabetic patients.

Another Approach

Dr. William Philpott made an interesting observation. Certain foods will elevate the blood sugar in specific individuals more than will other foods of similar composition. His logical suggestion was to test each food commonly eaten by a diabetic patient and eliminate all those which cause a significant rise in blood sugar. Unfortunately, the results with this approach at the Atkins Center have not been especially dramatic. We have recently switched to getting our information from the cytotoxic test, which measures the reaction that the ingestion of specific foods provokes in the white blood cells and is much easier to perform. (A full discussion of the test and food allergies is presented in the subsection Testing for Food Allergy in the next chapter.) As you will see shortly, what you eat and how it affects your system can result in changes in your energy level, mood, tension, nervousness, and the like.

7

...

HYPOGLYCEMIA
Everybody Has Some

I almost feel that I must begin this chapter with an apology to the readers of my previous books, for in most of them I have written at great length about hypoglycemia, also called low blood sugar. One of the books, *Dr. Atkins' Superenergy Diet*, was all about hypoglycemia.

Yet, in the context of what this book is really about — Has orthodox medicine failed us to the point that we need a new medicine based on a different model? — there is no condition that better shows both the weakness of the orthodox approach and the need for a new medicine.

I want you to follow along with me as I develop this premise, for it will shed light on my whole thesis.

How Common Is It?

Let's start by getting this fact straight. Hypoglycemia, in the form of hypoglycemic reactions, is *extremely common*. Not in 20 percent or 40 percent of the population, as its more enthusiastic proponents claim, but in the majority of the population. I'm speaking about *changes* in energy level, mood, mental alertness, headache, shakiness, faintness, crankiness, hunger, tension, nervousness, and the like that occur from time to time, and change from hour to hour, bearing some relation to when or what the person has eaten. Why don't you ask the next ten people you meet if they have ever detected any of the above sensations in themselves and you will get some idea of just how common is the hypoglycemic response. If you find that nearly everyone admits to some of these symptoms, then you will see why I always say, "Hypoglycemia is a little like height; everybody has some."

Contrast this with the official position of orthodox medicine that hypoglycemia is extremely rare, if it exists at all. There are numerous physicians who proudly announce, "I don't believe in hypoglycemia," and act accordingly. And there are hundreds of thousands of patients with bona fide by-any-and-all-criteria hypoglycemia who have been treated by those very doctors. Talk about medical mismanagement! Here you see it on a grand scale. These patients have gone through the medical mill — hospitalizations, CT scans, tranquilizer addiction, psychiatric admissions, shock therapy, and more — all because their physicians were too obstinate to admit that the obvious was obvious. I should know, I've treated them afterward. I can go to my files right now and pull out several hundred charts of people who have had this experience.

The Key Question

Now, the main question to be answered here is, Why? Why is there such a polarized difference of opinion as to whether a specific condition even exists? This book deals in controversy, but generally the controversy is over how to approach a given medical problem, not over whether the problem exists.

The Answer

In the first place, there's a little of the apples-or-oranges confusion. I'm talking hypoglycemia, the response; they're talking hypoglycemia, the disease. But in point of fact, hypoglycemia is a response. Calling it a disease by asking if the diagnosis can be proven sets up a totally arbitrary distinction that has no real meaning. The reason for this is that no one has agreed on criteria for establishing the diagnosis. Certainly, the glucose tolerance test, which is the most appropriate way to diagnose the condition, does not offer any natural boundary line that can serve as a cutoff point to divide the hypoglycemic from the nonhypoglycemic. There will always be true hypoglycemic responders who fall into the "normal" classification and apparently normal responders who meet the hypoglycemia criteria. I have personally reviewed more than twenty-six thousand glucose tolerance tests on my patients and I'm struck with the large number of patients who are borderline responders.

If the glucose tolerance test cannot establish a diagnosis, what good it is? I still think it is an extremely valuable test — not to establish a diagnosis, but to suggest a course of action.

Let's take a moment off to review a case history. This case history will be very much like hundreds of others we've handled at the Atkins Center. In fact, more than half the medical "horror stories" I have heard have been related to the mismanagement of hypoglycemic responders.

Jack Holmes

When Jack Holmes, age forty-three, came to see me in July 1985, he was a successful salesman who owned his own company, traveled around the country, led a very active life, and had been trying to figure out for more than twenty years why he was so tired. He had been to eight doctors in that time span. It seemed to Jack that it was fair to think at least one of them would have had something useful to say about his condition.

What actually happened? Well, he had been given eight standard physicals and been told eight times there was nothing wrong with him. One or two of his doctors had asked him if he was unhappy with his job, if he and his wife fought, if he had any reason to feel depressed. Jack told them he wasn't depressed, he was *tired*.

Over the course of two decades, he had gotten absolutely no help! Most of his physicians suggested he should eat well and get enough sleep. A few wondered if he wasn't overworking. Jack wasn't convinced by that, since he hadn't noticed that he felt any better on weekends or vacations than at other times.

"The last doctor I went to, an internist, noted that I weighed 195 [Jack is six feet tall] and told me to diet down

to 175 and I'd feel fine. The way he fired that off the top of his head and then sat back down behind his desk looking as though he'd solved the problem didn't sit well with me, so I said, 'Doc, you don't know what you're talking about. You're telling me I'll feel good if I weigh 175? Well, listen to this — when I was twenty years old I weighed 168, I was boxing, I was in great shape, and I was still in a doctor's office complaining about fatigue!'"

We gave Jack a glucose tolerance test — which none of his doctors had even suggested. His resting glucose level was 95. After a glucose solution was administered, the level shot up to 190 within half an hour and went down to 52 after three hours — as good an indication of hypoglycemia as you're likely to see. I put him on the low-carbohydrate diet and our standard vitamin regimen.

Jack had always had cravings for high-sugar treats like ice cream sundaes and slices of apple pie, but the prospect of putting a lifetime of exhaustion behind him kept him strictly on the diet. "I felt the difference almost immediately," he said. Three weeks after I first saw Jack Holmes, he told me that he hardly ever felt tired anymore, and some joint stiffness that he had been suffering from was gone.

Jack had also had a problem sleeping at night, usually waking up after two or three hours. His other sleep problem was that he *did* fall asleep during the day, usually an hour or two after every meal. That, of course, was hypoglycemic fatigue, and on a low-carbohydrate diet he certainly didn't have a problem with that. His night sleep got better, too.

There was nothing complicated about Jack's course *once the diagnosis was made*. It was simply a classic case of hypoglycemia, and when he severely restricted his carbohydrates, his fatigue vanished because his blood sugar never fell off the edge of the table anymore. His food cravings largely disappeared also, although he told me he still occasionally dreams of that piece of apple pie. His weight, which had been 204 pounds on his first visit, fell after three months to 182.

Jack occasionally went off the diet, and he soon grew used to experiencing an almost total relapse into fatigue when he did. On one occasion, he went with an employee to a Mexican restaurant in Manhattan and then dropped the man off on the way home. A few minutes later he stopped at a red light.

> *"The next thing I remember was a policeman tapping me on the shoulder and asking me if I'd had too much to drink. I had conked right out waiting for the light to change."*

For Jack Holmes, the main difference now is, "My life has become much pleasanter." Like most former hypoglycemics, he has found it more satisfactory to restrict his carbohydrates than to live with fatigue.

This case history and the hundreds of others that parallel it indicate that low blood sugar is an extremely easy condition to diagnose — if only the physician would recognize the symptoms — and it's even easier to treat.

Occasionally we see patients who have been correctly diagnosed as hypoglycemic and who follow a standard hypoglycemic's diet, yet who fail to get the expected improvement. But a good 95 percent of the patients will, just like Jack, experience a steady, uncomplicated improvement, with all the symptoms vanishing within a few weeks.

Of the 5 percent of hypoglycemic responders who don't improve, most are fruit and fruit juice consumers. They fail to recognize, until we point it out to them, that 50 percent of the sugar in fruit is glucose, the very substance whose tolerance test they have just flunked. Cutting out fruit (as well as lactose, the milk sugar) will usually solve their problem.

Hypoglycemia is not a fatal disease, not a progressive disease; in fact, it is not a disease. As I said, it is a response. Yet the widespread failure to diagnose it correctly has led to untold suffering, even chronic mental disease. The reasons behind this phenomenal nondiagnosis just happen to be the very shortcomings of orthodox medicine that are a theme of this book.

The War Against Hypoglycemia

In 1973 the Endocrine Society, the American Diabetes Association, and the AMA issued an unprecedented joint position statement to the effect that hypoglycemia was an extremely uncommon disease.[1] For doctors the statement carried the implication: "You'd better believe this or else." Since then the peer-pressure campaign has intensified, with many doctors who diagnose hypoglycemia being accused of quackery by the AMA's hit men.

Why? What is it about this condition that causes the hackles of the AMA to rise?

Medical Self-worship and Economics

I can think of a couple of causes. The first is the furtherance of the medical mystique that orthodox physicians are so attached to. The one privilege that physicians have by law is the power to prescribe medicines. Therefore, that's the privilege they enshrine. Their worship of medicine becomes a worship of medicines.

But what of hypoglycemia? It is simply a nutritional disorder caused by a faulty diet and corrected by a proper diet. The prescription pad has no place here. What the doctor can do, so can someone's spouse, or — and here is where it hurts — so can a lay "nutritionist" with a correspondence course degree. Doctors don't like that one bit.

The second cause, sad to say, is economics. Ever since the medical establishment decided to accept financial support from the drug industry, it has come to feel that its interests are indistinguishable from those of the big pharmaceutical houses. And since medical journals, medical societies, and research and educational programs are all largely funded by the drug industry, they're not entirely mistaken. To a large extent, this dependence and identification came about innocently over a long period of time. However, it has become so institutionalized that today one can hardly see that there is a conflict of interest of heroic proportions.

But is there anything about the existence of reactive hypoglycemia that poses a threat to establishment economics?

You bet there is!

How to Understand the Role of Economics

Just ask yourself this question: What would be in the pharmaceutical industry's best interest and what would not? An awareness that many of our problems come from a prevalent condition that we can correct ourselves, without drugs or any medical attention except advice, certainly isn't. That's taking us much too far from the intervention of the Great White Fathers and their prescription pads.

Hypoglycemia, which demands self-help, not intervention, is an ideologic thorn that could create a core around which the self-help-based Health Revolution might shape itself. Nothing could be more dreaded by the medical establishment. The symptoms of hypoglycemia are nature's way of telling you: "It's time to get your act together, Charlie. If you don't like your symptoms, don't cause them." Big industry has no role to play in that dialogue.

What Causes Hypoglycemia?

Now that we have dealt with the problem of why low blood sugar so often goes undiagnosed, let us assume that you are troubled by its symptoms and need some help with the basics. We touched upon some of them in the last chapter.

In the first place, hypoglycemia, or low blood sugar, is named wrong. It should be dubbed "excessive secondary reaction to sugar." The body's primary reaction to the intake of sugar is for the level of sugar in the blood to escalate; the secondary reaction is for it, chiefly under the influence of insulin, to drop. When that secondary reaction is exaggerated, the blood sugar falls too rapidly or to too low a level, either of which can cause symptoms. A further cause for symptoms derives from the body's efforts to "brake" the rapid fall by the sudden release of counterregulatory hormones, principally adrenaline and its relatives. Anxiety attacks, cold sweats, palpitations, headaches, nocturnal awakening, and nervous tension are symptoms probably related to the adrenaline reaction, while fatigue, faintness, inability to concentrate, sugar cravings, confusion, and memory symptoms are thought to be due to the lack of a readily available brain fuel, namely, glucose.[2]

How Do Hypoglycemics Get Well?

The most important principle to keep in mind is that sugar is the proximate cause of hypoglycemia. Hypoglycemia, by the way, does have a first name — reactive.* This implies the fact that the fall in blood sugar is a reaction to what you take in. In most cases, the culprit is a glucose-containing food.

Most cases respond to a sugarless diet (this also means no caffeine or alcohol). Usually the simple carbohydrates (sweets, fruit, and milk) have to be eliminated, at least in the beginning of dietary management. Both of the basic diets used at the Atkins Center qualify; in fact, they were created for the express purpose of stabilizing blood sugar.[3] It must be emphasized that a sugarless diet is not a *cure* for reactive hypoglycemia; it is merely a way of bypassing the problem.

Why Do We Use Nutritional Supplements?

There is some evidence that reactive hypoglycemia is a symptom of an acquired metabolic error, such as a relative deficiency of one or more vitamins or minerals. Accordingly, part of the nutritional protocol we follow is to provide generous amounts of the B-complex vitamins, since most metabolic processes in glucose metabolism are mediated by one or more members of the B complex. Also, the four minerals used in the diabetic protocol must be provided (zinc, manganese, chromium, magnesium).

In difficult cases, there are a few nutritional tricks that may help. One is the use of the amino acid L-glutamine. (Amino acids are protein building blocks.) Glutamine acts like a sugar and can actually serve as a metabolic fuel for the brain, in which instance it acts in a fashion similar to glucose. I have found it useful for patients who crave sweets (or alcohol). In doses of 500 to 1500 milligrams at a time, its effect can be very gratifying. It is especially useful in cases in which the craving for sugar makes the initial phase of "getting with" the diet difficult.

*There are dozens of other types of hypoglycemia, with a variety of causes, ranging from insulin-secreting tumors of the pancreas, to insulin overdosage, to a variety of endocrine imbalances. But over 99 percent of cases are the garden-variety reactive hypoglycemic response, which is the only type we will be discussing here.

The other trick for controlling difficult blood sugar problems is the use of glycerine (or glycerol). Glycerine is the carbohydrate part of fat. It can attach to three long chains of fatty acid and form a triglyceride, a substance better known to dieters under the name "ugly fat." But as a separate substance, glycerine has a metabolic effect of its own. Taking an ounce at exactly the time you feel your hypoglycemic symptoms can counteract your low blood sugar and directly relieve your symptoms. Many of my patients have found this useful little trick a godsend, but it should not be overdone.

And If You Still Have Symptoms?

If you are still symptomatic after all of the above has been properly tried, then the chances are that the diagnosis is incomplete. We must assume the presence of food intolerance, colloquially but inaccurately also referred to as food allergy.

Food intolerance produces just about the same symptoms as reactive hypoglycemia, but it can be distinguished from the latter by the timing (it most often comes on within hours after eating) and especially by which foods cause it. When you are intolerant of a food, your reactions may even be mediated by changes in blood sugar, according to Dr. William Philpott, author of *Victory over Diabetes*. This means that starches (complex carbohydrates) or even proteins might cause the characteristic blood sugar elevation-then-fall. Of course, this would provoke the same symptoms that a simple sugar would produce in a hypoglycemic.

The overlap between these conditions is immense. Using the results of the cytotoxic test, we have come to the conclusion that almost everyone (but especially hypoglycemics) shows intolerance for *some* foods.

Ideally, therefore, most patients should be on blood sugar stabilization *and* food-intolerance avoidance, but our experience has been that 80 percent of low-carbohydrate dieters will improve simply with the low-carbohydrate rule. Identifying food allergy is really essential in only 30 percent. That's because a food intolerance is most common to a high-carbohydrate type of food. Nevertheless, I think some aspect of food-allergy testing is extremely useful to all my patients who are looking to find that "perfect diet."

Testing for Food Allergy

If we start with the premise that there are, for each of us, foods that cause us problems, and that we should learn to avoid, it is no less than amazing how many different ways we have to discover what those foods are.

First and foremost is our personal discovery of connections between foods and symptoms. Whenever we notice that certain unpleasant symptoms invariably (or very often) follow our consumption of certain foods, beverages, or combinations, then we learn about these food intolerances from that greatest of all teachers, experience. (Even as I write this, a sick morning-after headache is currently convincing me that I can never again eat in a Chinese restaurant.)

Other ways to discover our food intolerances include pulse testing; kinesiology (muscle testing); direct observation after sublingual provocation (i.e., placing the suspect food under the tongue, one of the major techniques of the original clinical ecologists); blood glucose elevation (Philpott's technique); immunoglobulin testing (especially IgG, or immunoglobulin G); EAV (electro-acupuncture according to Voll) and electrodiagnosis (a very good system based on measurable electrical potential differences transmitted through acupuncture meridians); and a variety of systems based on the dissolution of the granules of the white blood cells, called granulocytes. The last studies fall under the heading of cytotoxic testing and have provided most of the information the Atkins Center has used in patient management.

Cytotoxic studies do not include the testing systems for true allergy, which is the limited area handled by most board-certified allergists. These allergies are mediated by just one of the immunoglobulins, called IgE, also known as reagin. They are identified by skin tests (scratch and intradermal testing) and by IgE-measuring blood tests such as the RAST test. We also employ these tests in certain patients at the Atkins Center (those whose total IgE levels are high on the initial screening test), because they are certainly among the most accurate. But from a food-intolerance standpoint, they simply don't cover all possibilities.

In other words, some food intolerances very significant to a patient's health are not IgE-mediated; that is, they are not "classical" allergies. So standard allergy tests miss them.

Theorists in the field of clinical ecology, the expanded view of allergy adopted by Complementary Medicine, describe the mechanism of these non-IgE food allergies as follows: Each food has its own protein structure, characteristic of the biologic class it derives from. If the food is eaten beyond the capacity of the upper gastrointestinal tract to digest it completely, the proteins will not be completely broken down into their *individual* amino acids, but will remain as *chains* of amino acids called peptides. These peptides are of a size that can be transported through the wall of the intestinal tract into the blood stream, yet they are just a little too complex a molecule to be recognized by the white blood cells as normal.[4] Therefore, the white cells (the neutrophilic granulocytes, to be exact) set upon them to digest them. In doing so they release an enzyme that causes their granules to dissolve, which phenomenon is the one observed by the technician in the cytotoxic test process.

The cytotoxic test, developed by the husband-and-wife team of William Bryan and Marian P. Bryan, of St. Louis, is based on a blood test. The technician mixes the cell containing "buffy coat" of the patient's blood onto slides containing concentrations of the various foods or chemicals to be tested. After a suitable period for incubation, the technician studies the configuration of the granulocytes under a microscope and notes the degree to which their granules have dissolved. This can be estimated in terms of marked, moderate, slight, or no reaction. The result, according to the Bryans, will correlate with the degree of food intolerance that the patient has *at that moment* to each of the substances tested.

Despite the rather meticulous published research on cytotoxic food testing by the Bryans and others, the test has engendered considerable criticism as being inaccurate and as not correlating well with the "allergy" state of the patient. Accordingly, other tests, based on the actual measurement of IgG response to each food, have been developed to get a very similar type of information.

With a good technician, the results of the cytotoxic test can be quite accurate and reproducible. The test has the advantage of being less expensive than most of the others; therefore, it is readily applicable for routine testing. Its bottom line is a very happy one. If the doctor uses it to steer the patient away from the general classes of foods to which he or she shows the greatest intolerance, as well as from the specific foods to which the reaction was quite striking, then four out of five patients will be obviously benefited. We use it most successfully for fine-tuning a diet whose primary objective is to stabilize each individual's blood sugar response.

And If That's Not Enough?

Remember, low blood sugar is not usually a diagnosis, it is a response. And even less often is it the only diagnosis. You may be sure, then, if you still have "low blood sugar" symptoms, that there must be another diagnosis as well, one which still has to be discovered. In such instances, I generally suspect some chemical or environmental sensitivity, heavy metal poisoning (especially mercury), a systemic yeast infection, a blocked metabolic pathway, some hidden allergies, or some "medical" condition, still undiagnosed. If this is the case, you, my friend, really do need to find a complementary physician. The game of helping you can be won only by someone who has the full deck to play with.

8

...

CANDIDA ALBICANS
The Complementarist's Diagnosis

Since the Complementary Medicine I propose is based on causation, I now wish to call your attention to another aspect of causation beyond the nutritional connection we have been discussing.

We must deal with the matter of *iatrogenic causation* — problems that derive from our medical practices. The next two subjects meet with extreme professional resistance because they carry with them the implications that the professional practices of medicine and dentistry may have themselves contributed to the causation of disease.

I submit to you as the first example of iatrogenic causation the "epidemic" of *Candida albicans* infections, whose symptoms can be as diverse as arthritic pains, hair loss, constant colds, memory loss, fatigue, allergies or food sensitivities, intestinal bloating, and depression.

How I Learned About Systemic Candida

I learned about the yeast organism *Candida albicans* in medical school, and subsequently I have advised hundreds of my female patients on how to relieve their yeast, or monilia, vaginitis. But just about seven years ago, I was taken aback by one of my patients, who informed me she was being treated by a respected nutritional colleague for a *systemwide* candida infestation, without any microbiological proof that she had it. When she asked my opinion of that line of pursuit, of which to that point I had no awareness, I was inclined to pooh-pooh the entire approach as being patently without merit. But I reminded myself that such a response would make me guilty of displaying the very trait that I find so deplorable when used against innovative medicine — authority's use of the expert's mantle to denigrate something it actually knows very little about. So I graciously replied: "That's an interesting theory; I had better learn more about it if I hope to advise you correctly."

Well, I didn't get around to that until another year went by, when one of my nutrition-oriented colleagues caught my attention after one of our dinner meetings. "By the way," he said, "I'm now seeing two former patients of yours. They didn't do so well with you, so I went over them. I found they had candida, put them on nystatin, and they're doing great now." You can bet I learned about systemic candida in a hurry.

I was aware that Orion Truss, M.D., of Birmingham, Alabama, had initiated the concept that this familiar yeast organism was contributing to a lot of previously undiagnosed symptomatology. I read his book *The Missing Diagnosis*[1] and followed it up with *The Yeast Connection*, by William Crook, M.D.[2] Then I began to look at the same patients I had been treating all along with a somewhat expanded understanding of what may contribute to their symptoms. Before I tell you what I learned, let me offer you a little background.

Candida — The Basic Understanding

We tend not to consider the health function played by the microorganisms that live in our intestines. But there are more than four hundred species of indigenous resident bacteria in constant competition in our intestinal tract. Health in this case is achieved by keeping them in equilibrium so that no organism dominates the balance of these intestinal flora. Usually this balance is maintained by the resident bacteria, but there are both internal and external stresses that often disrupt the equilibrium.[3] When the imbalance causes an overgrowth of yeast organisms over the normal bacteria of the colon, the most frequently overgrown yeast is *Candida al-*

bicans. When *Candida albicans* ("the yeast organism") occurs as an overgrowth in the intestinal tract, it produces an imbalance (disease) that can affect so many people in so many different ways that the term *the missing diagnosis* applies. That term refers to the fact that these symptoms are the complaints presented by millions of patients who will never be correctly diagnosed. Most people, including orthodox physicians, who have heard of *Candida* or *Monilia albicans* think of it only as causing thrush, an oral or vaginal yeast infection. However, this is but the very tip of the iceberg.

Systems Affected by Candida

There are three major systemic tracts most often affected by *Candida albicans;* the gastrointestinal tract (intestinal bloating, particularly of the large intestine, poor absorption of vitamins and minerals, food allergies and sensitivities, nausea, diarrhea); the urinary tract (urinary frequency, burning, pain, swelling, odor); and the respiratory tract (localized and diffuse pneumonia, emphysema, bronchitis, chronic sinusitis, postnasal drip).[4]

The most specific of these symptoms are bloating, inability to tolerate vitamins taken orally (especially those derived from brewer's yeast), and food sensitivities to yeast- and mold-type foods. Candida causes a high rate of food intolerance. There are also generalized body symptoms such as weakness, forgetfulness, and depression.

Candida overgrowth seems to be more prevalent among women who take birth control pills;[5] however, no one is certain why this occurs. Others susceptible to this type of infection are diabetics, people who use antibiotics, people who have poor diets (especially those heavy in sugar), women who douche excessively (local thrush only), and those who consistently have strong emotional flare-ups. These factors cause changes in the body that affect the balance of the varied bacteria in the intestinal tract.

An External/Internal Illness

The imbalance in the yeast colonies that causes this broad range of illnesses can come about in a number of ways. The most usual manner of acquiring candidiasis is through the use and/or overuse of antibiotics. We all have a candida population to begin with, but it is also possible to aggravate candida growth through sexual relations. It is assumed that an influx of yeast is passed on to the recipient, causing a rapid increase in his (or her) existing *Candida albicans.*

In addition to the gastrointestinal, urinary, and respiratory tracts, candida can affect the skin or nails, areas which are *external* to the body. For the most part, *Candida albicans* does not cross gastrointestinal membranes. It is not truly *systemic,* though we continue to use the term; rather it stays where it was introduced to the body. The vagina and mouth are ectodermal structures, meaning they represent an infolding of the external surface of the body. Thus, it is possible to think of the gastrointestinal tract, the main locus for candidiasis, as external. Think of the intestinal tract as a tube running the length of the body, with the mouth as a funnel and the rest a tube extending to another funnel, the anus. You can see that it is, in a sense, external to the rest of the body. The mouth, esophagus, stomach, and intestines run *through* the body rather than throughout it. Rarely do we see candida in the blood stream. When an organism is not blood-transmitted, it cannot technically be viewed as a systemic organism. The term *systemic candidiasis* refers to those infrequent severe infections where it is transmitted through the blood stream; the general candidiasis we most often see is correctly termed *mucocutaneous* (pertaining to the skin and mucous membrane).

For all candidiasis's physical effects, often the most painful are its mental ones. Candida patients often have a psychological make-up that the experienced clinician learns to recognize. Most are neurotic, seemingly hypochondriacal, negativistic, spacy and confused, easily defeated, and seemingly reluctant to get well. This may be the consequence of a long series of frustrating interactions with physicians who failed to grasp their problem. Combine this with hypoglycemia (which most candida sufferers have concurrently) and multiple food intolerances and chemical sensitivities to a shifting array of substances (which candidiasis makes them prone to), and you have a condition capable of *causing* neuroticism. The psychological effects of the disease are often misdiagnosed as a psychoneurotic illness and treated with psychoactive drugs instead of an appropriate anticandida regimen.

Just How Common Is It?

Well, let me say this. In the five short years that I have been pursuing the diagnosis of candida overgrowth as a generalized medical problem, I have been led, by studying the responses of my patients, to the conclusion that more than one quarter of my patients must be treated as presumptive cases of this form of *Candida albicans*. Remember, these are basically the same patients I had previously been treating for something else. This change may be due to more than a personal discovery or awakening. It may be in part due to the probability that, since the 1920s, the incidence of candidiasis has been increasing, owing to very specific identifiable factors.

Why Am I Seeing More Candida?

The apparent epidemic of *Candida albicans* overgrowth can be blamed on several very contemporary factors. The number-one factor is our diet, particularly our intake of sugar. Just as the use of sugar, when added to yeast, helps make bread rise, so does sugar increase the effects of yeast in the body. The greatest increase in our sugar consumption took place in the 1920s, and its predominance in our diet has continued until most recently. There is ample evidence that sugar intake correlates with *Candida albicans*.[6] Even the AMA in an editorial of December 12, 1986, conceded that candidiasis was on the rise and that in many instances diet was an effective treatment.[7]

Second, you will recall that in the 1940s and 1950s the era of antibiotics began. With it, a more compelling factor was added to this yeast invasion. It has been well established, and will be discussed at length in this chapter, that antibiotics, especially those taken by mouth, cause overgrowth of *Candida albicans*. Then, in the 1960s, came the Pill, which has also been demonstrated to cause this yeast overgrowth in women.[8]

The Mercury Connection

The fourth reason may be the most important cause of all — dental amalgams. Since I am devoting the next chapter to the discussion of the mercury toxicity problem, I simply want to emphasize one point here. Mercury impairs the immune system in a very specific way, and that impairment may be exactly what leads to candida overgrowth. The research of Dr. David Eggleston provides some evidence of the way amalgams may affect the immune system. Dr. Eggleston's research showed that removing and/or inserting silver dental filling brought about a dramatic change in T-lymphocyte levels. ("T" distinguishes those lymphocyte cells derived from the thymus. The T cells are critical to normal immune functions. They regulate practically all cellular and humoral immune responses.) He showed that in one patient, *removing* six fillings *increased* the T cell concentration by 55.3 percent. Reinsertion of four fillings *dropped* these cells 55 percent.[9] More research of this type is needed to prove that impairment of the immune system by mercury can lead to candidiasis.

One other connection is known — *Candida albicans* (and other microorganisms) has been shown to convert the ordinary toxic ionized mercury vapor to a substance called methyl mercury, which happens to be ten times more toxic than elemental mercury, and which can be retained in brain tissue for eighteen to twenty-two years.

Reasoning from what is known about the causative factors — sugar, antibiotics, oral contraceptives, and dental amalgams — we might suspect that *Candida albicans* overgrowth must have been on the rise for better than six decades. It is only now that we are beginning to diagnose and see it for what it is, a disease, or imbalance, that most often is set off by antibiotics. And, as you see from that short list, three of the four leading contributors to its causation stem from the noblest professions. Thus, candidiasis surely qualifies as an iatrogenic illness (illness caused by orthodox medicine).

Candidiasis Is an Alternativist Diagnosis

I have presented to you a story of an illness — a typical example within the paradigm of orthodox medicine. Mucocutaneous candidiasis is a disease caused by a microorganism, diagnosed by laboratory testing, studied by pathologists and microbiologists, treated by antibiotics (albeit different ones from those which cause it) and other pharmaceuticals, managed in hospitals, written about in medical journals and texts. Yet, its prevalence is being denied by orthodox medicine. Complementary Medicine, meanwhile, has recognized it as one of the major clinical problems that it must deal with.

Candidiasis, much like hypoglycemia, has run afoul of the bitter we-or-they schism between the two warring medical philosophies. Just in the past few years, doctors who diagnose and treat candidiasis are being targeted by orthodoxy's odious antiquackery campaign. And now I am beginning to hear stories of patients whose claims for third-party reimbursement are being denied after review by their insurers' 100 percent orthodox medical advisory boards, simply because of their diagnosis.

The question we must try to answer is, Why? Why is candidiasis, once it exists beyond the genital organs or the mouth, no longer a proper diagnosis for a patient of a "real" doctor?

Before we struggle with the knotty answer to this one, let's review a couple of typical cases and see how Complementary Medicine approaches them.

Gloria MacNeil

Gloria MacNeil first came to my office on August 3, 1983, complaining of arthritis, especially the pain in her hands. She had been frightened by the fact that over the previous five to six weeks she had lost twenty-five pounds. Two other things had also happened: Her hair was beginning to fall out, and she was suffering memory lapses.

"I am sixty-seven and I know I'm getting older, but I certainly don't think that any of this is because of old age. Something is wrong, but no one has been able to tell me what it is."

Gloria gave me additional information. She was allergic to many things, suffered annually from hay fever, and had been going to an allergist for ten years. Because of her allergies, she had been on a rather stringent elimination diet for all of this time. While on the diet she felt very well.

In the last year or two she had been ill and had been treated with antibiotics. During this time she also began "cheating" and eventually fell off her diet. Worth emphasizing is the fact that she now found that she was no longer capable of tolerating vitamins that previously had been a part of her health regimen.

> *"At first I thought that perhaps there was something wrong with the types of vitamins I was now taking, so I switched manufacturers. I also checked to see if the vitamins were made from brewer's yeast, which I know causes me allergy problems. I went to my family doctor, who doesn't believe in vitamins. He also happens to have a pharmacological degree, and as you can imagine he said, 'Taking vitamins is a dead end, they won't help you. Stop taking them.'"*

Gloria continued with her story, indicating that nothing had helped — nothing her family doctor did, nothing the allergist did. She kept getting worse. It was at this point that she decided to come to me.

Gloria was given our comprehensive physical examination, including a glucose tolerance test. Her blood sugar level went from 90 to 210 in the first half hour, and dropped to 53 by the third hour (which I interpreted to indicate both hypoglycemia and borderline diabetes). Since she could not take vitamins by mouth, I gave her a vitamin-and-mineral drip (an intravenous infusion, including vitamin C, magnesium, B_6, B_{12}, and the rest of the B complex, etc.). To remove most potential food sensitivities and provide needed energy, I also placed Gloria on a low-carbohydrate diet with certain vegetable additions.

WHY I SUSPECTED CANDIDA

Two facts in Gloria's medical history made me suspect that she was suffering from *Candida albicans* overgrowth: She reported a gradual worsening of her symptoms after antibiotics, and she suddenly showed "allergic" reactions to vitamins taken orally.

On September 19 Gloria returned, indicating that although she felt somewhat better, all of her symptoms were still present. Since we were not set up at that time to do blood cytotoxic evaluating, I had Gloria take an electro-acupuncture test (Voll technique), which although less reproducible, is capable of identifying food sensitivity and has the advantage of being instantaneous. I learned that Gloria had a strong reaction to grains, beans, and brewer's yeast. Here was another clue, yeast sensitivity. The findings correlated with my impression that candidiasis was behind Gloria's complaints. The test also indicated a moderate reaction to nuts, corn, and wheat. These foods were immediately removed from Gloria's diet.

THE EXPANSION OF SUCCESS

She returned on October 25, saying that she was feeling a great deal better; she had more energy, and the arthritis was gone except in her hands. She also said that she was no longer having bouts of memory loss and her hair loss was markedly less. These improvements led me to believe that Gloria might not need anything more than this nutritional therapy, so I continued her regimen of vitamin drips two times per week.

On November 21 Gloria returned, looking healthier.

"I feel splendid. The drips seem to be helping."

All of her symptoms were rapidly disappearing, and even her hands were getting better. Gloria was on this protocol for the remainder of the year.

On her January 1984 visit, a trace mineral analysis (done from a hair sample) found her to be low in chromium, magnesium, and iron, but since Gloria still could not take vitamins orally (a sign that she still had candida overgrowth), I continued her vitamins and minerals by injection, increasing the amount of vitamin A, plus the deficient minerals. When she returned on February 10, she said she was better but still not 100 percent.

HOW THE CYTOTOXIC TEST HELPS CANDIDA PATIENTS

At this point, the center was set up to investigate food intolerances more accurately by way of the cytotoxic test. This showed Gloria to be strongly reactive to oysters, eggs, shrimp, oranges, parmesan cheese, almonds, sesame seeds, prunes, and wheat, and moderately reactive to corn, white flour, cane sugar, lentils, and peas. I not only explained to Gloria the need for avoiding the foods to which she was reactive, but I also decided the time had come to start her on specific anticandida treatment. She was begun on nystatin, 2 million units a day. (Nystatin is discussed in detail later in the chapter.)

At her March visit Gloria said she felt better, and her arthritis was almost completely gone from her hands. I increased her nystatin dose to 5 million units. On her next visit Gloria indicated that when she took more than the 5 million units, she felt nauseated, and so she ended up taking between 3 million and 5 million units daily. A few months later, a repeat cytotoxic test showed that most of her food allergies were corrected, except those to cheese and mustard.

Gloria had an excellent summer, without hay fever. Her allergist, noting that she was doing well, encouraged her to continue on her regimen. This was the first summer since her first attack ten years before that Gloria did not have a single bout with hay fever. Then, during the summer, Gloria noticed a small rash. Attributing it to the nystatin, she stopped taking it. She also went off her diet, eating cheese with crackers, coffee, and apple pie. By the time I next saw her, she had been off her diet and her nystatin for over two months. Not unexpectedly, she returned with an arthritis flare-up.

Gloria wanted to know whether the nystatin withdrawal had led to her flare-up. I told her that her problem was more likely to be the apple pie. *Candida albicans* is yeast, I reminded her, and is drastically affected by sugar. In case I haven't mentioned it before, there are two groups of people who should avoid sugar: those who breathe, and those who live.

Gloria returned several weeks later, stating that the flare-ups had disappeared and she had no intention of going back to sugar.

To reinforce her decision, I pointed out three specific reasons for her to stay away from it: her food sensitivity, which may be a trigger for her arthritis; her diabetic type of hypoglycemia; and her yeast infection, which feeds on sugar.

Gloria is still not cured. She still gets flare-ups in moldy and dusty environments, or whenever she goes off her diet. But she sails through most days without a single one of the symptoms that brought her to us.

Judith Camaratta: Candida Plus Low Blood Sugar

Judith Camaratta first came to the center on February 16, 1984, reporting that within the last few months she had had two bouts with double pneumonia.

> "No one else has been able to help me. I feel sick all the time. I have constant sore throats and my glands are always swollen. I am tired all the time and I am frightened at how forgetful I am becoming. My doctors tell me it is either my hypoglycemia and/or a generally run-down condition and it will have to have run its course. I can't wait!"

Judith had recently been in the hospital for a battery of tests, but "they didn't find anything other than my hypoglycemia."

This was one case in which orthodox medicine had diagnosed hypoglycemia. However, when I learned that her doctor had given her Inderal because of her low blood sugar, I was shocked, although I should have known better. "How can they use drugs when a diet will do?" I thought. (The Inderal, a beta-blocker, was being used to suppress the adrenaline response to low blood sugar.) I was even more shocked when I reviewed Judith's previous diet. It included skipping breakfast, having cake four times a week, and consuming fruit and fruit juices daily.

Our workup confirmed the hypoglycemia. In the glucose tolerance test, her blood sugar went from 80 to 110 in the first half hour and dropped by the third to 42. Her weight was 149 pounds and she stood five feet three inches tall.

WE START TREATMENT

I placed Judith on the low-carbohydrate diet and gave her the nutritional supplements that have become standard at our center. Although low blood sugar had made me suspicious that she had *Candida albicans* infection, I did not then institute any specific treatment.

Her next visit was approximately one month later. She was down to 141¾ pounds and was in ketosis (that is, the body was burning its fat for energy), as we had intended. Although her energy had increased, none of her symptoms disappeared; so I ordered a cytotoxic test. The test revealed a high food sensitivity to vinegar, along with cheese, molds, beef, chicken, cane sugar, corn, mushrooms, and wheat, as well as to the candida organism itself. This is just the sort of profile we get typically in candidiasis patients. The cytotoxic test provided enough indirect evidence — sensitivity to all tested mold and fermented items (vinegar, cheese, mold, mushrooms), plus wheat, the most frequent co-offender.

I insisted that Judith stop all the foods to which she was sensitive, as well as sugar, yeast, and mold products and their derivatives.

On her next visit she reported:

> *"All of my symptoms are still there but are so much less that I know I am getting better."*

SPECIFIC ANTI-YEAST THERAPY

Since I was more certain about the diagnosis, and since Judith was only partially better, I decided to try to kill off some of the intestinal yeast overgrowth. So I prescribed nystatin.

When Judith returned for her next checkup, her weight was down to 138 pounds and she was still in ketosis. She said:

> *"I really feel great. There is a dramatic change. Although I had started feeling somewhat better and had more energy, it was nothing like now. Oh, by the way, I forgot to mention I no longer am so forgetful."*

By September 1984 I added caprylic acid and my Antioxidant Formula to Judith's regimen. Judith's appearance matched her comment that there had been continued dramatic improvement on every front. Every symptom she had was now gone. "I know I am healthier."

I asked her how she knew.

> "Well, what's most unusual is that anytime my daughter has a cold — this is even before I had these problems — you could bet that I would soon get it. But Nancy has now had a very bad cold for weeks. People in my office are suffering from colds and I haven't caught anything. I just don't get sick anymore! It is too good to be true. Before, I was physically and mentally in a state of distress. I can't compare it to anything. It was just so bad! Now I'm on top of the world! I again enjoy being with my daughter and work. That's probably the best part. I'm thirty-five and I was feeling like an old woman, but now I'm back and I don't intend to have it changed."

What These Cases "Prove"

I have just told you of the cases of two patients out of the thousands whom I have treated for candidiasis. I didn't "prove" anything. Add on another 998, and it still won't prove anything. But it sure is gratifying to be able to help patients who weren't getting anywhere with their medical problems and to see them finally proclaim their wellness.

The fact that nothing has been scientifically "proven" means this: There will be other women (and men) similar to Gloria and Judith, hundreds of thousands of them, who will seek help from their mainstream physicians and will get no more help than my two got before they came to the center. Their doctors will not go on a search-and-destroy mission against generalized candidiasis because it is not a proven illness.

To too many physicians, *unproven* means *disproven*.

What Can We Learn from These Cases?

Both women had been treated by traditional, concerned, and careful physicians at accredited hospitals, yet neither patient was recognized to be suffering from *Candida albicans* overgrowth. What happened?

Basically, the symptoms were not those expected by the orthodox clinician, who, in diagnosing candida, looks for "classical" vaginal or oral itching or rashes. The physicians were the victims of educational narrowness, as indeed they must be if they read and accept only the orthodox literature.

Without a mindset for this condition, based on an awareness of the prevalence of *Candida albicans* imbalances, there was not enough in the presenting histories to lead a doctor to this diagnosis. It was only because of my awareness of this illness and its symptoms, plus my familiarity with the cytotoxic test, that I was able to make the proper diagnosis.

The use of the cytotoxic test is an example of an important factor to orthodoxist and complementarist alike: diagnostic instrumentation. Each matches the diagnostic efforts to his intent. The orthodoxist seeks a diagnosis that will permit him to intervene for the patient's benefit; the complementarist seeks to teach the patient to intervene in his own behalf. Orthodox instruments are geared for major deviations from normalcy. Complementary clinicians have a series of diagnostic tools that lead to nutritional changes and give us information lost to orthodoxy. The glucose tolerance test is a second example of a diagnostic instrument given different emphasis by orthodoxist and complementarist. Like the cytotoxic test, it is helpful in directing the clinician to the diagnosis of diet-related disorders.

What the Complementarist Looks For

The most specific symptom of generalized candidiasis is intestinal bloating, a swelling of the lower abdomen. If that bloat is aggravated by beer, bread, pasta, sweets, or juices, then it is an even more specific indicator. High on the list of contributors to candida susceptibility is a history of antibiotic use; the more courses in a lifetime, the more likely is the diagnosis.

Also, the past or present use of the Pill makes the diagnosis more likely. Other common symptoms are general malaise, weakness, forgetfulness, moments of depression, hair loss, even joint pains that are similar to arthritis. Often the hypoglycemic patient develops a sudden general run-down condition beyond what his hypoglycemia typically causes. A good clue is provided whenever one reacts adversely to taking vitamins orally. Almost 90 percent of those individuals who cannot tolerate vitamins orally have *Candida albicans* overgrowth. We always ask whether our patient has become highly sensitive to yeast and fungus products or products containing them, for example, yeast and yeast breads, beer, mushrooms, cheese, mustard, vinegar. To this list must be added sensitivity to inhaling mold spores; this means discomfort in haunts such as bathrooms, basements, areas with wet leaves, summer beach houses, and so forth. Last but not least, we always look for the presence of dental amalgams.

Why the List of Symptoms?

I've recited the list of symptoms not because I'm teaching you to play doctor, but because I know there must be a goodly number of you who have this problem and I want you to begin to take steps to get some effective help. Should all of that take place, and you get to the point where you know candida is your problem, you may then want to know how we treat it at the Atkins Center.

The Therapeutic Trial

I trust that you will notice that in the cases presented, I violated a cardinal rule of standard medicine — I treated without a fully established diagnosis. I did that for the reason that the response to the treatment (nystatin) would indicate the diagnosis. This is called a therapeutic trial. The complementarist can afford to use a therapeutic trial as his modus operandi because he uses mainly health enhancers. Here, the worst thing that can happen is nothing. Using a drug like nystatin is an exception, albeit a *relatively* safe one.

Remember, I began by presenting diet and nutritional substances that could only prove beneficial, regardless of the specific diagnosis.

Beyond all the general advantages of low dietary intake of sugar and the stabilization of blood sugar that seems to benefit all of us, there is a specific advantage in low-sugar and low-carbohydrate dieting for the patient with a systemic candida problem.

Which Is the Best Diet for Candida?

Many of you are aware of another pendulum swing in our culture — the swing between high- and low-carbohydrate diets. In the seventies, low-carbohydrate diets were the rage; in the eighties, high (complex) carbohydrates were more favored. *All the while, human physiology has remained remarkably constant.*

The truth is that each of us has a different metabolic make-up and differing clinical problems, plus a personal roster of specific food intolerances. The time has come for us to learn *dietary principles,* not specific diets.

Clinical experience by the aforementioned Dr. Truss and Dr. Crook and many others meeting at the several Yeast-Human Interaction symposia has provided considerable agreement that systemic candidiasis patients must avoid sugars (including fruits), alcohol, high-starch items, most grains, and dairy products, plus foods that are themselves fermented (vinegar, for example). In other words, the anti-yeast diet is very similar to the low-carbohydrate reducing diet I first wrote about in 1972.

Low-Carbohydrate Proponents Are Quite Comfortable with the Yeast Diet

But this makes my vegetarian-oriented nutritional colleagues squirm a little. It does serve to bring us all a little closer to a different-strokes-for-different folks orientation for custom-tailoring our patients' diets.

The inescapable fact is that a low-carbohydrate regimen is particularly effective in controlling yeast infections. As I mentioned earlier, in the making of bread, a small amount of sugar added to the yeast-flour mixture greatly enhances the rising effect of the yeast. Well, in the intestinal tract sugar serves as an ideal "culture medium" for the growth of *Candida albicans*.

Empirically, that's just what we see, also. A sugar-restricted diet does help our candida patients, perhaps more than any other aspect of our therapy. To appreciate this point, one has only to observe the experiences of dozens of our patients whose case studies I might have presented who, having gradually improved after months of our combined therapies, just happened to go on "vacation" binges of sugar-eating. The majority of these patients reported to me, somewhat sheepishly, that most of their symptoms had returned!

As I rethink the reasons for my patient successes achieved in the sixties and seventies with the Atkins Diet, I now feel they are often explained by postulating the correction of a candida condition. I particularly believe that the thousands of patients whose gastrointestinal complaints clear up promptly on carbohydrate restriction are, for the most part, people who have a significant candida problem.

Specific Therapies Against Candida

As you refer to the two cases above you may be struck with the fact that I used a pharmaceutical preparation, nystatin. "You're supposed to be against drugs and now you're using one," you might protest. "How do you square that one?"

That, my friends, is exactly why I felt compelled to shift ideologically from alternative medicine, which is totally exclusive of orthodox medicine, to Complementary Medicine, which welcomes all the healing arts. Sometimes the best available agent is a pharmaceutical. (I haven't yet defined the term *biologic medicine*, which I espouse very highly. Nystatin actually is a biological.)

Nystatin has become the preferred medication against candida because it is both safe and effective. Nystatin is a mold derivative and can cause allergic reactions in mold-sensitive individuals. More often, the apparent bad reactions that the more sensitive patients have are due to a die-off reaction. Called the Herxheimer reaction, this occurs when large numbers of yeast cells die in a short time and the toxic by-products set up further immune reactions. This die-off is really a good sign, but it must be controlled. I do this by starting with a small dose of nystatin (let's say, 500,000 units) and gradually build up to 4 million to 8 million units.

Nystatin has the further property of not being absorbed systemically from the intestinal tract. This means it will act specifically only within that area and will not cause systemic reactions. That can also be a disadvantage when it is necessary to treat the vagina, bladder, mouth, nose, or other areas outside the gastrointestinal tract. Orthodox medicine does offer other drugs that do that, but all include a greater risk of toxicity.

The Caprylic Acid Story

My favorite specific therapy is not a drug. It is safer than nystatin, but less effective. It is a naturally occurring short-chain fatty acid called caprylic acid. For purists, this provides an effective *nutritional* treatment. I frequently start a patient on caprylic acid and then augment it with nystatin to produce a complementary effect.

My Texas colleague John Parks Trowbridge, M.D., has written an excellent book called *The Yeast Syndrome,* in which he details the above as well as some other effective therapies such as the herb taheebo (pau d'arco), acidophilus, and some homeopathic remedies. For those who want to learn more on this subject, I heartily endorse his book.

The Atkins Center Approach

I hope you have gathered that we use a multifaceted approach. First and foremost is the low-carbohydrate, low-yeast diet individualized to avoid major food intolerances. Then we replace the normal flora of the intestine with acidophilus and/or bifidus cultures. Often we use homeopathic dilutions of candida. Always there is a program of nutritional supplements (more about that in a minute). The specific therapy with caprylic acid and nystatin will, of course, play its role.

In addition, we like to take care of the allergic aspects of the problem by giving neutralizing dose treatment against the yeast organisms. This is an approach that has spun off from orthodox teachings in allergy. The usual allergy approach is called desensitization; in this, the allergist starts the patient off with a safe dose and gradually builds up the dose, by small increments, until, a year or so later, a mature state of immunity finally exists.

The Neutralizing Dose Technique

Here the doctor or his technician performs a series of intradermal tests using decreasing dilutions of the yeast or mold to be tested. They will raise wheals (hives) in the area where the antigen was injected just under the skin. But somewhere along the line, as serial dilutions are given, there will be one dilution that is simply too dilute to raise a reaction. The concentration found thus is the neutralizing dose. This concentration can be given as a shot, or as we do, as drops for under-the-tongue use. This puts the patient at the same point he would be after a year's desensitization, except that we get these results after an hour's testing.

Sounds great, doesn't it? So why do orthodox allergists reject it under the usual buzzword of "unproven"? Simply because they are quite comfortable with what they have already been taught and have come to terms with the fact than in allergy, "not everybody gets better."

Nutrition to the Rescue

If you'd like to know what nutrients we emphasize in treating candida, pay attention. First of all, specially formulated vitamins are usually required, because candida patients do not tolerate brewer's yeast very well. The most common vitamin source is brewer's yeast.

Most constituents of the B-complex vitamins are important, so that we include a yeast-free form of B complex. The B vitamin biotin is especially interesting here. In large doses, it seems to have a direct antigrowth effect on candida. I use between 5 and 15 milligrams (5000–15,000 micrograms) daily.

I will be, as we go along, extolling the virtues of omega-3 (EPA) and omega-6 (GLA) fatty acids. Both are very important here. The entire roster of antioxidant nutrients is also clinically quite useful. Beta carotene is particularly valuable.

Among the minerals, I usually include magnesium, zinc, and manganese. Add all these to the diet specifics and you can see the comprehensiveness of the nutritional approach.

Look How Complicated Our Program Is

Orthodoxy, when it is imaginative enough to think of the candidiasis diagnosis, treats very simply. The patient is given the appropriate antibiotic, period. "Why is their medicine so simple and yours so complex?" you ask.

Doctors who treat with drugs do learn of their dangers. And they learn how treacherous are combinations of drugs. Thus a proper drug protocol would, out of prudence, be the simplest. In contrast, doctors working with nutrients soon learn about the essential teamwork of the nutrients. As Dr. Roger Williams, dean of nutritionists, has said: "A nutritional program is only as good as its weakest link." And a system based on balancing everything must be complex; there are so many things to keep in balance. Thus a complementarist knows he must touch all the important bases.

I hope I have shown you how, from diagnosis to treatment regimen, dealing with candida as a systemic illness demonstrates the advantages that Complementary Medicine has over the simplistic approach currently used by mainstream medicine. We complementarians suspect the existence of the condition because we listen: we support the nutrition of the patient; we concentrate on the underlying causes; we support the patient's immune system; and we use only medications from which the patient can receive the maximum benefit in relation to the lowest risk.

9
. . .

MERCURY AMALGAM TOXICITY
What Have Our Dentists Wrought?

There was a time, not very long ago at all, when I, upon seeing a patient's report of high mercury levels (typically, it would show up on a hair trace mineral analysis report), would question the patient about possible industrial exposures, and then about his or her consumption of tuna and swordfish. So preposterous was the notion that the dental profession could be negligent enough not to check out its number-one cavity-filling substance for possible toxicity that the idea of a dental cause for mercury toxicity never even entered my mind!

But once a mind is trained to consider iatrogenism (the belief that disease is *caused* by doctors, or in this case, dentists) as the pandemic of our century, the unthinkable becomes obvious. *Most mercury poisoning is caused by dental amalgams and most of us have (or have had) these amalgams.*

Our Dental Amalgams Can Poison Us

Mercury is a heavy toxic metal that can affect every organ system in the body. The source of mercury that we're discussing, more often than not, is our dental amalgams. (Mercury is mixed with the silver the dentist puts in your teeth to make it more malleable.) It enters our bodies through the lungs and the gastrointestinal tract and eventually traverses every part. This inorganic mercury, which eventually is changed to methyl mercury and is stored in fat tissue, goes on to attack the brain and nervous system when it reaches toxic levels. The *acute* mercury toxic state, which occurs from a single large exposure, causes specific symptoms such as vomiting, diarrhea, inflammation of the lungs and the mouth lining, metallic taste in the mouth, and unconsciousness. The *chronic* toxic state, which represents poisoning that occurs from exposure to small quantities over a longer period of time, causes a gradual toxicity. Chronic mercury toxicity is insidious, like a pile of children's toy blocks balanced precariously until the moment when the last block knocks the pile over.

The organs involved in chronic mercury poisoning include the nervous system, brain tissue, cardiovascular system, kidneys, connective tissues, and red blood cells, as well as the allergy mechanism.[1] This constant sneak attack can gradually wear down immune function and lead to a variety of degenerative diseases. When the immune system breaks down, the body's responses might range from mere discomfort to potentially acute disease states, such as asthma or cardiovascular irregularities.

How We Check: The Mercury Vapor Test

At the Atkins Center, in addition to the hair trace mineral analysis, we use the mercury vapor test. The latter is performed by a cute little gadget that gives an on-the-spot digital readout of the mercury content in the air sample at the tip of the instrument. We place the tip end in the mouth near the molars (but not touching), and just like a silent Geiger counter, it locates mercury leaks in a minute. When those tests are positive (as they are over 50 percent of the time), we go on to search for mercury in the blood or urine.

Often enough we find high levels of mercury in the hair, blood, or urine of people who have no teeth or no fillings. Obviously, there must be other sources, and one is the diet. I then question patients about their intake of tuna and swordfish.

I would like to present you with two examples of mercury-related conditions that went undiagnosed. The diagnosis of mercury toxicity is confusing because the doctor can too easily diagnose the condition presented to him by the patient without recognizing its relationship to mercury toxicity.

Carol Drury: Too Many Symptoms

"I hadn't realized the dental work I was having done affected my medical problems until after I had my amalgams removed."

Carol is an internationally known artist who came to the Atkins Center in June 1983 because she had symptoms for which her physician could find no cause.

"Because of the numbness in my hands and fingers, my doctor said I had arthritis and he placed me on an arthritic medication, Naprosyn. I was on it for one week and felt so ill I went off it."

She was also sent to be tested for cancer when she complained of a constant sore ache under her armpit, but no cancer turned up. Then, because of constant crying episodes, she was sent to a psychiatrist for several years.

Carol had been to see many physicians and was even diagnosed as hypoglycemic at a well-known clinic, a rarity in orthodox circles. She got some assistance from a chiropractor who helped make her aware of the nutritional aspects of her health. However, she continued to have many symptoms: numbness in her hands and fingers, especially on the left side, aching under her arm and in her breast, spells of extreme drowsiness after eating, stomach pains, and difficulty concentrating. She was suspicious that she might have some food allergies because of the definite reactions she had after ingesting certain foods.

Carol did not have a weight problem. Her GTT (glucose tolerance test) confirmed the presence of low blood sugar. Her hair analysis indicated high mercury, as well as high copper and low zinc. At that time, 1983, I was not yet oriented to the dental aspects of mercury toxicity. What I did note, however, was that Carol consumed five cans of tuna fish per week. I told her to stop eating the canned tuna, and to follow the no-sugar Meat and Millet Diet. Her supplement program consisted of our Basic Formula, augmented with extra niacinamide, vitamin B$_6$, vitamin C, and PABA.

CAROL BENEFITS FROM NUTRITION ALONE

At five weeks her somnolence was gone and her stomach symptoms responded to acupuncture. By September, Carol announced that she was feeling "one hundred percent better" than when she started. In truth, it was not 100 percent because she still continued to have food reactions, cold extremities, a dull ache under her armpit, and a sore left breast.

> "When I looked through my daily logbook, I noticed that every time I had dental work done my left side would bother me, I'd get an earache, and have shooting pains in the extremities on my left side."

At this point, I placed Carol on a mercury-mobilizing regimen (that is, one to help flush the mercury from her system) consisting of high doses of vitamin C, selenium, glutathione, and cysteine. After three weeks on this program, her urinary mercury recovery was 48.7 nanograms per twenty-four hours, well beyond the upper limits of normal. ("Normal" in this instance is an arbitrary number, 20 nanograms, which is inappropriate since the normal amount of mercury in the body is zero.) By that time, I had been properly enlightened to the fact that most mercury poisonings are due to "silver" dental fillings, so I recommended that Carol have her amalgams tested. In recounting her story to a staff member, Carol noted:

> "When Dr. Atkins suggested I have my amalgams tested, my family dentist refuted the amalgam issue and went out of his way to show me all the literature put out by the ADA [American Dental Association] negating the issue."

There the matter rested momentarily. Meanwhile, my staff also tested her for cytotoxic food sensitivities and we found she was intolerant of grains, fermenting agents (yeasts and molds), sugar, and tomatoes. We reformulated her vitamins to eliminate all traces of brewer's yeast and placed her on a rotational yeast-free diet. By March 1984, her cold extremities had improved dramatically.

A MERCURY DENTIST'S EXPLANATION

At this time, I urged her to see my referral dentist for amalgam problems. The decision was made to go for amalgam removal. "Considering Carol's high urine mercury and mercury vapor test," the referral dentist recounted, "and the fact that she was already on a good diet and supplementation, I felt, after consulting with her, that it was appropriate to remove the mercury amalgams from her mouth. This was done quadrant by quadrant, removing fillings with the largest negative currents first."

In addition to performing a mercury vapor test, dentists with a similar orientation will also test patients for current potential. The current generated from restorations is measured in microamps, tooth by tooth. "This is done," the consultant explained, "because amalgam fillings with higher currents are breaking down more rapidly. Let me show you the perfect analogy between the mouth and a car battery. When you have different metals in an electrolyte solution, one metal is the positive terminal, the other metal is the negative terminal. In the mouth, every amalgam is different, due to its composition — this depends on how it is mixed and prepared by the dentist, and on the effects of moisture when the filling is replaced. The technique is never duplicated exactly. Remember," he went on, "the saliva is a solution of electrolytes and thus provides all the elements to make a battery cell out of the mouth. As in a battery, there are currents produced from certain fillings. Some currents are stronger than others. Although the readings will differ from time to time within the same person, the relationship between a high reading and a low reading will always remain the same."

Carol's big improvement did not come until after her amalgams were removed. Why don't I let Carol tell the ending of her story?

"Once the dentist began to remove my amalgams I began to improve. I actually went through a return of all the symptoms — nausea, stomach pain, body aches and

pains — after the second quadrant was removed. I couldn't believe how all the symptoms correlated with my dental work.* By the time all my amalgams were removed and replaced, my symptoms ended. My food allergies were gone, my brain cleared, my stomach pains were gone. This didn't change the fact that I still have hypoglycemia, so I must stay on my diet."

Monica Flanagan Has Made the Rounds

"As a teenager I developed many allergies, my teeth were terrible, I had constant cavities, and I developed palpitations. There were times when my body would shake so violently that I thought I was going to die."

When Monica visited the Atkins Center in 1985, she was slightly overweight. In her mid-thirties, she hoped to become an actress and singer but her myriad symptom complaints frustrated her ambitions. Among her symptoms were violent palpitations, constant diarrhea, intestinal spasms, back pain, low energy level, weight gain, and insatiable hunger. The rest of the list was so long she ran out of space on the symptom form we use. She had been placed on many drugs, starting at the age of ten, when she had an appendectomy that resulted in a kidney infection. The list of physicians she had seen since then read like a medical directory, while her list of medications read like a pharmacy shelf: numerous antibiotics, Corgard, Tagamet, Mylanta, prednisone, birth control pills, Anaprox, and more.

In August 1985, we began to unravel Monica's seemingly complicated problems. She was placed on the Atkins low-carbohydrate diet and the following supplements: Basic Formula, Antioxidant Formula, extra manganese, magnesium orotate, calcium orotate, oil of evening primrose, phenylalanine, octacosanol, extra vitamin

---

* Aggravation of symptoms during amalgam removal is a common finding. Although distressing, it indicates that the procedure is warranted. We are currently considering the possible advantages of coordinating the dental work with EDTA chelation therapy (see chapter 14) administered on the same day.

B_{12} and B_6, extra folic acid, and PABA. Because she could not tolerate the entire vitamin program at first, we had to build up her intake bit by bit. Her candida profile was positive, so Monica was also given a homeopathic concentration of *Candida albicans* and was placed on caprylic acid. She exhibited positive reactions to candida, brewer's yeast, mozzarella, crab, and other foods on her cytotoxic test. Because she had elevated IgE levels, we tested her for allergy. She developed wheals to yeast and mold with intradermal testing, and so we gave her sublingual drops in the same concentration that neutralized her skin reaction.

HOW WE FOUND MONICA'S MERCURY

Monica's glucose tolerance test was normal. Her hair analysis showed low manganese, magnesium, and calcium levels, but the striking finding was a considerable elevation of her mercury level. Her mercury vapor test showed an elevated mercury vapor on the left side. During the next two months, Monica began to lose weight more easily, and she noticed she could go longer stretches (up to four hours) without feeling hungry. Her diarrhea stopped once she was on the low-carbohydrate diet. She reduced the dosage of the Corgard she needed for palpitations, but she could not get off it completely, and she still felt exhausted. At this time, we recommended that Monica go to our dental consultant to check her mercury amalgams and see if their removal was necessary. In October, Monica began to have her amalgams removed and replaced with nonmetallic composite fillings. The amalgams were removed by quadrant, or section.

> "After my second quadrant was removed I found that my palpitations had stopped; I no longer had to take the Corgard."

In early November, Monica, now completely free of medications, noted that her dysmenorrhea (painful menstrual periods) was also better.

> "I do get nervous before an audition, but it's a more normal nervous. I've begun singing again and my chest does not pound at all. Even my energy level is up."

After all the amalgams were removed, Monica received a series of six vitamin C drips, in order to remove some tissue residuals of mercury, utilizing the heavy metal binding (chelating) ability of ascorbic acid. She was also on the full regimen of vitamins.

> *"Once I was on the vitamins, I noticed that I had no pain upon waking; I no longer had everyday back pain. Toward the end of my dental work, I decided to start an aerobics class and I broke down crying when I realized I could do it. It had been such a long time since I could do exercise."*

Monica's problems got somewhat better with our initial diet-and-supplement approach, but her problems were not solved until her amalgams were removed. The diet regimen, vitamin supplementation, and allergy testing helped her weight problem, hunger pains, intestinal spasms, and diarrhea. Once the mercury amalgams were removed, her energy level changed, back pain improved, and best of all, she was able to discontinue the medication she needed for palpitations.

What These Two "Anecdotes" Can Teach Us

In these two cases, as in the majority of cases, the hair analysis, which was positive, was more helpful in pointing us toward the mercury problem than the blood levels, which were negative. This suggests that the hair mercury levels may correlate better with the clinical situation than does the blood mercury. The quantity of mercury recovered in the urine seems to be an even better indicator of mercury mobilization by diet, antioxidant nutrients, dental rehabilitation, homeopathic mercury, or chelation. Although amalgam removal does nothing to remove the mercury that is already fixed in cells, the body, once the source is removed, is better able to get rid of the cellular mercury, as chronicled by the rise in urinary mercury levels.

The Rationale of the Antimercury Nutrients

"Mercury-protocol" nutrients, such as selenium, glutathione, cysteine, and vitamin C, have a special affinity for mercury and will form a complex with it, allowing it to be extracted from the tissues it is fixed to.[2] Urine and blood serum are tested before and after the mercury-releasing protocol, which was devised by the late Dr. Carlton Fredericks. If we find that urine or blood levels rise significantly after three weeks of the regimen, we continue the supplementation until the levels begin to fall. Another method used to pull mercury out of the body is through chelation therapy (chapter 14).

When we re-examine our discussion about the differences between orthodox medicine and Complementary Medicine, we will be struck with the fact that the diagnosis and management of patients with mercury toxicity fits comfortably in the realm of complementarianism, yet would be a misfit in the area of orthodox medicine.

Why Orthodoxy Has Trouble Dealing with Mercury

The key point here is the difference in the systems used to understand patients. Orthodoxy likes to proceed in a linear, stepwise fashion — first establishing a diagnosis, thus placing the individual in a diagnostic category, and then treating him in a manner identical or similar to others in the same category. The treatment follows a protocol established by statistical analysis; thus, the doctor treats his group member patient by playing the percentages. In contrast, the complementarist, who succeeds by achieving balance and treats by rebuilding weakened aspects of his patients, is not as concerned with the diagnosis as with the causation of imbalances, particularly those he can identify and change.

Now add to that understanding the awareness that mercury toxicity is not a complete diagnosis but, since it affects so many of the body's organ systems, a contributor to a variety of diagnoses and the cause of a variety of imbalances, and you will immediately see why Complementary Medicine can work with this concept and orthodoxy cannot.

That's why Monica collected diagnosis after diagnosis from her lengthy list of mercury-related conditions, but no one diagnosed the mercury toxicity. Once a diagnosis was arrived at, her doctors searched no further. The complementary approach, in contrast, begins with the premise that all adverse influences on a patient should be identified. "Therapy" is directed toward correcting anything that could cause an imbalance.

How Mercury Does Its Damage

Heavy metals, such as mercury, are toxic to the body primarily because they knock out vital enzymes in the body's metabolic pathways. Enzymes are made up of long chains of proteins (amino acids), and they are vital to the body's functioning: They serve as catalysts to every specific biochemical reaction. Without them, plant or animal life could not take place. Mercury, in particular, has an affinity for the enzymes of the sulfhydryl group, and these are its primary victims.[3] Sulfhydryl-containing amino acids are those in which the element sulfur replaces the usual carbon in certain key spots. In this way, mercury can inhibit the enzymes necessary for cholesterol formation, which is important for the production of vitamin D, bile salts, and the steroid hormones;[4] or it can inhibit the action of cysteine, which functions as an antioxidant and free radical scavenger, improves the immune system, and aids in the repair of DNA.[5] Sulfhydryl groups are also involved in the formation of hemoglobin.

Mercury and the Immune System

Amalgams interfere with the immune system.[6] In the previous chapter, I noted that antibiotics affect the immune system, resulting in a *Candida albicans* overgrowth. According to some medical scientists, amalgam contamination suppresses several aspects of the immune system in the same manner. Others have found that mercury attacks our lymphocytes (the body's immune fighters).[7] This, in turn, leads to chronic recurrent infections, colds, and other immune problems.[8]

Industrial Sources of the Mercury Problem

A 1981 study reported in the *Journal of Dental Research* showed that mercury is released from amalgams through the act of chewing.[9] Researchers showed that the blood level of mercury went up during chewing and returned to a baseline level when the subjects stopped chewing. In addition, previous in vitro studies have shown that amalgams increased cell cytotoxicity.[10]

To be sure, not all mercury is from the dental source. Other sources may be found in industrial areas where mercury is used in manufacture of thermometers (this is why I absolutely forbid my patients to chew on their thermometers!), electronic batteries, paints, some cosmetics, and pharmaceuticals such as mercurochrome.

Industrial mercury toxicity is attracting increasing attention in establishment circles, even though they are being suspiciously quiet about the real threat — the mercury we carry with us *wherever* we go. For instance, the National Academy of Science in 1981 reported on a study investigating mercury as an environmental pollutant. The report concluded:

> In view of the toxicity of mercury and the inability of researchers to specify the threshold levels of toxic effects on the basis of present knowledge, all such [mercury] contamination must be regarded as undesirable and potentially hazardous.[11]

The mercury issue is an environmental health problem that has been recognized by federal and state authorities. The Environmental Protection Agency and Food and Drug Administration have set limits for mercury products released into the air and water; its use in paints, pesticides, and pharmaceuticals has been limited.

Something Is Fishy

Guidelines have been set for allowable mercury levels in foods, especially fish. However, the way in which these guidelines are supervised leaves room for error. Fish are caught and samples analyzed, but the average level of mercury arrived at does not necessarily correspond to the level that might be found in an individual fish. For instance, in the case of swordfish, mercury levels can vary from fish to fish depending upon the size of the fish, or where it has been feeding. The larger the fish, the greater the concentration of mercury if that fish has been feeding in a polluted area. How many of you can remember the mercury scare of 1953? This classic example of mercury poisoning took place in Minamata, a Japanese fishing village. Inhabitants of the village ate fish contaminated by organic mercury that came from a chemical plant. The poisoning became known as Minamata disease. It caused widespread nervous system damage and death. Children born to those afflicted with the disease were almost invariably mentally retarded or deformed.[12]

When one of my patients' lab reports comes back with elevated levels of mercury in the blood or urine, the case is officially reported to the New York State Health Department, which thereupon proceeds to investigate every possible source of industrial mercury contamination — but not the possibility of contamination by way of the dentist's office. Yet virtually every one of the scores of patients I have reported on is a homemaker or white-collar worker whose only other possible mercury exposure might be staring at a thermometer.

The ADA's Safety Precautions

Does the American Dental Association have any concern for the danger of mercury? You bet it does — for the dentist. It has set strict guidelines for disposal of mercury in dental offices. The scrap mercury that is left over from amalgam filling is to be placed in a sealed container, because vapors can be released into the office. These ADA authorities recognize that mercury is quite a toxic substance and must be stored in a safe place. Why do they think a safe place is inside their patients' mouths?

The Issue Is for Real

I hope I have convinced you that those of us who are trying to raise your awareness of the importance of the mercury/dental amalgam problem are not just whistling Dixie. This issue is important because researchers have not been able to determine at what threshold levels mercury is a contaminant. Each body reacts differently. The search for mercury toxicity must become a routine practice in a doctor's office and the avoidance and removal of amalgam must become a routine practice in a dentist's office.

The American Dental Association Position

As a physician concerned with the welfare of the patient, not the doctor, I have had to take on the AMA on many occasions. I didn't think I'd ever have to take on the ADA — that's not my table. But look at the latest position statement on this subject made by ADA spokesman Richard Asa:

> Amalgams have been used for 160 years in this country and have been put in 100 million people. There is no legitimate credence to support adverse claims of the safety of amalgams. . . . A small segment of the population, estimated at less than 1 percent, may be allergic to mercury — but we must emphasize that allergies should not be confused with toxicity.[13]

In other words, your only concern must be with an *allergic* reaction; the fact that mercury is directly toxic is not relevant.

Now, isn't that just like a trade union protecting its membership? Doesn't it appear to you that they simply cannot admit their profession has been wrong on such a grand scale? Doesn't it remind you of another one of those stonewalling jobs we've become so familiar with lately? In view of the overwhelming evidence that the mercury is getting into our systems, it looks to me as if they're busy covering their assets.

10

HEADACHE
Prevention Is the Cure

W e have been and will be scrutinizing the differences between the existing medical practices and my proposed
Complementary Medicine in a variety of diseases, some of them
very serious. But to get the real flavor of the distinction between
the old and the new medicines, you may profit from analyzing their
widely differing approaches not to a disease but to a symptom. It
is a symptom so prevalent and so debilitating that it has achieved
disease status, and even has evoked the development of dozens of
clinics dedicated solely to its management. I'm speaking, of course,
of headache, a symptom known from firsthand experience to virtually all of you.

The Headache Clinic Phenomenon

In the old days (until a decade or so ago), headaches were treated
by the victim's self-prescribed use of aspirin or some slightly more
glorified painkiller. This was the man in the street obeying the
axiom "If it ain't broke, don't fix it, and when it does break, patch
it up." If the headache-patching came too often, or didn't provide
enough relief, the victim would see his family practitioner, who
would in turn handle it with better painkillers, with or without an
attempt to clarify the diagnosis.

So when a few forward-thinking hospitals introduced the idea of
establishing clinics devoted solely to the management of headache

patients, I thought: "What a wonderful idea! Now headache victims will have the advantage of being studied and treated by doctors who, through their experience, will know how to approach their problems." But, alas, that experience has, in my opinion, provided very little real advantage for their patient-clients.

The Reason for Their Shortcomings

All headache clinics to date have been constructed on the orthodox medical model, which has meant:

- overemphasis on anatomical diagnostic testing (CT scans, etc.)
- almost total refusal to seek the cause of headaches by pursuing dietary connections
- failure to seek the specific responses that make one individual different from another, using diagnostic pigeonholing instead
- emphasizing treatment with symptom-relieving pharmaceuticals, rather than prevention, in the large majority of cases
- considering relief of symptoms with medications, rather than absence of both symptoms and medications, to be a satisfactory end result

Who Am I to Criticize?

I am offering the above critique not as a rabble-rouser, intent on fomenting dissatisfaction with the establishment, but from the vantage point of a practicing physician who has treated more than a thousand patients complaining of frequent headaches, and has seen the headaches eradicated in over 90 percent of them — not by a drug, or even a vitamin combination that works therapeutically, but *by preventing them, after learning what causes them.*

The facts seem unmistakably clear. The proper treatment of headache lies in its prevention, and, with some notable exceptions that I will go into momentarily, prevention can almost always be achieved.

Types of Headache

Complementary Medicine seeks the *cause* of the imbalance that causes a headache. Of course, there are different kinds of headaches. There are headaches that are musculoskeletal in origin, headaches that are due to traction (pulling) on pain-sensitive structures, and headaches of the vascular, or throbbing, pulsating, variety. Each of these major categories has a distinctly different implication.

Muscle-Tension Headache

This one is said to be the most common variety, although in my experience I do not see it as often as the vascular headache. The key question one must ask is: Is there a throbbing nature to the pain? If the answer is "No," or "I'm not sure," then chances are the headache is of the muscle-contraction variety. Our center is one of the rare medical groups that have a chiropractor on staff who examines patients as part of the initial workup. Muscle headache patients benefit consistently from some musculoskeletal manipulation. Our acupuncturists may also help here, as may acupressure specialists. Machines producing healing wavelengths, such as ultrasound, diathermy, or the electro-acuscope, also provide useful therapies.

When headaches are chronic and recurring, the chances are greater that the discomfort is in fact caused by misalignments of the musculoskeletal structures and amenable to manipulative therapies. If health is balance, and disease is the absence of balance, that principle surely applies to our body's structure as much as its biochemistry.

Traction Headache, the Most Dangerous

Now, suppose something serious enough to distort the anatomy of the brain and its structures were going on. If that were to cause a headache, what would it be like? It would tend to be increasingly severe and relentless, and it would not go away with the usual remedies of diet or anatomic manipulation. The most feared headaches are caused by space-occupying lesions, such as hemorrhages or brain tumors, or by infections like meningitis. These headaches are due to pulling (traction) on pain-sensitive brain linings or to inflammation. The fear of "missing the diagnosis" leads to the almost routine ordering of sophisticated and expensive laboratory procedures such as brain CT scans whenever neurologists or headache clinics are consulted. I am reluctant to pass judgment on this practice, since it can be lifesaving, but when it turns out to have been unnecessary, as it usually does, it succeeds in raising the cost of medical care.

My plea here is to reserve such testing for severe headaches that don't go away after trying the simple, straightforward therapeutic approaches we will be explaining in this chapter.

Chronic Vascular Headache, a Diet-related Disorder

Now that you have been warned of the possibility that headache can be a serious symptom, let's move on to the happier subject of the garden varieties of throbbing headaches, or sick headaches, that we can, nine times out of ten, get rid of — if we're wise — not by a symptom-controlling drug therapy, but by prevention based on a heightened awareness of what causes them.

Vascular headaches have been classified and reclassified by headache "authorities" dozens of times. Classic migraine, common migraine, cluster headaches, histamine headaches, and many more have been described, each with certain unique features.

But at our center, we have found it more fruitful to consider all vascular headaches to be *toxic* headaches and have set about trying to isolate the toxic factors. Once these factors have been removed by diet control, or, if they cannot be entirely removed, have been mitigated by vitamin and nutritional supplements, the toxic headache is generally cured or controlled.

The Headache-Diet Connection, Orthodox Style

Since headache has been one of my pet concerns (the Atkins Center is planning to open a nutrition-based headache clinic), I have studied the medical literature and editorial comments of the leaders in the field in recent years. One cannot help being aware that in this area, too, there is an ongoing ideological struggle over the role of diet in headache.

Although the research of Ellen Grant, reporting in *Lancet* in 1979, clearly sounded the clarion call to tell the world that food intolerances were behind *most* migraine episodes,[1] the academicians simply weren't buying. Admitting some food-related headaches — induced, for example, by tyramine-containing foods such as cheese, by caffeine use and withdrawal, by chocolate, ice cream, and a smattering of other foods — they steadily defended the party line that most headaches were *not* diet-related. This left them free to devise some ingenious combinations of pharmaceutical agents that demonstrated a proven superiority to placebo when used by a group of headache victims. That is, a significant proportion of these patients showed *some* improvement on these drugs. That's a far cry from the nearly universal success proper dietary maneuvers have had in freeing people of headache.

Our Results

I've alluded to our total success in nine out of ten instances — as long as the diet is followed. You can imagine, then, quite correctly, that I might have hundreds of case histories to choose from. Most of them do not make interesting reading; they are simply people who complained of frequent throbbing headaches, who were put on the appropriate sugar-stabilizing, food-intolerance avoidance programs, and who returned after two or three weeks stating, "I don't get headaches anymore."

But let's follow a few examples in greater detail so that you may see how individualized the approach must be.

Roberta Stein

"You have to understand the miracle of this. Every day of my life I woke up with headaches. I had painkillers by my bedside so I could take them as I woke up. Before

*Atkins I was a drug addict and wound up going to a psy-
chiatrist. . . . Now I function, I think, I am clear-headed."*

Roberta Stein came to me after suffering with migraine since she
was fifteen years old. She had been seeing orthodox physicians,
who effectively turned her into a drug addict.

In addition to her migraine, she had stomach, esophageal, and
ulcer problems and wondered whether they were related to her
migraine, or her medications. She had already put herself on her
own form of low-carbohydrate diet about three weeks before she
came in for her first visit, and she had experienced a significant
decrease in the number and duration of attacks. So she was "pre-
sold"; she wanted to see what other treatments I could give her in
addition to the diet that seemed to be working.

In telling her story, Roberta told me first of all that her weight
had shot up from about 135 pounds to 157 pounds during the previous two years, which coincided with her having given up cigarettes. Over the three weeks of her diet she had started to lose
some of that extra weight.

During the years she had suffered migraines, Roberta had been
prescribed Demerol, Percodan (which coincided with the development of her ulcer), Valium, and morphine suppositories and injections. The heavy use of these narcotics brought on psychotic
episodes. One day while on narcotic medication, Roberta was driving, and she imagined — simply hallucinated — a car coming head
on toward her. She swerved to avoid the car that wasn't there and
wrecked her own car, injuring herself. After this she consulted a
psychiatrist, but after a number of sessions he recommended that
she continue on the painkillers, insisting that the pain, and not the
narcotics being administered in the attempt to kill the pain, was
bringing on the episodes.

The day of our consultation, Roberta was taking codeine, Per-
cocet, and Valium. In the recent past she had been given Cafergot
(a combination of ergotamine and caffeine typically given migraine
patients) and propranolol (a beta-blocker). The use of a beta-blocker
is an innovative pharmacologic approach; it inhibits the ability of
the brain to react to adrenaline and noradrenaline (in this instance,

the blood-vessel-dilating effect of adrenaline is one of the suspected instigators of migraine attacks).

None of these medications had any effect on Roberta's pain.

Roberta is an example of a patient who had visited one of the well-respected orthodox headache clinics, one of the first to be opened here in New York City. Though the clinic's doctors took some dietary and environmental factors into account — eventually banning chocolate and sugar from Roberta's diet — they did not deal with the idea of administering glucose for tolerance testing, and steadfastly refused to make other substantial changes in Roberta's dietary or nutritional routine. Instead, after a complete battery of other types of diagnostic testing, they began prescribing more painkillers. They did come up with the contribution that Roberta was lactose sensitive, and took away the six to eight cups of coffee and tea with milk she had been drinking each day.

Our screening lab tests showed she certainly was hypoglycemic, that she was mildly anemic, which we attributed to profuse menstrual bleeding, and that her serum calcium was low, which may have been related to the elimination of dairy products from her diet.

I immediately removed Roberta from all medication. I put her on a strictly low-carbohydrate diet, gave her instructions to take our standard vitamin formula plus two tryptophan tablets each night at bedtime, an additional 3 grams of vitamin C, and 500 milligrams of B_6.

A mere ten days later, Roberta came back to me, and said, "I feel fantastic. No headache. My energy is better. My sleep is better."

One can speculate as to why Roberta's headaches went away so quickly, but my experience suggests that it was the sugar-stabilizing effect of the low-carbohydrate diet, which can prove very helpful for the common type of headache that is caused by hypoglycemia. The same facts can be explained by the hypothesis that Roberta had undiagnosed allergies to some of the various carbohydrates that were eliminated by the new diet. Vitamin C, which has the capacity to block certain chemical transformations (nitrites to nitrosamines, for example) may also have contributed to our mutual success.

Over the next few months, she did have an occasional headache, which she described as very mild and nondebilitating, and she continued to lose weight. But over the long run, Roberta became a difficult case from a behavioral point of view. Periodically, she lost the will power to stay on her diet. When she deviated from her diet, her weight would increase and she experienced mild headache and ulcer symptoms. She then eventually would return to her diet and the symptoms would clear.

Roberta is a typical example of a patient whose single case history can teach a basic lesson. In this case, we learn that a low-carbohydrate diet can be all that is needed to correct recurring headaches. The fact that Roberta's headaches returned with virtually every diet deviation provided the replication that ruled out coincidence in her case. To be able to generalize, all that is needed is to see how often individual headache cases can be corrected by the same simple dietary maneuver that worked for Roberta.

Our next case illustrates a different point.

Margaret Dempsey

When Margaret Dempsey first came to me in August 1984 she told me she felt "terrible" most of the time, and that she was "not a nice person to be around." She was overweight, had a hard time sleeping, and was constantly anxious and cranky. I asked Margaret to describe her chief complaint, and she ended up describing what sounded to me like classic menstrual-related migraine. She said she had a severe PMS (premenstrual syndrome) cycle that lasted a good part of the month before, through, and immediately following menstruation (which severe PMS can do, in spite of the "pre" in premenstrual). These menstrual problems were usually accompanied by severe headaches, which she described as migraine, with nausea and cold sweats.

For the past five years, her physician had prescribed Elavil, Dalmane, and Librium, drugs with powerful psychoactive side effects. She told me that since taking the medications she had felt like "a total fruitcake."

The most significant finding in Margaret's battery of tests was that she was hypoglycemic. I put her on the standard low-carbohydrate diet. And most important, I concentrated on the nutritional supplements I find useful in treating premenstrual syndrome and menstrual-related migraine. This meant the basic multivitamin formula, plus extra B_6, folic acid, niacin, B_{12}, vitamin C, manganese, magnesium orotate, calcium, and tryptophan. To this regimen was added three times the usual dose of oil of evening primrose, the major dietary source of gamma-linolenic acid (GLA).

The very next month, September, Margaret reported that neither the severe premenstrual symptoms nor the migraines had occurred. And between her menstrual periods, there was no more anxiety or crankiness. She told me,

> *"I just felt like a new person — just, you know, just living in another body, but this one I should own! Before, I always felt depressed. Now, never! Before, I was a total fruitcake. Now I feel like a Cadillac!"*

What These Cases Reveal

I trust that you will go beyond the superficial impression that these are just two "anecdotes" about patients whose headaches are connected to either their diet or their menstrual cycle and that you will see these as examples drawn from a large tabular study of approximately a thousand headache patients. From reviewing the case records of that number of patients who complained of headache at the Atkins Center, it is clear that between 80 percent and 90 percent of them were considerably improved by our system of *prevention*. Our preventive precept is elementary: *Find out what causes the headaches and stop doing it.* The clues to causation most often lie in blood glucose dynamics or in the field of allergy/intolerance that complementarists call clinical ecology.

Prevention Versus Drug Therapy

Now, let us suppose that one of the better headache clinics were to publish its results on treatment of headache patients, using its system, and that it, too, could demonstrate that better than four out of five of its patients were "significantly improved." Which treatment protocol would you choose for yourself?

Let me help you answer that. The headache clinic, assuming it was proceeding along the path all the other orthodox clinics have embarked upon, would employ a drug or some combination of pharmaceuticals — some variation of the present theme of pain-killers, anti-inflammatory agents, beta-blockers, antidepressants, vasoconstrictors, muscle relaxants, antihistamines, or other agents that work by blocking some enzymatic pathway the body customarily takes. They work by relieving the symptoms, not by removing the cause.[2]

Most of these medications are powerful ones, and many are likely to cause side effects.* If the side effects are unpleasant ones, I'm sure most people would opt for the complementary *prevention* system, which causes no side effects except the not inconsequential problem of not being able to eat what you used to eat and still love.

But suppose that the proposed medicine combination has no side effects. Imagine that you are like some of those wonderful smiling people in the TV commercials who merely pop a pill and beam: "No more headache!" What's wrong with your continuing with the medication?

This Is a Sticking Point

Here is where I have had to talk myself blue in the face to convince thousands of my patients (not just headache sufferers, but almost everyone) that there is something better than feeling fine "on your medicines." I have a strong personal conviction of the truth of the axiom "*A person without symptoms and without medications is far healthier than a person without symptoms who takes medications.*"

To me that is self-evident; but it is not so to many of my patients. Drug-taking, even when no unpleasant symptoms are produced, still means exposure to risk. Oftentimes the harmful effects of drugs are insidious, and oftentimes they are so delayed that the cause-

---

*The term *side effects* is really a misnomer. Most effects of a drug are as much a part of the drug's action as the specific effect that affords the symptomatic relief to the patient. They, too, are direct effects of the drug's enzyme-blocking action; they are not incidental. The correct term for side effects should be *unwanted direct effects*.

and-effect relationship to subsequent illness is missed. No one, not even the doctor who prescribes the drug, can say with certainty that some later illness — let's say a bone marrow deficiency, an autoimmune disorder, or cancer, or just plain lowered resistance — was not, in some small way, caused by some enzymatic blocking agent administered a decade or two before.

So, I'll ask you again: Which treatment sounds better to you, prevention or drug therapy? You may be surprised, but the answer I would like is "Perhaps one, perhaps the other." Even a 90 percent success rate is no consolation for the one person in ten who doesn't get better. Whereas I obviously believe that all people who can "cure" their headaches by never getting them in the first place should do just that, there will be some for whom only pharmaceutical intervention will work. For them, the brilliant discoveries of establishment medicine may provide the difference between suffering and sanity.

Treating Headache at the Atkins Center

Two cases cannot begin to show you the approach we use at the Atkins Center. It might serve better to describe our protocol. As I explained, we emphasize prevention based on finding the cause and then avoiding it. This means we must do a lot of detective work, as well as some educated trial and error. Even those who follow the peer-reviewed (orthodox) medical journals have been exposed to what I feel are the two main connections between vascular headache and diet: low (or unstable) blood sugar and individual food intolerances. For this reason our protocol almost always involves a glucose tolerance test plus a cytotoxic test.

Both Roberta and Margaret, along with about two of every three of my vascular headache patients, demonstrated hypoglycemia on their GTT. The appropriate low-carbohydrate diet will, just by itself, correct a majority of headache patients' problems. When that simple strategy does not work, a search for individual food intolerances will work just as often as it did for Ellen Grant's patients in London. For us the best and quickest instrument for detecting which foods are the culprits for which people is the cytotoxic test.

More detective work, if needed, would involve rethinking the possibility of musculoskeletal imbalance (of the type we seek in muscle-contraction headaches) or in looking for environmental chemical toxicity or allergies. If we don't identify a cause by our testing, we continue our causation approach through educated trial and error. This means avoiding the suspected environmental factor to see if the headaches disappear and/or reintroducing it to see if the headaches come back.

One Study

I might mention that I have seen hopeful signs that orthodoxy will soon have to consider food intolerances as a headache source. The prestigious medical journal *Lancet* published a very interesting study in October 1983, prepared by J. Egger and four other physicians at the Hospital for Sick Children in London.[3] Using eighty-eight children with a mean age of just under ten years, all of whom had had migraine headaches at least once a week for the previous six months, Egger began to adjust their diets to see if food allergies could be responsible.

The British doctors put each child on a diet of one meat, one carbohydrate, one fruit, one vegetable, and vitamin supplements for three to four weeks. If a child improved, other foods were re-introduced one by one; if not, a new diet was tried. The result: 93 percent of the eighty-eight children became headache-free once their food allergies were discovered and the foods were taken out of their diet. Most of the children had had reactions to several foods, seventeen had been affected by only one food, and one child had reacted to twenty-four foods and was symptom-free when all those were withdrawn. Cow's milk, eggs, wheat, chocolate, and oranges were all foods to which more than twenty of the children responded. Interestingly enough, sugar affected only two. I attribute that to the fact that sugar wreaks its havoc through another mechanism, namely glucose and insulin dynamics.

Egger and his associates next took forty of the children *and did a double-blind study of their food reactions,* using a savory- or sweet-base placebo with the control group. The results were exactly the same as those in the first, uncontrolled study.

The doctors were, let's hope, delighted. We know they were astonished, because, as they admit in their article, they had undertaken the study with the intention of proving, once and for all, that the dietary hypothesis was a false one. Instead — under the unblinking scrutiny of a double-blind study — they provided the finest experimental demonstration of the correctness of Complementary Medicine's theory of headache causation that I know of.

Of equal interest in Egger's study was the fact that other problems common in this age group were both found and corrected by change of diet, including abdominal pain, behavior disorder, epileptic fits, asthma, and eczema.

Beyond Causation, What?

Complementarists have a nutritional pharmacology that is safer than the usual drug therapies.

Several nutrients are effective in rendering toxic headaches less toxic. For example, vitamin C is a great protector. We have mentioned the protection it affords against headaches based on nitrates. It also acts as an antihistamine, and this may be particularly valuable in chronic cluster headaches. The fact is, we don't even know a fraction of the mechanisms whereby vitamin C, one of our major protectant vitamins, does its job. To evaluate the benefit of a nutrient such as this, it is grossly inappropriate to predict its effects from what is known of its mechanisms; it is far better to be empirical and observe the results it provides.

I can't help, at this point, recalling a radio debate I had one morning with Dr. Gabe Mirkin, one of the outspoken adversaries of the clinical nutrition movement. I suddenly became aware of the common error in logic he consistently demonstrated as he carried mechanistic thinking to an absurdity.

Mechanistic sophistry runs something like this: "We all know that vitamin C works by means of mechanism X. That mechanism plays no part in condition Y. Therefore, vitamin C could not possibly work in this situation." Shocked as I am at such a bypass of logic, I realize that this blend of erudition and ignorance takes place far too often among advocates of the mainstream position.

What Else Works?

Bottom-line thinkers have noticed that toxic headaches can be prevented or ameliorated with bioflavonoids, of which I have found the most effective one to be quercetin. I find pantothenic acid, and especially a derivative called pantethine, to help in the prevention. Then I employ the entire spectrum of antioxidant nutrients (vitamin E, selenium, cysteine, glutathione, and others — see page 218 for a discussion of antioxidants).

I have discovered two ways of avoiding my now infamous Chinese restaurant headache: (a) before eating, take 2 quercetin, 3 pantethine, ½ teaspoon of vitamin C, and 2 antioxidant tablets, or (b) order Mexican food.

Sometimes we help a migraine patient by prescribing tryptophan. The rationale here is that many migraine patients become serotonin-depleted; tryptophan quickly restores this neurotransmitter. At other times the answer lies in providing GLA, especially if the headache is part of the premenstrual time frame, as it was in Margaret's case. Just as often, the answer is in providing the omega-3 fatty acids, and the choice then becomes EPA. A study by Dr. Charles Glueck of the University of Cincinnati College of Medicine demonstrated that taking 15 grams of a commercial fish oil preparation containing EPA each day lessened the frequency of headaches by more than half.[4]

Or, and here is an example of how the complementarist has more resources than one who is simply a nutritionist, one may prescribe herbal preparations. Most of my successful herbal experience centers around the herb feverfew, whose success has even been documented by a double-blind study of E. S. Johnson's appearing in the *British Medical Journal*.[5] I think you can see from this that headache control provides support for one of the most basic principles of Complementary Medicine: *All healing arts can and should be made to complement one another*.

Complementary Medicine must, therefore, have a knowledge base that gives mastery of all of the aforementioned techniques. It will still stand apart from the drug-oriented system of its orthodox predecessor. Nutrition techniques come first. Pharmaceuticals are a last resort; and in headache control, they are rarely necessary.

11

. . .

FEMALE PROBLEMS
The Nutritional Approach

I f you are interested in studying the differences between ortho-dox medicine, alternative medicine, and their sophisticated offspring, Complementary Medicine, you may well be fascinated when you use as an example the field of gynecology (women's disorders).

Like all other specialties, gynecology has a surgical side and a medical side. Uniquely, more than any other specialty, the medical side depends on a knowledge of endocrinology. In other words, it is more related to the delicate glandular balances that control a woman's reproductive cycle as she changes day to day, month after month, and as she blossoms into full womanhood and subsequently loses her reproductive capacity. Because her hormones, her estrogen, progesterone, luteinizing hormones, lactating hormones, and adrenal and pituitary factors are all substances normally present in the body, the gynecologist is, even by his orthodox medical training, a practitioner of orthomolecular medicine, since he treats by regulating the concentrations of these substances. It is no wonder, then, that the nutritional principles that affect these hormone levels are being discussed by orthodox practitioners, and they are not being rejected. Dr. Neils Lauersen, author of *Premenstrual Syndrome and You*,[1] recommends B_6, magnesium, and GLA and yet remains a respected member of his hospital staff. Gynecology may well be the only specialty in which such a seeming paradox exists.

But there's a dark side to gynecology, too. When a doctor is trained to be a gynecologist, he is actually trained to be a gynecological surgeon. And there may well be the rub. When you go to your gynecologist for an opinion, you may fail at first to recognize that he is wearing two hats — one is that of a consultant (who makes recommendations) and the other is that of a surgeon (who performs operations). When, in the role of consultant, he outlines your plan of therapy, he plans it sincerely to the best of his training and ability. The problem is that when surgery looms as a possibility, one answer he gives is worth seventy-five dollars to him (or whatever he gets for that office visit) but the other is worth five thousand dollars (or whatever he gets for doing the surgery). If his medical belief system is geared toward justifying the incorporation of surgery into the game plan, it goes a long way toward helping him overcome his rather staggering economic commitments. (In New York State, for example, he may be paying sixty-five thousand dollars a year in malpractice insurance alone.)

In 1984, according to the National Center for Health Statistics, 664,000 women in this country underwent hysterectomies (removal of the uterus and usually the cervix), and 498,000 underwent oophorectomies (removal of the ovaries). Nora Coffey of the HERS Foundation (Bala-Cynwyd, Pennsylvania) notes that the real number is even higher, because not all hospitals are included in the statistics.[2] In a speech before the Women and Cancer Conference (October 1985, New York City), Coffey stated that "sixty-six percent of these operations were performed for suspected cancer; yet cancer of the cervix or uterine cancer occurred in only four percent of these women." As far back as 1971, a New York State study reviewing unnecessary surgery concluded that 43 percent of the hysterectomies performed were not justified.[3]

Contrast the American experience with that in England, where the technique for paying the physician is done on a per capita fee basis. The patient pays the same amount of money whether or not she gets sick and sees the physician. Thus, the most profitable patient for an English physician is one who enrolls in the program but remains well and never visits the doctor. The result? English gynecologists perform only one-third as many hysterectomies as their American colleagues. Yet both read the same journals and have access to the same information.

Complementary Medicine's Approach

If orthodox medicine, with its emphasis on organ removal, does not have all the answers, then what about alternative medicine? Unfortunately, present-day alternativists, who offer acupuncture, herbal preparations, homeopathy, manipulations, and the like, can help only a modest segment of the gynecologically troubled population. What is needed is an approach that deals with the cause of most of a woman's disorders — the gradual unbalancing of her glandular system — and specifically, a *nutritional* method for rebalancing the endocrine system.

Nonetheless, even within Complementary Medicine, orthodox gynecology for a long time remained the primary treatment mode for most women. The alternatives couldn't deal specifically enough with the delicate balance between estrogens, progesterones, luteinizing factors, and the like. Not, that is, until the pioneering contributions of Carlton Fredericks, Ph.D., who was until his recent death the acknowledged patriarch of clinical nutrition.

Fredericks's contribution was this: He devised *nutritional* protocols for overestrogenized women and for those with low-estrogen conditions. Now one could modify the hormonal equilibrium for women who were out of balance without prescribing hormones! Add to this the pioneering work of Dr. David Horrobin, who demonstrated the importance of prostaglandin E_1 (and thus the need for GLA) in restoring a woman's hormonal balance, and once again nutrition becomes the crown jewel in a new Complementary Medicine.

Now let's look at some specific examples of the way we at the Atkins Center apply these principles in the most common women's disorders we treat.

First of all, we have been able to identify three basic protocols, or treatment plans — an estrogen-elevating system, an estrogen-converting (lowering) system, and a balancing system based on GLA. There remains to be discovered a fourth protocol, one that would stimulate the development of an increased level of progestational hormones, but one for which we have not yet found a nutritional system of intervention.* The table shows where they apply.

* It has been suggested in a study by R. S. London ("The Effect of Alpha-Tocopherol on Premenstrual Symptomatology: A Double-Blind Study," *Journal of the American College*

Three Treatment Systems and the Disorders to Which They Apply

Estrogen-Increasing Protocol	Estrogen-Converting (Estrogen-Decreasing) Protocol
menopause (some symptoms)	uterine fibroids
secondary amenorrhea (loss of menstrual periods)	endometriosis
	fibrocystic breast disease
primary amenorrhea (never had menstrual periods)	breast cancer
	menorrhagia (excessive menstrual bleeding — some types)
loss of libido	
atrophic vaginitis	
infertility (some types)	
osteoporosis	
cervical dysplasia	

GLA (Balancing) Protocol
premenstrual syndrome (PMS)
ovarian cysts (some types)

From the time Dr. Fredericks joined us at the Atkins Center as our director of Nutrition Services, we had ample opportunity to put his theories to the test. We were concerned not only with whether these nutritional concepts could affect women's health dilemmas but how consistently and to what extent. Since I was at first skeptical of the ability of nutrition alone to modify an endocrine imbalance, I was rather pleasantly surprised to learn that the majority of our patients experienced clinical improvements similar to the case histories I am about to describe. Here are a few typical examples of how a nutrition-based Complementary Medicine has affected the lives of patients.

---

of Nutrition 3 [1984], pp. 351–56) that giving vitamin E in a dose of 150 IU (international units), not more or less, does have the effect of increasing progesterone levels. If this is borne out by future studies, it will be one of the few examples of a "therapeutic window" in nutrition. The term applies to an effective dosage range limited by both upper and lower borders.

Virginia Russell

"All of a sudden I was told I had a fibroid. . . . The doctor suggested Provera, and if that didn't work, then surgery — a D and C [dilatation and curettage] — and possibly a hysterectomy in the future."

Virginia, a nurse on a gynecology floor at a large metropolitan hospital, knew enough to recognize that a change in her menstrual pattern needed investigation, and she knew who the "best" gynecologists were. So when her periods began to come closer together, to the point that they came twice a month, she saw her gynecologist, who found nothing and told her to come back in a few more months. She did, and this time, November 1984, he found she had a fibroid tumor the size of an orange.

Fibroids are benign tumors in the muscular wall of the uterus. They are common and are only rarely precancerous. Their main threat is increased menstrual bleeding, thereby causing a chronic iron-loss anemia. For many women, a fibroid growth in the middle years is a normal occurrence. Many women are not made aware of the fact that fibroids usually stop growing and may even regress as one enters menopause.

Virginia was visibly shaken and upset with the course of treatment prescribed for her.

"I was in shock. . . . I don't smoke, I don't drink, I ate good foods."

The doctor sent her home with Provera.

"Being a nurse, I pay attention to labels. I knew already it was a dangerous drug; after looking it up I was shaking. I felt going on a hormone does not solve a problem, it masks the problem and could make it worse. Even though I'm a nurse and I tell people to take drugs, I feel patients have the right to question why they are taking the drugs, they have the right to know."

Virginia told the gynecologist that she had decided not to take the Provera. Years before, Virginia had been introduced to homeopathy, so she knew she had other choices. The doctor did not argue with her and said, "Fine, if that's what you want to do."

Virginia came to see me in December 1984. In addition to the fibroid in question she had other problems. For instance, she was very overweight and had a history of many efforts at weight loss and regaining. I placed her on a very-low-carbohydrate diet, as well as the estrogen-converting fibroid protocol. Most fibroids are associated with estrogenic overactivity. In addition, Virginia received our Antioxidant Formula, extra vitamin C, and bioflavonoids, zinc, vitamin E, and oil of evening primrose.

Dr. Fredericks's estrogen-converting method employs a group of nutritional compounds called lipotropic factors. The major lipotropes are choline, inositol, and methionine. We placed Virginia on 1500 milligrams of each daily.

Virginia began to lose weight. In April of 1985 she was tested for the presence of candida because of bloating and because of the frequency with which candidiasis occurs in fibroid patients. The tests showed that her immunoglobulin levels to candida were elevated, and she was placed on a candida protocol consisting of acidophilus, caprylic acid, the herb pau d'arco, and a homeopathic candida preparation. She was also tested for food intolerances and as a result she had to further restrict her intake of certain whole grain foods.

Virginia continued to lose weight, and in May of 1985 she returned to her gynecologist for another examination. At this time, the doctor told her the fibroid had shrunk to the size of a smaller orange.

> "I was so excited, I jumped off the exam table and said, 'Don't you realize what we're doing, we're doing this without drugs.'"

Her doctor acknowledged that he was happy for her but showed no interest in the protocol we were using at the Atkins Center.

Three months later she again returned to her doctor. This time she was free of the tumor! There was no sign of the fibroid!

When Virginia reported this last encounter with her gynecologist to me, I was fascinated to hear of his lack of interest in learning how it was done. After all, fibroids aren't supposed to shrink away to nothing; if they did, how could one justify all those hysterectomies?

Virginia's enthusiasm was not dampened. She kept bringing up the subject of this new system for shrinking fibroids to her colleagues, but no one seemed to be interested in it. Those who did comment pointed to the fact that it took her a whole year to get rid of the fibroid and "look at the expense."

I must admit I am not surprised at the responses Virginia got from her gynecology ward co-workers. The belief system that surgery is appropriate permeates the entire profession, and the nursing staff is no exception.

Rhonda Eisman

"I was beside myself. I had pain in the lower abdominal area, pain in the pelvic area, and pains in my back. My gynecologist, internist, and surgeon found nothing wrong, but the pain would not go away."

In September 1984, it was this pain that sent Rhonda to the hospital, where she was diagnosed as having endometriosis.

Endometriosis is a condition in which uterine lining tissue (endometrium) occurs in abnormal locations in the abdomen, especially the pelvic area. The endometrial tissue is very sensitive to the presence of estrogen. Many studies have shown that endometrial tissue has the capacity to turn cancerous with high levels of estrogen. Endometriosis can cause severe pain and sometimes hemorrhage. Oophorectomies and/or medical treatment with danazol (a drug that suppresses estrogen levels) are considered the most effective treatment in the orthodox world.[4]

Rhonda went through surgery to remove an endometrial cyst on her right ovary. But she continued to have pain after the operation. Her gynecologist told her, quite surprisingly, that the problem was not gynecological. Two more doctors and three different types of drugs later, Rhonda's pains continued, beginning on her ovulation day and lasting for two agonizing weeks every month.

When I saw Rhonda in August 1985, I placed her on a low-carbohydrate diet (she was a little overweight and her GTT showed a hypoglycemic response). We used an estrogen-lowering protocol similar to the one Virginia was treated with. That means she got choline, methionine, inositol, primrose oil, and vitamin E, to which we added the Antioxidant Formula, vitamin C, bioflavonoids, and — based on information gleaned from her hair analysis — zinc, manganese, and chromium.

After just over three months, it was Rhonda's day for a return visit. "I feel better in so many ways, but I'm a little confused," Rhonda told me. "My pain usually starts at midcycle and from then on it's 'crunch time' until my period comes, and this month nothing is happening."

"Did you ever consider that you might be getting better?"

Well, Rhonda's pain finally did come, and it lasted just one day. Her next three cycles were nearly painless.

Rhonda adds:

> "I'm doing well on the low-carbohydrate diet; I seem to react poorly to carbohydrates. It's incredible. I have no pain from the endometriosis, my personality has changed, and my husband says I'm back to the old me again. At one point I was depressed and feeling sorry for myself. People would say 'Enough, already.' I'm taking everything that is natural and my body is working for me. My husband cannot understand why most physicians are so ready to use drugs. There are alternatives, and I hope other women can realize this."

Please bear in mind that endometriosis usually causes more and more suffering until the distraught patient ends up on the operating table, where she may or may not get complete relief from suffering. Our records, as of mid-1987, indicated that we had used the de-estrogenizing protocol on about fifty patients with a variety of conditions as listed in the table earlier in the chapter. The results were good enough (62 percent clearly improved, 16 percent subjectively felt better, 22 percent no better) that we could begin to entertain the notion that we had an effective nutritional intervention.

I was curious enough to order a search of the medical literature for further supportive evidence. Nothing! Zip! Not a word! Then I called on Dr. Fredericks, whose protocol this was anyway, and who had been using this system for forty years.

"What's the scientific basis of your de-estrogenizing protocol with methyl donors?" I asked, the latter term referring to the use of choline, methionine, and inositol.

"I don't know for sure," he replied. "The impetus was a series of studies in the thirties and forties indicating that the liver is the essential organ necessary to convert the most active form of estrogen, estradiol, to the much less active form, estriol. It doesn't seem to deal with the process of methylation. But choline, inositol, and methionine were, and still are, the best nutritional agents I know of for supporting liver function."

Well, there you have it from the man who, until his recent passing, was the nutritional Chairman of the Board. If there are any gynecological researchers in my audience, take this information with my blessing. I think it will make a good scientific paper. Meanwhile, as an empirical physician, I am going to continue to use this protocol — and try to improve upon it. From an orthodox point of view it may be unproven, but it has helped a lot of women and hasn't hurt anybody yet.

Case-Study Analysis

In dealing with hormonal problems, the orthodox gynecologist has many tools to work with. He can prescribe estrogen, he can administer progesterone, he can use estrogen-lowering drugs, and he can use other hormones that indirectly affect the woman's glandular balance.

The nutritionist has the advantage that when he does something nutritionally he is not risking side effects. He has the disadvantage that his nutritional precursors cannot always create every specific hormonal variant that he desires.

An example of this nutritional nonspecificity is that he can provide the nutritional precursor for estrogenic hormones by providing its basic structure, the sterol ring (which derives from the much-maligned cholesterol). But the sterol ring also happens to be the building block for progestational hormones, adrenal substances, and male hormones. All of this may not be what the doctor ordered, so he must take another tack. As you have seen, the ability to deactivate estrogen provides the nutritionist ample opportunities to help. And his ability to enhance estrogen provides even more.

Estrogen Pros and Cons

In the days when I treated only overweight patients and patients with blood sugar problems, I developed an antipathy for estrogen which had nothing whatever to do with its role in causing an increase in the incidence of some types of cancer. My major concern over many years has been the disastrous effects that estrogen treatment has had on blood sugar levels. I have taken at least six hundred female patients off estrogen therapy, which is a common mode of treatment for menopausal problems (about which, more later), because of the disabling symptoms mediated through low blood sugar. Estrogen therapy can have the following effects on blood sugar levels:

- convert low blood sugar into lower blood sugar levels
- convert asymptomatic hypoglycemia into a symptomatic hypoglycemia
- cause even higher blood sugar levels in the diabetic

In other words, it aggravates our already excessive insulin response to our diet's carbohydrates. Orthodox gynecological medicine, which promotes the use of estrogen preparations, has challenged this viewpoint. It is neither proven nor disproven, and the risk-versus-benefit ratio of estrogen therapy still remains a hotly debated question.

One reason for the uncertainty about estrogen's effect on blood sugar is that it lowers blood sugar in some women and raises it in others; these effects then tend to cancel each other out in a mathematical analysis that lumps everything together. This is one of the weaknesses of present-day medicine — lumping diverse individuals into a single, mathematically analyzed group and drawing conclusions about the group, not about the individuals within it. Furthermore, much of the research usually relied on was done over too short a period of time. It can take up to two years for significant changes in blood sugar to take place.

I was not happy about the use of estrogen therapy, although it is still valuable in the treatment and prevention of osteoporosis. When osteoporosis is a woman's major problem and low blood sugar is not a problem, then estrogen administration may be appropriate. However, when blood sugar problems are the focus, the physician has some difficult decisions to make. That is why I was compelled to find an alternative treatment for osteoporosis and other conditions associated with menopause. I studied the biochemistry of estrogen and was struck with the fact that one of the vitamins of the B complex, folic acid (folate), increases estrogen response. This was also found to be true of PABA, which is part of the molecule of folic acid and which Carlton Fredericks noted was "probably the active entity in the interplay of that vitamin with estrogen."[5]

Armed with the knowledge that in treating other conditions some physicians have been using folic acid in higher doses than the U.S. government would allow (Kurt Oster was using 60 milligrams for heart patients and reported no problems),* we began using higher doses in women with certain menopausal complaints. At the Atkins Center, we have used the high-folate protocol hundreds of times. It seems to provide an estrogen-like effect without the estrogen risks. Before I continue with a more detailed discussion of menopause, estrogen therapy, and especially osteoporosis, allow me to select one case hisory to show you how folic acid can work as an estrogen substitute.

Bessie Turner

Bessie Turner is a fifty-two-year-old energetic woman who works part time and is very involved in community work. When I first

---

*For reasons that I have always asserted were flimsy at best — and at worst, a deliberate attempt to weaken vitamin therapy — the U.S. government limits the dosage of folic acid in a nonprescription pill to 0.8 milligrams. Meanwhile, the Canadian government freely allows the sale of the 25-milligram form over the counter.

met with Bessie, she complained of menstrual cycle problems. Her periods were getting "fewer and far between." Her menstrual cycle had been irregular for the last two years, and her period had stopped six months prior to our meeting. She had begun having hot flashes at that time, at first a few but then more frequently, and she was experiencing violent mood swings.

> *"The hot flashes began to drive me crazy. Normally, I'm a very nice person, and my husband didn't know what to do with me."*

She also felt depressed and irritable.

I placed Bessie on a low-carbohydrate diet after results of a GTT showed her to be a reactive hypoglycemic. In addition, I placed her on the following supplements: 800 IU (international units) of vitamin E, 2 grams of vitamin C, 1500 milligrams of PABA, 6 capsules of ginseng, 3 cups of tea made with dong quai, and an herbal preparation called Ovatone. I also wrote prescriptions for 20-milligram tablets of Megafolic (one of the formulas we use at the center), which when taken three times daily would provide 60 milligrams of folic acid, and for 600 milligrams of vitamin C.

After the first month on the diet and nutritional regimen, Bessie was feeling better and had lost weight. "I'm down to a size fourteen now," she related. After the second month, there was further improvement and weight loss. However, after the third month, Bessie panicked. She called to tell me she had menstrual bleeding.

"Well, when you go to the fountain of youth, you have to expect all the disadvantages of youth," I said. Bessie responded, "Come on, I haven't had a period for nine months." I told her to wait till next month to see what happened. She reported getting a more normal period the following month, but the flashes were gone. The monthly periods are not permanent and eventually Bessie will go through menopause.

An interesting phenomenon took place in the midst of Bessie's treatment program. Her hot flashes returned. I stopped the folic acid and the flashes went away. A few months later the flashes came back. I resumed folic acid treatment and the flashes went away. I can only speculate on what happens; apparently, the system has to stay in balance, and when folic acid is taken too long the return of the flashing can be the result of an imbalance in either direction. I have seen this phenomenon a few times. What I've seen most often is an improvement, with the flashing subsiding when folic acid is administered. There is also improvement in the dry, atrophic vaginal mucosa typical in menopause, and many women show a renewed manifestation of their sex drive.

I am amazed at the paucity of research confirming this rather evident use of folic acid as an estrogen substitute. Only in the matter of cervical dysplasia (a precancerous change) in women on oral contraceptives has the effect of folate been reported upon, and here a 10-milligram dose was extremely effective.[6] I am confident that the next decade will witness a considerable number of studies proving the value of folic acid for estrogen replacement.

Menopause and Its Symptoms

A woman is considered to be in menopause when she is amenorrheic (she doesn't get her menstrual period) for more than a year after age forty. Statistics have shown that 50 percent of the female population are in menopause by the time they reach age fifty. Some signs and symptoms usually associated with menopause, such as hot flashes, osteoporosis, and painful intercourse, have been related to estrogen deficiency. The most common medical practice is to use estrogen therapy to treat these symptoms. But menopause may bring with it other symptoms, such as headaches, mood swings (especially depression), irritability, cravings, insomnia, and cardiovascular problems. These symptoms are probably not directly related to a deficiency in estrogen, but rather are really hypoglycemic reactions aggravated by the endocrine imbalance created by the cessation of ovulation, which is central to menopause. This means that the dietary/nutritional program I described for low blood sugar (chapter 7) should work in those cases. And it does.

How Does Osteoporosis Connect Here?

I agree with the prevailing opinion that osteoporosis is closely associated with menopause, based on the significant fact that bone loss begins to occur within the first three years of menopause. Osteoporosis is an extremely common condition and seems to progress with age in women (in whom it is *nearly universal*), as well as in men. It is characterized by bone loss associated with a reduction in bone density. This results in a shortening of stature, due to a forward curvature of the spine, and an increased susceptibility to fractures.

It is still not fully known why osteoporosis develops. Most of the research of the last twenty years provides strong evidence that both estrogen deficiency and lack of dietary calcium are contributing causes.

The real brouhaha is over whether or not postmenopausal women should be given estrogen-replacement therapy to prevent or reverse this disabling bone condition. This is a typical unsettled medical controversy that has attracted highly vocal proponents and equally vociferous critics. And the rift extends through alternativists as well. The reason for the controversy is that estrogen's success has been equivocal and its side reactions tend to affect systems the gynecologist or bone physiologist is not likely to look at. Because of its relationship to calcium absorption, estrogen has been reported to be effective in slowing the rate of bone loss in postmenopausal women. At the same time, other studies have failed to demonstrate that it could prevent fractures.[7] Estrogen proponents point to research that clearly suggests that the body makes more efficient use of dietary calcium when estrogen is present.

Is There Another Approach?

At the same time the defenders of estrogen therapy have been espousing their cause, the complementary physicians have been looking into the nutritional, dietary, and herbal aspects of osteoporosis. The complementarian recognizes that there are ways to avoid osteoporosis without resorting to estrogen drugs.

Calcium, being an element, cannot be made in the body and must be obtained from dietary sources. Calcium requires vitamin D in order to be absorbed into the blood. Vitamin D must be provided through the diet or by exposure to sunlight. Other important minerals in bone are phosphorus, magnesium, and, to a lesser extent, silicon. Calcium and phosphorus have an inverse relationship in the body. Too much phosphorus can actually lower calcium levels and cause eventual bone loss. Unfortunately, high levels of phosphorus are found in many refined and processed foods. Phosphorus, in fact, is one essential nutrient that the astute nutritionist has to de-emphasize. Ninety-five percent of us take in too much phosphorus and should look for ways to reduce our phosphorus intake.

The key to treating osteoporosis may not be calcium, but rather the mineral magnesium. Despite the fact that calcium and magnesium are competitors at a cellular level (most heart patients are learning of the importance of having magnesium dominate calcium to stabilize heart rhythm and protect against coronary vessel spasm), they bear quite a different relationship to each other where blood and bone concentrations are concerned. In the blood, calcium and magnesium fluctuate together; that is, a higher level of one will bring about an increase in the other. In this instance, magnesium can be used to raise calcium levels more efficiently than can calcium by itself. Accordingly, the Osteoporosis Formula for nutritional supplementation at the Atkins Center provides almost as much magnesium as calcium. It also provides vitamin D,[8] vitamin A, silica, zinc, and chondroitin sulfate; and for reasons discussed above, it certainly contains folic acid.*

Is Estrogen for Everyone?

One lesson I want to get across is the concept that, among women, two basic metabolic types can be discerned. One tends to be thin, relatively underdeveloped. This is the low-estrogen type. Such women respond well to estrogen therapy and may even do well on estrogen after their menopause. Of course, they also do well on folic acid.

But the other type — typified by women who physically may be overly developed and tending toward overweight (particularly in

---

*Folic acid may also work by converting the toxic intermediate homocysteine into methionine, which it does effectively. (L. E. Brattstrom, "Folic Acid Responsive Postmenopausal Homocysteinemia," *Metabolism* 34 [1985], p. 10737.) Homocysteine is known to contribute to osteoporosis.

the upper body), who often have high levels of triglycerides and insulin, and who tend toward blood sugar disorders — represents an already overly estrogenized type. All these tendencies are aggravated by estrogen. These are the women for whom estrogen should probably not be prescribed. For them, the Megafolic approach may prove to be a better solution if estrogen therapy seems necessary.

In each case, using folic acid provides the doctor and the patient with a technique for accomplishing what estrogen therapy hopes to do, without subjecting the woman to the adverse effects of estrogen. These effects are such that I advise discontinuing estrogen for many women, especially patients known to have (or who show a possibility of having) any of the following problems:

> cardiovascular disease
> diabetes
> hypertension
> high triglycerides
> high cholesterol
> tendency to weight gain
> candidiasis
> stroke
> unwillingness to stop smoking (the cardiovascular effects are
>   multiplied)
> fluid retention
> liver disease
> breast cancer
> fibrocystic breast disease
> thrombophlebitis
> thromboembolism
> unexplained vaginal bleeding
> unexplained menstrual disorders
> uterine fibroids
> endometriosis
> gallbladder disease

I also recommend against estrogen if a woman suffers any of the hypoglycemia-related symptoms and disorders:

fatigue
mood swing — depression, anxiety
irritability
panic attacks
cravings
seizure disorder
headaches
schizophrenia, confusion, or other mental disorder
palpitations (mitral valve prolapse)
bloating
multiple sclerosis
peptic ulcer
irritable bowel syndrome

Is it any wonder, then, that I hardly ever prescribe its use?

There are still women who have none of the above problems and who, because of hot flashes, painful intercourse due to atrophic vaginitis, osteoporosis, previous surgery, or symptoms already shown to be relieved by estrogen, should be prescribed estrogen. In those cases, I prescribe it in conjunction with folic acid, PABA, zinc, and vitamin E, so that I can prescribe the lowest possible dose. Its safety factor seems to be enhanced by using it along with a progesterone-like hormone. Dr. Penny Wise Budoff, in her book *No More Menstrual Cramps & Other Good News*,[9] provides the lay reader with a convincing argument why estrogen is much safer when progesterone is added to it.

But don't think that Complementary Medicine's contribution to womanhood is limited to raising or lowering estrogen activity. The most prevalent women's complaint of all depends on a different nutritional system, and it can be corrected virtually at will! I'm talking about premenstrual syndrome (PMS), a condition that affects from 20 to 60 percent of all menstruating women, according to whose statistics you read.

What Is Premenstrual Syndrome?

As the name implies, PMS is a very disabling cluster of symptoms that a woman notices every month at the same time, before the onset of her menstrual flow. It usually begins from two to ten days before the onset of menses. Common symptoms often associated with PMS are irritability, breast soreness, edema (water retention), weight gain, sugar craving, headaches, depression, and tiredness.

PMS is another one of those prevalent conditions that encourage the development of specialty clinics devoted entirely to the one subject. (Headache is another good example.) The fact that there are PMS clinics opening up all over the country implies that there are at least some doctors who feel that the condition is quite treatable. Contrast this with a statement made recently by a medical writer for the *New York Times*, who said, "The answer is absolutely not known."[10] The effect of this was to discourage women from seeking readily available help, when what the author really meant was: "I don't know what the treatment is." One of the most universal characteristics of orthodoxy in medicine is a fiercely immodest chauvinism, which brings with it the tacit assumption: "If we don't know the answer, then no one else possibly can." The problem is compounded when the media, given to an unquestioning science worship, accept this arrogant nihilism as incontrovertible fact.

In point of fact, PMS is a pussycat. During the very month this statement appeared in the *New York Times*, the Atkins Center saw twenty-six PMS patients and twenty-two showed dramatic improvement. The following case history is typical of the many PMS patients we treat.

Veronica Chandler

"My life was a nightmare. I lost control; I felt so miserable I wanted to crawl into a hole."

When Veronica visited the Atkins Center she was fifteen pounds overweight. She complained of a loss of mood control prior to her menstruation. She also had tremendous cravings for chocolates at that time and would gain four to seven pounds the week before menstruation. Her own gynecologist explained that she had premenstrual tension and offered her tranquilizers. She tried the tranquilizers and found they turned her into a zombie. Another gynecologist suggested that she go on progesterone. After taking the progesterone for two months she felt better, but the cravings started to reappear, along with intense feelings of irritability, by the third month of the drug therapy.

VERONICA'S DIET-RELATED DISORDER

At the Atkins Center, Veronica was given a glucose tolerance test, which showed that her blood sugar level peaked at 180 milligrams percent and then dropped to 52 at the third hour. All the rest of her tests were normal except the cytotoxic test for allergies and food intolerances. She showed sensitivity to candida, yeasts, molds, and dairy products, cottage cheese in particular. Corn, wheat, onions, and grapefruit were also foods she reacted to. This was interesting since Veronica was constantly on a diet that included cottage cheese and grapefruit just about every day. When she binged, she ate lots of chocolate in all forms (cake, cookies, ice cream) or she went for popcorn.

"I was amazed to find out that the foods I ate were the foods that I was sensitive to," noted Veronica. When she went on the Atkins Diet (low carbohydrates), she felt it hard to stay on; she had a very hard time staying away from sugar. "Although I still craved sweets, I craved them less. Dr. Atkins had told me that I wouldn't notice an improvement until the second month of my period and I must stay away from sweets," Veronica recounted to my nurse. During her first menstrual period, which was only fourteen days away, she did not notice much of a difference except that her mood appeared to be more stable. She related, "When my period ended I noticed my energy level was better and I could follow my diet more easily." By the second month she had no mood changes and her period passed effortlessly, though she still had some bloating. During the following six months Veronica had no PMS symptoms at all.

"However, when Christmas arrived, I went for it all. I blew it! Cake, cookies, mince pie, eggnog, the whole shooting match. When my premenstrual period arrived soon after, I was reminded of every symptom I had ever experienced. That taught me — or at least I hope it did."

THE RATIONALE FOR VERONICA'S TREATMENT

We placed Veronica on a low-carbohydrate diet because of her blood sugar instability and her overweight. When she lost fifteen pounds, she was put on unlimited use of allowable low-carbohydrate vegetables and one cup of those starchy foods that she did not react to on her allergy test. Interestingly, a recent study has shown that PMS patients ate more refined sugar, refined carbohydrates, and dairy products than women who did not suffer from PMS. The study also found that nutritional factors such as the B vitamins, zinc, manganese, and iron may play an important role in the cause of PMS.[11]

Veronica was placed from the outset on a vitamin regimen of L-glutamine before meals (if she felt a sweet craving), oil of evening primrose, vitamin B_6, magnesium orotate, zinc, and manganese; she also took Antioxidant Formula, folic acid, and vitamin B_{12} sublingually. After four months of the vitamin regimen, the primrose oil was reduced, as were some of the other nutrients. When it became apparent after all symptoms except the bloating cleared up, I addressed the candida issue. Veronica was put on caprylic acid, acidophilus, plus drops for mold and yeast in the neutralizing concentrations.

The "Big Picture"

Veronica is now marked in our tabular results in the 100 percent improved category. She does not have PMS anymore. Our tabular figures indicate that a result like this takes place 64 percent of the time. Some benefits occur in another 24 percent of our cases.

Our success rate with PMS is remarkably like that of a large study of over 150 women who had previously not responded to treatment and who were then simply treated with evening primrose oil.[12] For this reason, plus our own specific experience, I can only conclude that the provision of adequate amounts of GLA, which the primrose oil supplies, is the single most important key in managing this condition. Dr. David Horrobin, the GLA guru, writes that "biochemical studies have clearly shown that women with PMS . . . are less efficient than normal at converting linoleic acid to GLA."[13]

Since GLA, as a nutrient, provides no risk whatever, this conclusion is inescapable: If a woman has PMS and has not been treated with proper doses of primrose oil (or black currant seed oil, which also contains GLA), then her physician has just plain muffed it.

The fact that one out of eight PMS patients has not improved suggests poor dietary compliance or our failure to recognize all of the chemical allergies and hidden food allergies. In other words, the patient may be eating something she shouldn't be. PMS is very much a diet-related disorder.[14]

Dr. Abraham's Contribution

The problem in dealing with premenstrual tension is that no two cases are alike. Veronica Chandler had her own set of symptoms, which may have also been influenced by her own allergies and candida problem. Each patient needs an individualized program even though many have some symptoms in common. Dr. Guy E. Abraham of the UCLA Department of Obstetrics and Gynecology has analyzed and organized a way for physicians to diagnose premenstrual syndrome and thus treat it.[15]

Dr. Abraham divides premenstrual syndrome into four subgroups. Each subgroup contains a list of symptoms common to women who fall into each group. They are described in a brilliant and inspiring chapter of the book edited by Dr. Jeffrey Bland, *1986 — A Year in Nutritional Medicine*.[16] I use the word *inspiring* because it meets the rationalist physician's intellectual demands for the specific facts he needs to begin to make clinical use of nutrition. For example, women suffering from symptoms of anxiety, irritability, and nervous tension beginning at midcycle and getting progressively worse as the cycle approaches menstruation are in the subgroup PMT-A. (Dr. Abraham refers to PMS as premenstrual tension). Women in this subgroup are found to have hormonal imbalances.

Women who experience weight gain fall into Dr. Abraham's PMT-H subgroup. The *H* stands for *heaviness*. I prefer to call it PMT-B, for *bloating* (and for better alphabetizing). Symptoms such as premenstrual weight gain, water retention, and abdominal and breast tenderness are experienced by women in this subgroup. Dr. Neils Lauersen, who uses this classification also, notes that 60 percent to

66 percent of PMS sufferers belong in this subgroup.[17] Some women may be ingesting more salt in their diet or there may be a hormonal imbalance in aldosterone, an adrenal hormone.

In the PMT-C subgroup (the *C* is for *craving*), researchers have shown a positive correlation between PMS cravings and stress-related feelings. Symptoms exhibited by this group can be fainting, fatigue, palpitations, and headache. Hypoglycemia is induced by a rise in insulin levels due to the increased sugar intake. Women who are in this subgroup and are under stress require more energy and find they have an increased desire for sugars.

Women in Dr. Abraham's subgroup PMT-D will exhibit symptoms of depression, withdrawal, and suicidal feelings premenstrually. Anxiety and irritability, which are symptoms associated with PMT-A, also appear in this subgroup. In addition, other complaints by the women in this group may be confusion, incoherence, lethargy, and difficulty verbalizing. Dr. Abraham feels that "pure PMT-D may be present in less than three percent of PMT patients."[18] Part of the problem may be related to a hormonal imbalance from midcycle to menses, when progesterone is at higher levels than estrogen. Interestingly, Dr. Abraham notes that a nutritional deficiency causes this subgroup to surface. Such a deficiency can contribute to stress and hormonal imbalances.

What Dr. Abraham's findings indicate is that women with PMS cannot all be treated in the same way. Dr. Lauersen notes that most women will need changes in diet, supplementation, counseling, exercise, stress relief, and medication if it is indicated. With an adequate source of GLA, however, medication (usually a progesterone-like substance) is rarely required.

Obviously, there is a need for a new approach, because PMS is affecting more than 5 million women. We have been so pleased with our success in the complementary treatment of PMS that we plan to open a PMS subdivision at the Atkins Center. At this center we will combine the services of a nutritionist, a gynecologist, a chiropractor, an acupuncturist, an internist, and our allergy (or clinical ecology) unit. This is a good example of how Complementary Medicine is supposed to work. When done right, all the healing disciplines can be made to complement one another, working in harmony to a single purpose.

PART II

. . .

Cardiovascular Disorders

12

. . .

HEART DISEASE AND
THE HEALTH REVOLUTION

There are two main reasons a major portion of this text discusses the management of heart patients. One is that I am a cardiologist and I have been treating heart patients for three decades. The other is that this is the most pressing medical problem in all Western countries and the one most likely to lead us all to our demise.

I have pointed out that clinical nutrition is not taught at any level of an orthodox physician's training — school, hospital, or postgraduate — and from that I draw a rather disconcerting premise: *An orthodox cardiologist, even if he is chief of service at a medical school, is probably not the best person to be treating a person with heart disease.* That privilege is better handled by a capable complementary physician, because nutritional therapies are his stock in trade. And these nutrition therapies are what really can create wellness by *rebuilding* the heart, not merely blocking its disease manifestation.

But Orthodoxy Preaches Heart Nutrition

To be sure, orthodox physicians do deal at great length with nutritional principles. Restrict fats, or salt, or calories, or cholesterol, they say. However, not only are their general principles sometimes wrong, but because they have yet to learn the specifics of nutritional therapy, they do not, cannot, deal in the details that make all the difference. If you are now going to an orthodox cardiologist, I believe I can prove my point. Ask him if he has a working knowledge of the cardiovascular benefits of omega-3 fatty acids, prostaglandin E_1 precursors, magnesium orotate or aspartate, L-carnitine, coenzyme Q_{10}, L-taurine, garlic, bromelain, or even lecithin, vitamin B_6, or the antioxidant nutrients. The real truth is that he darn well *should* be using this kind of nutrition, because these agents have real and powerful effects, as I intend to show you in the pages that follow.

The Diet Part of Nutrition: How to Succeed in Cardiology

I'm not sure I know how to define success in medicine. If it is to be defined as accumulating lots of money, then I'm a modest success. But if it is defined as having helped improve the health of thousands of patients, then I certainly have been a successful cardiologist.

But anyone who reviews my voluminous documentation of these patient successes must be thunderstruck, as even I am, at the degree to which these successes have been achieved by guiding patients toward new eating patterns.

Most of my patients have been freely consuming eggs, butter, cream, beef, shellfish, and other foods interdicted as high-cholesterol or high-fat. They have been avoiding white bread, gelatin desserts, fruit sherbet, juices, bananas, white rice, pasta, margarine, and other foods often encouraged on a "heart diet." My ideal diet for heart patients is virtually the opposite of that recommended by the majority of both orthodox and alternative authorities.

Once this startling fact sinks in, you may place me in the uncomfortable position of having to respond to this statement: "If you're right, Dr. Atkins, then everyone else must be wrong."

Is There Only One Right Way?

In fact, some of you may recall the celebrated lawsuit in which I had to seek legal redress from a particularly outspoken proponent of an extreme low-fat diet who felt that his success gave him the right to accuse me of "causing" heart disease and a variety of equally horrible maladies. Only his untimely demise kept me from having my day in court, where I could show to the world the fallacy of assuming that one man's success automatically implies another man's failure. For example, if an American can reach the Orient by traveling west, it does not mean another cannot get there, quite successfully, by flying east.

One has only to use one of the basic premises of Complementary Medicine — "Look at the bottom line first" — to know that perhaps *both* approaches can be useful. The proper question, then, is not, Which of these diets works? but rather, Which works better, and for whom?

Until someone out there sees fit to do a study comparing both dietary approaches, *one against the other,* proponents of either viewpoint can say, as I am saying now, "It sure is obvious to me that mine works better." And I might add that I have the documented evidence of my experience with thirty-five thousand patients to back me up.

As a small aside, let me say about low-fat diets that though some benefits have been demonstrated from them, it's not quite clear that the benefits are the result of their low-fat qualities. All the way back to Dr. Norman Jolliffe's Prudent Diet in the 1950s, these diet plans have preached the avoidance of junk food, and that certainly does include sugar. Therefore, the success of these diets can't be used to *prove* the advantage of the restriction of fat. These *are* good diets to use against heart disease. It's not surprising. Sugar is such a bad actor for the heart patient that any diet without it will register very well on the cardiac management card.

Now, before I tell you how I treat heart patients, let me give you an overview of contemporary cardiology.

Four Major Categories of Heart Disease

There are many kinds of heart problems that I won't discuss here, for example, congenital deformities, rheumatic heart disease with a variety of tight or leaking heart valves, myocarditis, endocarditis, pericarditis, cardiomyopathy, and other problems. But there are four clinical problems that together concern 95 percent of the patients who seek help from heart specialists. They are hypertension (high blood pressure), congestive heart failure (this category may, in fact, be a consequence of several of the less common problems just mentioned), disturbances of heart rhythm (an endless variety of these), and coronary heart disease (also called ischemic heart disease).

The low-carbohydrate diet that now goes by the name of the Atkins Diet has well-established, documented, positive effects on each of these four main categories of heart disease.

The Low-Carbohydrate Diet's Advantages for Heart Patients

No effect of carbohydrate restriction is better documented than the fact that it consistently has a diuretic effect and causes an immediate salt and water loss. In case you don't believe the reams of medical literature on this subject, then try this experiment on yourself. Go on the diet and see how many more trips to the bathroom you take just forty-eight hours from now.

This water-excreting effect makes the diet fundamental therapy for both hypertension and congestive heart failure, two conditions for which diuretics are typically used. The most often confirmed medical fact in all my practice experience is the blood-pressure-lowering effect of any low-carbohydrate diet.

The control of heart rhythm is the result of the diet's stabilizing effect on blood sugar. By minimizing the rise and fall of glucose levels, the diet eliminates the body's need to use the heart stimulant adrenaline to raise quickly falling blood sugar.

The diet's effect on coronary artery disease, certainly the most important of the major cardiovascular disorders, is one which was first described over a half century ago, and probably represents a variety of mechanisms. I want to show you how it works. But first, let us understand the problem a little better.

13
. . .

CORONARY HEART DISEASE
The Death of Most of Us

Coronary heart disease has become the foremost disease in this country and the number-one killer. In America, that translates into 540,000 deaths per year. This life-threatening condition develops when the blood supply (and thus the oxygen supply) to the heart muscle is impaired. This happens because the blood vessels that provide nourishment to the heart (the coronary blood vessels) are blocked either as a result of a narrowing process called stenosis (due to plaque formation or atherosclerosis) or because they go into spasm.

Ischemic Heart Disease

Ischemic heart disease is the name doctors give to these coronary artery impairments. The term *ischemia* refers to an obstruction of the blood supply. As a result of ischemia, there is a breakdown in the delivery system of oxygen to the tissues. This often happens when severe stress, such as strenuous exercise, is placed on the heart. When the stress-induced deficiency in the heart's blood supply occurs, a pain signal is given off. The pain is usually experienced as a squeezing, tightening, crushing heaviness in the area of the chest called the precordium (meaning *in front of the heart*). The Latin name for pain in this area is *angina pectoris;* you have probably heard it called just plain angina.

What Is a Heart Attack?

Angina and heart attack are the two common manifestations of coronary artery disease. Both problems arise because of poor blood supply due to coronary artery narrowing or spasm, and both are considered ischemic heart disease (IHD), or coronary artery disease (CAD); but there is a difference. The distinction is that in a heart attack (myocardial infarction) some part of the heart muscle supplied by an obstructed blood vessel actually dies, whereas in angina, the heart muscle restores itself to viability. Angina often precedes a myocardial infarction. In a progressive case of atherosclerosis, the coronary vessel narrows gradually until it completely obstructs; this is called coronary occlusion, a term that was for many years considered synonymous with heart attack.

Complications of an acute myocardial infarction include the heart's failure to pump sufficient blood (congestive heart failure, acute pulmonary edema); shock (collapse of the arterial blood circuit with loss of blood pressure); grossly inefficient heart rhythms, such as the often fatal ventricular fibrillation; traveling blood clots (emboli); and blowouts of the heart muscle. These are just some of the ways in which heart attacks can lead to sudden and instantaneous death before the patient can even be brought into the hospital.

The Urgency of Angina

When a patient develops angina, an entire system of medical investigation is set in motion. This is because all physicians, orthodox and alternative alike, feel a responsibility to establish whether or not any tightening in the chest may be, in fact, due to the heart. Should the diagnosis of heart disease be confirmed, the patient will be sentenced to a restricted lifestyle and, in orthodox circles, a program of drug therapy and possibly surgery. Here we also see one of orthodox medicine's greatest strengths — the demand for and the ability to provide *an accurate diagnosis*. And with it, we have a compelling reason why the new medicine must include the best of orthodoxy together with the best of the alternatives.

Diagnosis

For more than forty years, the diagnosis of coronary heart disease depended almost solely on the findings of an electrocardiogram (EKG). The EKG shows characteristic changes most of the time but often gives misleading information. However, when the electrocardiogram is done while the patient performs a measured amount of exercise (called a stress EKG), it can be valuable in diagnosing insufficiencies of the coronary blood supply. When the stress EKG is performed on ischemic hearts, abnormalities may appear which do not show up on the resting EKG.

A major advance in understanding coronary circulation came some thirty years ago with the advent of an x-ray technique called a coronary angiogram. This became the recognized way to diagnose blockages. In this procedure a dye is placed, by way of a catheter, into the heart itself where it will be picked up by the coronary blood vessels. The outline of the vessels will be seen on the x-ray, so that the radiologist can note the degree to which they are narrowed or obstructed.

One problem with the angiogram is that the blood vessels appear normal if the angina is due to spasm. Another is that the doctor may be alarmed by a blockage he finds when in fact that area of the heart may be quite adequately served by collateral blood vessels (new ones that take over when a vessel is blocked). Failure to recognize the adequacy of collateral circulation may lead to unnecessary surgery.

The real drawback of the angiocardiogram is that because it is an invasive technique — that is, it "invades" the heart itself via an instrument (the catheter) — it is far too risky, especially considering that it is only a diagnostic procedure. Medical surveys show that one person in a thousand dies from the procedure and countless more suffer nonfatal but serious complications.

Contrast this with noninvasive tests now available in which the doctor can, without instrumenting the heart itself, find out whether the various areas of the heart are being adequately supplied with blood. The usual technique for noninvasive tests is to use a radioactive tracer — which produces less radiation than a chest x-ray — and to track its path through the body with a special camera.

There are a host of noninvasive tests — thallium scan, radionuclide cineangiogram (RNCA, first pass) or gated pool (MUGA), and others — and they are all preferable for the patient seeking nutritional or medical management. An excellent review of these noninvasive tests appears in the May 1986 issue of *Primary Cardiology*.

Is Heart Surgery the Answer?

For the person contemplating surgery, the angiocardiogram is the proper procedure. But who would contemplate surgery? This is a procedure which I think will just about be laid to rest by the end of the century. Most of the statistics recently published have shown that patients who have undergone heart bypass operations have fared no better, in the longer run, than those who were treated with nonsurgical techniques.[1]

The 1984 Coronary Artery Surgery Study (CASS), sponsored by the National Heart, Lung, and Blood Institute, followed 24,959 participants under sixty-five years of age who had either mild angina or one heart attack but no angina. Half were treated with drugs; the other half underwent bypass surgery (a coronary artery bypass graft, CABG). Those operated on showed no lifesaving advantage over drug therapy. In fact, those with mild angina without surgery fared better than the surgical group.

The Advantage of Heroics

This is not the place to discuss the heroics of managing a patient who is undergoing a heart attack, but I would like to underscore that in such circumstances it is far more appropriate to be treated in a well-equipped orthodox hospital, with its intensive care unit (ICU), than in a center where nutritional medicine is practiced. In the treatment of an emergency, nothing works quite so well as contemporary orthodox medicine. Its handling of coronary emergencies is the perfect example of why it deserves its reputation as a lifesaver. And orthodox medicine achieves its results through the use of heroics: drugs to stabilize heart rhythms or to correct heart failure or shock; balloons and enzymes to reopen the blocked blood vessels; emergency reparative surgery using heart-lung bypass equipment; and so on. Nutritional medicine still has an important role, but it works best after the patient is out of imminent danger.

However, you still may have only a fifty-fifty chance of survival, even with all these lifesaving options at hand. All cardiologists would agree that relying on heroics is unwise, and that the real treatment of heart disease lies in its prevention, rather than counting on the miracle of emergency treatment.

Drugs for Prevention?

Unfortunately, in orthodox medical circles prevention remains more pharmacological than it is nutritional. All agree on the need for lifestyle changes such as cutting out cigarettes, reducing stress, getting into a steady exercise program. All agree there should be attention to diet, although they may disagree over which diet is best. But the emphasis still remains on using drugs — drugs to reduce blood pressure, to prevent rhythm disorders, to prevent platelet clumping, to control heart rate, to lower lipid concentrations, to lessen the blood flow to the heart.

The net result is that patients often come in for a re-evaluation of their heart management program suffering more from their medications than from their underlying disorder. We've seen thousands of patients like that at the Atkins Center; let me give you one of many examples so that you can get the flavor of our approach to helping them.

Edward Weaver

On March 28, 1980, shortly after his fiftieth birthday, Ed Weaver walked into my office and told me, "I feel like a zombie." Ed was suffering from a heart condition manifested mainly as angina. Worse, the medication prescribed by his cardiologist was complicating his health problems. According to Ed, his life was a mess. As he later said, "I thought I was going to die."

Ed's difficulties, which included an enlarged heart, started in 1976. It was then that he began having severe chest pains (angina).

In 1978 tests revealed that his heart was getting even larger. A coronary angiogram was performed, which showed several blockages. Surgery was contemplated, but Ed was felt to be too poor a risk. Instead, he was placed on propranolol, a beta-blocker (beta-blockers reduce the heart's need for oxygen by reducing the heart rate); this weakened him so much that he needed nitroglycerine just to walk a block or two. Over the next two years, his heart tests showed progressive deterioration. His blood cholesterol level, 313, was elevated (a normal level would range from 150 to 225), as were his triglycerides, 196 (ideally, triglyceride levels should be below 100). He had tried dieting to eliminate some of the excess weight he had put on, but nothing worked.

Ed complained to his doctor that his health was not improving and the medication he was on made him feel emotionally depressed and just plain miserable. The doctor's response was that all-too-familiar phrase: You'll just have to live with your condition. So advised, Ed decided he had nothing to lose. He started reading about nutrition and vitamins. He was introduced to my book *Dr. Atkins' Diet Revolution*. When he asked his doctor's opinion of the diet, Ed was told, "He's a quack."

"I was at my wits' end. Nothing could be worse, so I began following the diet procedure in Diet Revolution *without my doctor knowing it. I went back to my doctor two weeks later and he discovered that I had lost approximately fifteen pounds. Both my cholesterol and triglyceride levels had also dropped. He said he didn't know what happened, but whatever I was doing to keep it up."*

With that offhand comment, Ed's doctor had quite unwittingly encouraged him to seek me out. Ed knew for himself, after experiencing such improvement, that a change was necessary. He came to see me, weighing 223 pounds, down from a high of 250 the year before.

ED BEGINS HIS CARE WITH US

At the time of his first visit Ed was taking 10 propranolol tablets a day (400 milligrams), 4 capsules a day of clofibrate (Atromid-S, a cholesterol-lowering drug), nitroglycerine, plus a long-acting nitrate. Ed had been dieting on his own, so that his blood tests revealed an already lowered cholesterol level of 255, triglycerides 112, and high-density lipoproteins (HDL)* at 45. The glucose tolerance test, which we order routinely on heart patients, revealed that he was an exaggerated responder to sugar. His blood glucose after administration of the glucose solution climbed to 170 and then dropped to 57 milligrams percent.

I immediately took Ed off his clofibrate. I reduced his propranolol from 400 milligrams to 200 milligrams in three weeks and to 20 milligrams in three-and-a-half months. I placed him on a personalized version of the Atkins low-carbohydrate diet. I also prescribed nutritional supplements, which included extra magnesium orotate, B_{15}, lecithin, 800 units of vitamin E, zinc, manganese, selenium, garlic, and cod-liver oil at bedtime.

ED'S GRATIFYING RESULTS

By September 2, 1980, six months later, Ed's weight had been reduced to 179 pounds. This table shows his progress at a glance.

	Before First Visit	3/2/80	9/2/80
Cholesterol	313	255	204
Triglycerides	196	112	93
HDL	—	45	45
Weight	230	223	179

Ed was so pleased that he decided he was too thin. His angina was gone. He had no pains. He felt better than he had for years. So he treated himself to some sweets, which led to a candy binge. This proved to be a huge mistake. Ed sheepishly reported that the sugar upset his system to the point that he had a "crying jag." He went back on the diet and the symptoms disappeared.

---

* High-density lipoproteins transport fats in the blood stream, including cholesterol, and are generally thought to be protective against heart disease.

THE DOCUMENTATION OF SUCCESS

By January 1981, Ed's treatments had him "feeling like a new man." He took up body building and returned to his first love, acting. All of these lifestyle changes produced no negative side effects. They improved Ed's sense of well-being to the point where I decided that it would be interesting to perform another heart examination; but this time, it would have to be noninvasive. I ordered a radionuclide cineangiogram (RNCA, the first-pass technecium 99 study). The results came back with a resting ejection fraction of 76 percent, and after strenuous exercise, a reading of 87 percent.* This sort of report was *better than normal;* most decathlon athletes would not score so well. The evidence clearly showed the reversal of coronary heart disease! Ed now visits the center two times a year for checkups. We have slowly moved his weight up to an ideal 190 pounds and it has remained constant for two years.

Ed still has problems, but they're not heart problems. When I saw him last, he asked me this burning medical question:

"Do you know a producer who has a part for an actor with great talent?
"When I look at my life before I met you and now, I know I would be dead if it weren't for you."

As you know, I always point out that the cases I present to you are typical of the many patients we see with a given problem, but in Ed Weaver's case, that is only partially true. In going from a coronary angiogram (the invasive kind) which showed many coronary vessel blockages, to a noninvasive angiogram showing better than normal function, we have documentation of heart disease reversal of a greater magnitude than I have ever seen before or since. If the same testing modality had been used both times, his case could have been written up in a medical journal.

---

* Ejection fraction is the measure of the percentage of the blood content of the dilated heart that gets pumped out in a single beat as the heart contracts. It is an important physiological measure of heart function. Generally speaking, the ejection fraction (EF) should increase with exercise; if it does not, that implies an insufficient blood supply to the heart itself (coronary insufficiency).

WHAT DID THE JOB

But in many ways, Ed is typical of all too many coronary insufficiency patients, who are suffering as much from their medications as from their illness. His dramatic improvement as he gradually shed his medication burden is typical of hundreds. The heart disease reversal he achieved is all the more striking in view of what Ed *did not* receive. There was no carnitine, coenzyme Q_{10}, bromelain, primrose oil, EPA, or chelation therapy. And, as I will be explaining, all of these are highly advisable procedures for the heart patient.

To me, and to Ed, the lion's share of the improvement has to be attributed to that low-carbohydrate diet, which nutritionally unsophisticated critics have repeatedly maligned as a "heart attack diet." I have observed this result so many thousands of times that I weep with frustration over my inability to penetrate the closed minds of persons who simply aren't interested enough to see for themselves.

It is a rare heart patient, indeed, who fails to benefit from our nutritional protocol, despite the fact that most of the world assumes otherwise. Indeed, I can assure you that I couldn't, in all conscience, take Ed and other patients like him off their medications if we didn't have the diet.

An Area of Mystery

The strange thing is that predictable as my success has been in this area, I'm forced to base my argument for this treatment purely on empirical results. I don't have a mechanistic explanation for the success the diet has with angina patients. *I don't know why it works.* There aren't many places in this book where I say that, but I do here. I don't know *why* the low-carbohydrate diet works for angina, but I've seen it do so over and over. And consistently, when patients have encountered a return of pain, they've admitted to me they went off the diet.

All my observations lead me to conclude that sugar is in some sense the culprit here. Heart patients who have been placed on our Meat and Millet Diet, which allows complex carbohydrates but no sugar, have experienced roughly the same benefits. And when backsliding patients have re-experienced pain, it has been after they have reintroduced sugar into their system. There are also some interesting general statistics that just might be indicative of something. For more than a decade — ever since the Atkins Diet became popular, in fact — the statistic called "death from heart disease" has been showing a decline. I'm not taking personal credit, but during just about the same time span, our national per capita consumption of sugar has been declining.

Are You Amazed at This Story?

Come on, admit it. This runs counter to what you've been taught. The real indictment is the one that must be hurled at those who have quite systematically taught you that such a result could never come from such a diet. The leaders of orthodoxy have rallied around the conclusions they have deduced and have declared: "Don't bother us with facts; we have already decided what's true."

In the next chapter, I will present two examples of patients similar to Ed, who have in addition undergone chelation therapy.

The success of chelation therapy, an orthodox medical therapy rejected only because medicine's leaders had figured on another answer, has contributed a lot to my present philosophy. The strength of Complementary Medicine is its willingness to accept politically rejected healing systems.

Let's see how it works.

14

CHELATION
A Wonder Regimen
for Coronary Disease

Let's start off with a little exercise in imagination. Pick the person you know best who comes close to fitting the following description: male, near the age of fifty, hardworking, some awareness of health issues, has quit smoking, tries to watch his diet, exercises as often as he can, even takes a few vitamins. Have you someone in mind? Now imagine this scenario:

Out of the blue, he suddenly develops a crushing pain in his chest and breaks into a cold sweat. He immediately gets to his doctor, who has him whisked off to the hospital, where blood tests and EKGs confirm that he has had a heart attack, or, as his consultant cardiologist puts it, an acute myocardial infarction. Fortunately, his vital signs stabilize and his four days in the ICU and next ten days in his hospital room pass uneventfully. Then the cardiologist insists that he get an angiocardiogram "so we can get a look at those coronary blood vessels." He agrees, and despite a few shaky moments when his heart rhythm goes out of control, survives the procedure well. The cardiologist returns for a serious talk.

"Your heart is healing well, but we did find an eighty percent blockage of the most important artery, the left anterior descending [LAD]. Statistics show this is a mean little sucker, and there are just too darn many people who get into real trouble with this artery — maybe have a second heart attack and die on the way to the hospital. Cardiologists agree that all these LAD people should have bypass surgery."

To shorten this story, let me say that our hero goes through bypass surgery with flying colors and prepares to resume his career four months later, in a more subdued manner, of course. His cardiologist prescribes a baby aspirin and customary doses of dipyridamole and a beta-blocker, to prevent complications. After a few months, our subject, a little tired and minus half his sex drive, notes that he has absolutely no heart symptoms and, surveying it all, happily concludes that he is "one of the lucky ones."

Not a Horror Story at All, Is It?

I have just described an everyday outcome for a person with a heart attack. His treatment was par for the course.

Yet, if that happened to you, one of my readers, I personally would be quite chagrined. For there is much more that, in my view, could have and should have been done (and perhaps much that need *not* have been done, including an angiogram and a coronary artery bypass graft).

From the previous chapters, I'm sure you have gathered that part of what should have been done was the prescribing of a very specific diet and a significant number of nutritional supplements, all designed to help reverse the underlying causes of heart disease.

But there is one further treatment, taken right out of the annals of orthodox medicine that, from the beginning, offered our subject his best chance of reversing his heart disease and perhaps of avoiding the need for heart surgery and medication. This treatment is the controversial and, among the pillars of orthodoxy, unpopular procedure called chelation therapy.

But I Haven't Even Heard Its Name . . .

Chelation (the name comes from the Greek word for claw) is one of the best-kept secrets in modern medicine. Tens of millions of people have never even heard of a procedure that is substantially more effective and infinitely less dangerous than bypass surgery.

The basic idea of chelation came from the fact that there are certain natural and synthetic substances — chelating agents — that bind certain elements, especially minerals, to them. Because of this, if a chelating agent is introduced into the blood system in solution, it will attach to many harmful minerals that have accumulated in the body and take them along with it when it is excreted. This property of chelation has been known for decades, and, as far back as the 1940s, it became the treatment of choice for lead poisoning.

I'll explain chelation in detail farther on, but for now what you need to know is that it improves circulatory function by removing metals such as cadmium, lead, calcium, and iron from the body, and that this is done by administering a synthetic amino acid, EDTA, by intravenous infusion into the body. EDTA then exercises its powerful attraction for loose, free-floating metallic ions in the blood stream and forms a chemical bond with them. And, as the EDTA passes from the body, it takes these toxic metals with it.

Margaret Hare

"I couldn't go out alone, and I certainly didn't dare drive."

Margaret Hare first came to me on June 9, 1983, sixty-two years of age and looking a great deal older. She had trouble walking. She had the mien and the demeanor of one suffering from chronic illness.

Margaret had been diagnosed as having angina in 1981. On one occasion, she passed out and had to be hospitalized. She had also been diagnosed as having hypoglycemia. "Everything took its toll," she said, "ending with my coronary in 1982." After her coronary, Margaret was sent to St. Luke's Hospital for evaluation as a possible candidate for bypass surgery. The doctors decided against surgery and placed her on drug therapy, including 3 nifedipine, 3 Corgard, and 3 Isordil tablets a day. She was regularly fed nitroglycerine through a skin patch. Her comments:

> *"I was on so many drugs, I was like a zombie. I couldn't take care of myself. If it weren't for my husband and two daughters, I don't know what I would have done."*

A year after her coronary and orthodox therapy, Margaret felt no better. So she came to me, weighing 128½ pounds at five feet six inches. Her blood pressure was high (152/96), as were her levels of cholesterol (331) and low-density lipoproteins, or LDLs (226).* Review of her past medical experience indicated that she had had a hysterectomy and had received chemotherapy. Even on the day of her first examination, Margaret suffered from angina. She said she usually had chest pains upon waking but they would disappear during the course of the day if she remained idle. If she attempted to walk for fifteen to twenty minutes the pains would usually return, and if she attempted to walk in cold weather the pain occurred without fail. More important, she was constantly tired, weak, and forgetful.

I placed Margaret on a low-carbohydrate version of the Meat and Millet Diet, which she began in mid-June. She obviously couldn't afford to lose more than five pounds at most, but carbohydrate restriction has such an advantage in managing the symptoms of angina and shortness of breath that I felt it was needed here. She was given the center's standard multivitamin formula, with additional garlic, magnesium orotate, and bromelain; I also prescribed our special Cardiovascular Formula, plus two tablespoons of lecithin, additional vitamins C and E, and extra zinc. (Details on our supplement formulas are in Appendix C.)

Because of the nearly universal success that coronary insufficiency patients have on our diet and nutritional regimen, I felt confident enough to tell Margaret that we would gradually reduce her heart medicine and that the first one to go would be the beta-blocker propranolol.

Margaret stared at me disbelievingly. "I'm having pain now and you want to cut down my heart medicine?"

"For two reasons. First, I want to do a noninvasive form of angiogram to evaluate the extent of your heart problem. In it, you will be tested before and after exercise. The beta-blockers prevent your heart rate from going up with exercise [that's their potential advantage], and we won't get an accurate test result.

"And the second reason is, well, you do want to be well,

---

*Low-density lipoproteins are carrier molecules for cholesterol and are generally associated with increased risk of cardiovascular disorders. Their optimal level is below 120 milligrams percent.

don't you? Then remember, medications are not used by well people."

Margaret gave a nervous laugh but did agree to begin a brand-new plan of treatment.

Approximately one month after her first visit, Margaret had been weaned from her propranolol and was given her first radionuclide cineangiogram (RNCA) test. It showed a moderate lack of arterial wall motion and 20 percent drop in her ejection fraction with exercise. This was the reverse of what should have been, since the normal heart increases its efficiency with exercise. The stress electrocardiogram confirmed the findings of the RNCA. Everything indicated coronary insufficiency.

As Margaret returned to the center on subsequent visits, we gradually increased her starch and carbohydrate allowances and continued to wean her from her medications.

On September 7, Margaret indicated that she was beginning to feel better. By September 21, I had removed her from all of her nitrates. She was still on a low dosage of Corgard and nitroglycerine. We then continued to reduce the dosage of all medications so that within the next two months, she would be off them completely. This would be the optimal time to begin chelation therapy. According to her response and physical examination, we had built up her stamina and cardiac function to the point where she was in a very stable condition. Yet, there was continued evidence of poor arterial blood flow.

Chelation with EDTA was now appropriate. Margaret began her chelation in October 1983. By November, her angina was markedly improved. She continued taking chelation treatments. By Christmas 1983, Margaret noted that, in her day-to-day activity, her angina was gone. For the first time in years, she was able to go out alone and do Christmas shopping.

> *"I felt so good, I couldn't believe it. I even noticed I was mentally sharper and didn't have those spells of forgetfulness anymore."*

On January 17, 1984, we re-evaluated Margaret and found that all of her lab results were moving toward the normal range. Her blood pressure had already normalized. By April 1984 Margaret was driving again and by May she was driving alone, wherever she wanted. She was working constantly around the house without feeling tired, even though she made sure to take a nap during the day. On one occasion while an interviewer was talking with Margaret, her husband interjected:

> "The change in one year is unbelievable. My wife is alive. She and I painted the twenty-by-forty swimming pool together. I've got me a young wife again."

In June of 1984, Margaret enthused:

> "You cannot believe the difference. When I first arrived, I couldn't carry my pocketbook, I often had to ask my husband to carry it for me. My family didn't think I was going to live and now I feel like a totally new person. You may see a difference between my first visit and now, but I don't think you understand the difference. I no longer think about death or life. I just live. There isn't anything I can't do, at least that's the way I feel. This week I have had two of my six grandchildren visiting me. One is three and the other is five. You will not believe this, but I was able to enjoy them the entire week and still feel great. I don't know how to thank you."

As this book goes to press, Margaret is still at the much-improved level I just described. She has not only had more years of *life* than were originally held out for her, but she has had years of *health*. We are currently working with some of the nutritional supplements we have found to have the most beneficial effects on her cholesterol reading, as well as on improving her exercise capacity.

Tim Delamare

On November 30, 1982, a tall, thin man of sixty years entered my office. At six feet one and 159 pounds, Tim Delamare, a chemist, appeared two or three inches taller because every inch of him was taut — there was no excess fat. Here was a veteran skier, mountain climber, and cyclist who had come to me because of coronary insufficiency.

About ten years previously, Tim had had a heart attack and was told he needed bypass surgery. He refused surgery and eventually, in 1979, found an alternative doctor who administered thirty chelation treatments and placed him on a low-fat, high-fruit diet. After thirty treatments Tim felt fine and discontinued his treatments and the diet, but he began to suffer from increased mental stress at work and home. When his symptoms began to return (his angina was more frequent and intense in the city than in the suburbs or at home), he went to an orthodox physician, who placed him on propranolol and nitroglycerine tablets. Tim's condition did not get better; he slowed down mentally and physically and "began worrying about life, job, and everything."

It was at this point that Tim came to me.

"I decided to return to what worked before. It couldn't be worse than what I am going through now."

HOW WE EVALUATED TIM

Tim had taken an RNCA in January 1979. With exercise, the heart widened rather than contracted; thus, the test revealed multivessel cardiovascular disease. When examined at the Atkins Center on his first visit, in late November 1982, he had a cholesterol reading of 325; triglycerides were at 189, HDL at 96, and LDL at 185. His glucose tolerance test suggested an early blood sugar imbalance. His problem, whatever it initially was, had become manifold. Tim had symptoms of cramps, angina, memory loss, general weakness and lethargy due to medication. As is so often the case with beta-blockers, his sex life had been drastically affected. Thus, our treatment would have to address all of these problems, attending to his iatrogenic symptoms as well as his underlying heart problems.

THE PRE-CHELATION TREATMENT

I put Tim on the Meat and Millet Diet and gave him our Cardiovascular and Basic formulas. To these formulas, because of his specific needs, I added 1000 milligrams of vitamin B_6 (more than I usually give), 1100 units of vitamin E, magnesium orotate, bromelain, bioflavonoids, L-carnitine, and chromium, plus mucopolysaccharides and 4 tablespoons of lecithin. The high dosage of lecithin was given as another layer of treatment for his LDL and cholesterol problem. No immediate change was noted, so I added calcium orotate and began reducing Tim's propranolol and nitroglycerine. It was at this point that chelation was begun.

HOW CHELATION CONTRIBUTED

By March, Tim's cramps were gone and his angina greatly reduced in both frequency and intensity. Over the weeks most of his symptoms reduced themselves and he said he felt better. I continued to increase the quantity of EDTA (per the chelation protocol) and reduced his propranolol to 20 milligrams daily. At this point Tim noted that his angina, which had been improving, was worsening. I continued all of the same treatments but held the propranolol at 20 milligrams until his symptoms, which had been controlled by the "beta blockade," adjusted to this lower dosage. When he indicated that the pains had stabilized and had even abated, I then more slowly reduced the propranolol until he was totally off the drug.

By May 1984, Tim's angina had disappeared, he was off nitroglycerine as well, and he enjoyed a full sex life. In May we gave Tim a second exercise RNCA. His ejection fraction was 63 percent at rest and 46 percent with exercise. The fall with exercise indicated continued heart disease, but the at-rest measurement had improved by 26 percent since 1979, which may be a significant difference.[1]

The test results helped confirm the obvious, that Tim felt much better than he had a year before. Tim had had to stop in his first RNCA test because of chest pains. He completed his last one without pain or dizziness. "I was only slightly out of breath — no more," he said. Today (1988) Tim is back skiing and mountain climbing. "I now walk for miles at a vigorous pace without symptoms. Before, I couldn't walk even a slow mile without pain." Tim is particularly pleased about how he feels about his job.

"You know, work had stopped being fun, but now I feel like my mind is sharper than ever. I attack chemical problems now and enjoy it as when I was a kid. I am in

an academic research setting and I used to dread going to work for fear I couldn't handle the mental stress any longer. Not now! Now, I am often there early and staying late. You know, when you have worked hard to become something and your ability to perform seems gone and then returns, and all the things you enjoyed doing physically you can do again, you feel like you have been born again."

Let's Look at the Record

The two cases I have just presented to you were not selected because they were the best examples of chelation responses in my entire practice. Rather, they were selected because they were so typical of the hundreds of patients I have treated in this manner.

Every working day, when I make my rounds and visit the chelation department of the center, I ask my medical associate: "How are the chelation patients doing?" His response is usually the same: "Just fine. No problems." When we analyze our entire experience with coronary heart disease patients on our chelation program, it breaks down like this:

improved	79 percent
no real change	13 percent
worse	8 percent

This improvement takes place in the kinds of cases in which there is no orthodox expectation of improvement except if the cases were previously mismanaged. In fact, Dr. Lawrence Krohn, who services a large segment of the cardiology community of Detroit with a high-resolution electrocardiography diagnostic technique, reported that only 20 out of 98 patients treated for coronary heart disease by orthodox treatments showed evidence of improvement with before-and-after testing, while all but 8 of a group of 56 patients treated by chelation therapy showed documented improvement when tested the same way.[2]

What Must It Take to Prove a Point?

More significantly, there are no examples in my practice of patients being made worse *by* the chelation. (Although 8 percent did worsen *during* the chelation, this represents a much smaller proportion than the approximately 40 percent who lose ground during standard management, according to the natural course of this illness.) None were hospitalized because of it and none died due to the treatment. Careful records of all chelation patients are kept by diplomates of the American Board of Chelation Therapy (of which I am one) and the results, nationwide, are remarkably similar. The current estimate is that ABCT diplomates and members of the American College of Advancement in Medicine have treated more than 500,000 patients with EDTA, with approximately an 80 percent improvement rate and an enviably low complication rate.

But, as you analyze the case histories of Margaret and Tim, you will see that, although both patients have obviously improved to the point that they, once cardiac invalids, are leading normal lives, there is nothing in their case reports that can serve to "prove" that chelation works.

The very strength of our overall chelation therapy protocol is what causes us difficulties in attempting to prove it effective. That is, we do so much more for a patient than administer EDTA. Who can say whether it is the chelation or the vitamin and mineral supplementation or the new diet that benefits the patient?

Heart Disease and the Issue of Proof

So, chelation goes on as an unproven therapy, which means that patients who opt for this form of treatment often have some difficulty getting reimbursement from their insurance carriers.

But when the shoe fits on the other foot, orthodoxy is unwilling to wear it. Cardiac bypass surgery, for example, was an unproven therapy for over a decade (now it is "proven" — proven to be of only temporary value among those who survive the surgery), yet there are no instances on record of any hospital's cardiac surgery unit turning down the thirty thousand to forty thousand dollars per case that the third-party carriers are all too willing to shell out.

More About Chelation and How It Works

The word *chelation* comes from the Greek word *chela*, which, as I mentioned earlier, means *claw*, and this describes the action of a chelating agent. The chelating agent is a "grabber" molecule. It grabs on to certain kinds of minerals and forms a compound with them with such affinity that the mineral can be pulled from its previous location. Although chelation is a natural process, the chelating agent that is used, EDTA, is not a natural product. The reason is that EDTA is a much more powerful chelating agent than those which occur in nature. Since we have to treat a very powerful illness, the arteriosclerotic narrowing of the coronary blood flow, we have found through experience that the powerful synthetic agent is required to get the job done.

A Brief History of Chelation

EDTA (ethylenediaminetetraacetic acid, or disodium edetate) was first synthesized by Franz Munz, a German chemist working on behalf of the chemical giant I. G. Farben Industries. It was introduced by Farben in 1931 as a substitute for citric acid in coating for cloth fibers. In 1949, EDTA was patented in the United States by the Martin-Dennis Company.

EDTA is better known to chemists than to physicians, because most of the more than five thousand published articles are devoted to its commercial applications in chemistry. One of the notable values of the agent is its precise nature and high predictability; it can be mathematically predicted how EDTA is going to act in the test tube and to what degree it will chelate. It is consistently used as a stabilizing additive to food, particularly canned goods. To confirm that, just read the ingredients list on your mayonnaise jar.

EDTA's first use in medicine was in 1941, when it was employed in treating lead poisoning, for which it is still recognized as the number-one treatment.

Chelation and Heart Disease

A decade later, serendipity struck. Dr. Norman Clarke, director of research at Providence Hospital in Detroit, noted that several patients he treated for lead poisoning reported that their angina went away. Thus began the research for employing EDTA chelation as a regimen for vascular occlusion.[3] Dr. Clarke's published studies set the tone for a decade of great enthusiasm over the prospects of using EDTA in cardiology.

At two major symposia in 1959 and 1960, chaired by Marvin Seven, M.D., dozens of cautiously enthusiastic papers written by the crème de la crème of academic researchers at several teaching institutions were read and published. The papers presented at those conferences served for a generation as the fountainhead of published knowledge about chelation therapy for a variety of medical conditions.

Then a very unusual event took place. Dr. J. Roderick Kitchell and Dr. Lawrence E. Meltzer, two of the researchers who had published five enthusiastic papers on a series of patients with angina and peripheral vascular disorders improving during EDTA therapy, noticed the obvious. During the first six months after their EDTA treatment, the patients showed further improvement, but subsequently backslid so that no lasting benefit remained. The backsliding, of course, took place because the effective treatment had been discontinued. This is tantamount to a diabetic getting worse when needed insulin treatments are stopped.

When Kitchell and Meltzer described their re-evaluation of the therapy in a 1963 paper published in the *American Journal of Cardiology*,[4] their editorial comments, rather than calling for a continuing use of chelation, instead contained only a statement of the futility of EDTA therapy. Why this ill-founded and illogical conclusion was published is known only to the authors, but medical historians feel that this paper, more than any other single event, held up research in this field for over twenty years.*

The Sponsorship Changes

There it would have died had it not been taken up by a small coterie of nonacademic, nutritionally oriented practitioners, who kept the treatment alive and perfected the protocol with nutritional

*This event is chronicled in great detail by investigative journalist Dr. Morton Walker in his book *Chelation Therapy* (1980).

techniques. In 1974, these chelation practitioners formed the AAMP, the American Academy of Medical Preventics (now the American College of Advancement in Medicine, ACAM), which over the next decade became America's pre-eminent organization in all of alternative medicine.

Unfortunately, as often happens in the early use of any new agent, the proper dosage had to be established, and in the process there were successes and failures.[5] Complications, including death, did occur when EDTA was administered too rapidly or in too large a dose. The main type of damage appeared to be in the kidneys; autopsies on those who died showed destruction of the kidney tubules that filtered the toxins. Originally, it was thought that EDTA itself was toxic to the kidneys. Shortly thereafter, researchers determined that the damage was actually done by the compounds formed when EDTA combined with toxic heavy metals such as lead and mercury. This sort of complication disappeared when a new treatment protocol was adopted, using a lower dosage and slower delivery time and checking kidney function after the first few treatments.

Suppose You Were Getting Chelation

Now let's imagine that you were a person who had a vascular problem or lead poisoning or some condition requiring chelation and agreed to take some treatment. What would it be like?

This is not a hospital procedure. It's going to take three hours in the doctor's office, and when you've finished with it you will be able to go to work, or even to play golf or tennis (assuming you could do that before). The treatment consists of a slow intravenous drip from a bottle of fluid that contains some very special ingredients. You will sit in a comfortable chair or lounge and the technician or the doctor will insert a tiny butterfly needle into a vein in your arm, then anchor it comfortably; over the next three hours, approximately one pint of sterile fluid will be dripped in at a rate of approximately one-half teaspoon per minute. Along with the chelating agent disodium EDTA (to which has been added enough magnesium to form a compound called magnesium EDTA), this bottle contains a variety of essential nutrients, particularly vitamins of the B complex and a considerable amount of vitamin C, which incidentally, is itself a chelating agent. It contains procaine, a pain-killer, so that the infusion will not sting, and the natural anticoag-ulant heparin, to prevent clotting in the vein. Afterward, the essential minerals that EDTA may have removed are usually added to the intravenous infusion, using the same vein and tubing.

Chelation Is Not Always the Same

Each individual chelating physician may have his own variation on the theme and may individualize each case. Some will give a lipid-lowering compound, containing choline, methionine, and inositol. Others may use the penetrating agent DMSO (dimethyl sulfoxide) to enhance the benefit. Others will use the intravenous vehicle as an opportunity to give some other needed nutritional agent on a personalized basis. My German colleagues report excellent results from adding a purified glycopeptide derived from the cytoplasm of fetal sheep hearts.

While this is being administered, you might be lounging around, chatting with other patients, watching television, reading a book or a newspaper, or simply dozing. Although most patients feel about the same after a chelation session, some report that they immedi-ately feel considerably stronger, presumably because of the lift provided by the B vitamins, while others report feeling drained. Most will get hungry, because one of the effects of chelation ther-apy is to cause a temporary drop in the blood sugar. That is why patients are instructed to eat something before and during the che-lation treatment. This procedure is repeated at intervals ranging from once in two days to once in two weeks. It is usually felt that chelation should ideally be administered every third day, but in point of fact most chelation patients, because of their busy sched-ules, agree to a once-a-week treatment schedule. Since a typical course of treatment involves twenty-five to fifty visits, this means that the full program may be extended over a six- to twelve-month time span, but this is appropriate for the majority of people who are not in acute distress with otherwise unmanageable symptoms.*

*Since cost is a concern to most people, let's note that the typical cost of a single chelation treatment may range from $75 to $100. A course of therapy therefore costs from $2,000 to

There's More to Chelation Than EDTA

This series of chelation treatments should never be considered the entire therapy. Some essential metals are removed from the body in the process of chelation. Therefore, the entire program must also consist of a program of nutritional supplements to be taken by mouth on a daily basis, and the prescribed diet. At the Atkins Centers, the diet is obviously similar to the ones that we have been discussing throughout this book. A program of exercise appropriate to the condition is also prescribed.

I have mentioned chelation as a treatment for coronary heart disease and heavy metal poisonings, but don't forget that it can be used for a variety of conditions, including other aspects of atherosclerosis, such as peripheral vascular disease (threatened amputations due to gangrene are often prevented), and cerebral vascular disease (memory loss and perhaps even Alzheimer's syndrome have been reversed).[6] Other physicians have used chelation in arthritis and in the management of a variety of other chronic illnesses.

How Orthodoxy Views Things It Cannot Explain

Once you have become familiar with the way in which orthodox medicine thinks, it will soon become obvious to you why the acceptance of chelation has had a rocky road. One of the weaknesses of the orthodox medical mentality is its overreliance on deductive reasoning. By this I mean it demands an explanation for any observed fact, and the explanation becomes more important than the observation. Many mechanisms have been proposed to explain chelation's effect, but none has been agreed upon; thus, orthodoxy has had difficulty accepting the procedure. As a matter of fact, orthodoxy refutes the fact that it works by knocking down some of the proposed reasons as to *why* it works. That's that mechanistic mentality I've mentioned before. So let me review some of the explanations of how chelation therapy works so that you may share in the confusion and understand why we need to look at *results*, *not explanations*.

$5,000. Compare this with the $6,000 to $8,000 balance due for bypass heart surgery *after* 80 percent medical coverage.

What We Know About the Mechanism of EDTA

Most heavy toxic minerals are divalent, that is, they carry two positive charges ready to link up with two negative ions. EDTA, when in the presence of divalent minerals, binds or attracts those minerals in such a way that it draws the positive charges to itself. The EDTA-mineral complex thus formed remains in solution. Such a solution, in the body, is now capable of passing through the blood vessels to the kidneys and out of the body. EDTA is best described as a pharmacologically neutral "escort" molecule that escorts divalent ions out of the body. Over the twenty-four hours after its use, chelating doctors are able to recover considerably greater than normal quantities of minerals in their patients' urine collections.

Divalent minerals, the kind that get tied up and excreted with EDTA, include the really toxic bad actors, such as lead, cadmium, aluminum, and divalent mercury; but they also include some essential elements, such as calcium, magnesium, zinc, copper, manganese, and other trace minerals. Thus the full chelation therapy protocol restores these useful minerals to their optimum level through nutritional supplementation and/or through direct administration of the mineral in the intravenous solution that contains the EDTA.

The Calcium-Magnesium Competition

Calcium and magnesium compete with one another through an ion exchange mechanism at the cell border, such that calcium favors contraction and magnesium favors relaxation of smooth muscle. The smooth muscle of greatest concern to the angina patient is that which governs the caliber (diameter) of the coronary blood vessels. Here a contraction, or spasm, can cause a lack of blood supply to the heart itself.

Recent research in cardiology points to the concept that the narrowing of the coronary circuit *by spasm* may be just as important a cause of angina and even of permanent heart wall damage as narrowing by plaque formation in arterial walls, the widely publicized concept that "explains" heart disease. The extremely successful category of heart drugs called calcium channel blockers is thought to work by preventing this type of coronary spasm.

International experts in cardiology add to this puzzle the fact that magnesium, especially as aspartates and orotates, works effectively on the coronary circulation, presumably by competing with calcium and relaxing the spasm. American medicine has not fully caught up with the magnesium story as yet, to be sure.

Now, EDTA certainly has a major affinity for calcium. The lowering of the serum calcium level is the most easily recognizable effect in chelation and is one of the main reasons for limiting the dose and speed of administering it. EDTA also has an affinity for magnesium, and losing this most valuable mineral would certainly be a major disadvantage of giving EDTA. Fortunately, chelation therapists avoid this problem by using the ABCT protocol, which calls for the inclusion of a fixed proportion of magnesium in the intravenous treatment solution. Thus, magnesium levels in the body will be conserved.

EDTA Removes Calcium

In point of fact, it was the decalcifying property of EDTA that the researchers of the 1950s proposed as the explanation of chelation's action. Simplistically, they proposed that the removal of calcium would widen the caliber of the blood vessels and thus reopen the coronary circulation. But this mechanism simply could not be confirmed.

However, there is one very important fact about calcium, which is that when a biologic reaction becomes calcified, it is no longer a reversible reaction and no longer subject to the possibility of change. An uncalcified arteriosclerotic plaque may be dissolved; a calcified one cannot. Thus, the rationale here is to decalcify the plaque so that it may subsequently be digested by various agents, as, for example, the enzyme bromelain. The original concept of calcium removal can be thus updated.

Chelation Removes Heavy Metals

But we should not ignore the original purpose for which chelation was used and that is the removal of heavy metals, because heavy metals themselves can play a role in causing heart disease. Blood vessels are not to be thought of as inert conduits for the blood; rather, they are just as biologically active as the liver or kidneys or any other vital organ. They depend on enzymatic activity, which can be destroyed by heavy metals because the heavy metals substitute for the catalyst metals that are part of enzymatic activity. When this happens the arteries are no longer viable. This mechanism may explain the effectiveness of EDTA, which, by removing the toxic metals, could then allow a return of enzymatic viability within the narrowed blood vessels.

More Mechanisms

There is another explanation for why chelation works — that iron and copper tie up antioxidants in the body, and that EDTA, by removing iron and copper, frees the antioxidants to protect against free radical damage.

To understand the importance of antioxidants, you first need to know something about free radicals — oxygen molecules with an unpaired electron in their structure. This imbalance makes these oxygen molecules highly reactive; they are constantly attempting to pair off with other molecules, and, to do so, they will attack any part of the body in which they find themselves.

These reactions are, at the molecular level, the cause of most degenerative disease, including atherosclerosis and cancer. Free radicals cause permanent cell damage; in fact, they eventually kill cells. And quite simply, when your cells are damaged, so are you. Where do these free radicals come from? Some are produced by the natural function of the body, but many are also the result of smoking, environmental pollution, improper diet, and exposure to radiation (including the radiation of the sun).

This isn't the place to go into the complex chemistry of free radicals, but protecting yourself against these molecules is one of the most basic steps toward good health. That's why the enzymes and vitamins that are called antioxidants (because they keep the unpaired oxygen molecules from running wild) are crucial. Vitamins C and E are among the most important antioxidants, and chelation is a sort of trusty bodyguard that watches over antioxidants and makes it possible for them to function.

What Does Orthodoxy Say?

I sincerely hope, if you are a heart patient, that by the time you have finished reading this chapter, you will be sufficiently enthused about this method of improving your heart function to contact your personal cardiologist and ask him: "I've heard about the benefits of chelation therapy; do you think it would be a good idea for me?" However, if you do, prepare for a blast from his verbal shotgun. If he is like 95 percent of the cardiologists I know, he will hit the ceiling when chelation is mentioned.

Orthodox medicine has a vendetta against chelation. As a matter of fact, when the delegates of the AMA met in Hawaii in 1984, they had hoped to pass a resolution condemning the use of EDTA for anything other than heavy metal poisoning. But thanks to the painstaking efforts of Dr. Garry Gordon, one of the founding fathers of AAMP, the resolution was watered down to a statement that EDTA's use in treating heart disease must be considered "experimental" and that further research would have to be done.

I'd Like to Pose Some Questions to You

Let's establish a couple of points. One is that EDTA is a synthetic chemical, first introduced by hospital-based doctors as a treatment for hospitalized patients, and it is totally within the paradigm of orthodox medicine.

The other is that the medical literature does contain some ten thousand articles about chelation, of which eighteen hundred were clinical studies (this means that the effects of EDTA in general medical conditions were studied). *Of these eighteen hundred articles, all but one described results as favorable to chelation therapy.**

Now that we have established that the attack on chelation cannot be for scientific reasons (all the clinical studies support its use), or for ideologic reasons (it's not a "different" kind of medicine), or for its newness (thirty-five years' experience on 500,000 patients), let me pose two questions: Why is chelation therapy anathema to the

---

*This information was established by a comprehensive library review compiled by Dr. Martin Rubin. It is available through ACAM.

medical establishment? and Why is chelation therapy a part of Complementary Medicine?

Three Answers for Why Chelation Is Anathema

The first answer, and I'll bet you're with me on this one, has to be "Money." Who loses if you win by getting healthy through nutrition and chelation? Well, the drug industry, the hospitals with cardiac surgery units, and those cardiologists too obstinate to adapt to a new technique. Now let me ask you: Who feeds the media most of what you learn about heart disease management? Answer: The drug industry, and those selfsame hospitals and cardiologists.

The second answer might be "Sponsorship." Recent history reveals that when chelation was abandoned in the 1960s because its orthodox adherents did not have the nutritional expertise to prevent the post-treatment backsliding, it was taken up by a group of nutrition-oriented practitioners whose successes served to take the treatment of heart patients away from the hospitals. The prospect of family practitioners getting better results than professors of cardiology was not relished by the academicians.

The third answer would have to be "Arrogance." Orthodox medicine is so lacking in self-criticism that it cannot even fathom itself as having missed the boat on anything. "If it were any good, don't you think we'd all be doing it?" is the mindless rejoinder I've heard orthodoxists apply to literally hundreds of different valid ideas.

Why Do Complementarists Accept Chelation Therapy?

But why is chelation a part of Complementary Medicine, even though it is not a natural technique? First and foremost, because it works. The pledge of the new medicine can only be: "We believe there is a validity to any true healing art. We hope to integrate all healing techniques into a workable system of patient management, and whatever works best and is safest, we must employ."

Second, Complementary Medicine has claimed the territory abandoned by orthodoxy in its self-annihilating demand for double-blind proof. The cutting edge of healing science belongs, by default, to orthodoxy's successor. *Orthodoxy is too busy proving itself to death.*

Orthodoxy is having a tough time with chelation. There are simply too many possible reasons for its effective action to allow armchair analysts to write it off without putting it to the test. My plea is this: Let's save the lives now and work out the explanation later.

15
• • •

CHOLESTEROL REVISITED

If I were to try to convince you that heroic treatments were the province of orthodox medicine, and that prevention was the neglected area left for the new medicine to deal with, many of you might think: "Hey, wait a minute. Look at the incredible campaign orthodoxy wages toward *preventing* heart disease. In fact, all our efforts to reduce our 'risk factors' are based on an orthodox concept."

Happily, all physicians, complementarists and orthodoxists alike, seem to agree that the coronary heart disease epidemic is best treated by prevention. The disagreement is over *how* that can be achieved.

I have no doubt that nutrition is the main method of prevention, but when the uninitiated deal with nutrition, the result can be just a bit simplistic. And what could be more simplistic than the idea that cholesterol causes heart disease and that the prevention of heart disease is achieved by avoiding cholesterol? Now, no scientist I know believes exactly that, yet a large segment of the public, having listened to a lot of scientific opinions, is somehow left with that idea.

How Important Is Cholesterol?

I guess I'm enough of a scientist to accept the validity of the many published studies, such as the one done on the residents of Framingham, Massachusetts, which have analyzed the likelihood of developing heart disease in terms of "risk factors." And, with some reservations, I do tend to go along with the concept that to reduce the risk factors is to help prevent heart disease.

Let's look at the facts as they have been presented to the public. The Framingham study, an ongoing study lasting thirty-plus years, was a huge research project to investigate the risk factors involved in heart disease. One of the first things the researchers discovered was that serum cholesterol (that is, cholesterol in the blood) correlated strongly with heart disease. As the study continued, and as other similar studies were analyzed, other correlates such as high-density lipoprotein and low-density lipoprotein ratios showed an even stronger statistical connection. Hypertension, cigarette smoking, and diabetes also correlated strongly with heart disease. Excess weight, lack of exercise, and type A personality (the hard-driving, anxious, ambitious personality) were minor contributors. What the Framingham researchers clearly failed to show was a correlation between diet and heart disease, and quite specifically between eggs, fats, or meat and heart disease. That is to say that, though they showed that the amount of cholesterol *in the blood* correlated with heart disease, they could not show that the amount of cholesterol *in the diet* correlated with heart disease. No one else has been able to show that, either. This is important, as you'll soon see.

Working in the Dark

The fact is that the exact manner in which, and the degree to which, cholesterol affects our cardiovascular system is a mystery to orthodox physicians and complementarists alike. Some scientists believe that cholesterol is just a marker, or indicator, of trouble, and that cholesterol levels are high in people with a tendency to heart disease *not* because the cholesterol caused the heart disease but because that which causes heart disease also causes the body to produce cholesterol. This would mean that lowering the serum cholesterol level independently of the other factors that had actually produced the heart disease would be ineffectual. Other scientists regard cholesterol itself as a major culprit. I won't be able to settle that debate in this short chapter, but I will provide you with a few things to think about.

In the meantime, I want to say very plainly that, in the absence of a clear conclusion, it is appropriate to be concerned about cholesterol. At the Atkins Center, we make it a point to treat every case of elevated blood cholesterol and, whether it is a cause or a marker, *we do lower it.*

What About the Wisdom of Nature?
Or, Cholesterol Can't Be All Bad

To those of you who believe everything in nature is for a purpose, I ask: Why do you suppose our bodies manufacture around 1500 milligrams of cholesterol per day? If you fail to eat it, your liver will simply manufacture it. This must mean there is an optimum concentration of cholesterol in the body just as there are optimal levels of blood sugar, blood pressure, sodium, potassium, or the like. If very high cholesterol levels are not good for you, neither are very low levels.

The fact is, cholesterol, a waxy, fatlike substance, is essential for good health. It is a major building block for the sterol ring, a complex chemical configuration that provides the basis for our sex and adrenal hormones, our myelin nerve sheaths, and our bile salts.

Two studies have been conducted to measure cholesterol in terms of overall life expectancy. In an American study, people with a blood cholesterol level of 200 to 225 milligrams percent lived longer than people with cholesterol levels of 150 to 200.[1] In an Israeli study, optimal cholesterol levels seemed to be closer to 180. Most likely, on a worldwide basis, the ideal cholesterol level will vary to some degree; apparently it is different for each culture.

So you see, I can't agree with the enthusiasts who preach that lowest is best. Very low cholesterol is more often associated with malignant and wasting diseases. I am happy when my patients' levels fall in the range of 150 to 225.

Now that we've established that cholesterol is essential, let's consider the picture of it most of us have come to accept.

Tell the Truth, Now . . .

How many of you understand the role of diet in development of heart disease in the following way? You eat lots of eggs and other high-cholesterol foods, plus lots of saturated animal fats, and this raises your cholesterol level. The excess cholesterol escapes from the blood into the lining of the blood vessels, where it gradually induces the formation of a raised area called a plaque in the blood vessel. The plaque caused by the cholesterol tends to build up as you consume more cholesterol, until some key coronary vessels get completely obstructed, and bingo, coronary occlusion — heart attack.

Is this the way it really works? Well, not quite!

Don't Free the Radicals!

If you were to talk to a contemporary pathologist whose field is atherosclerosis research, he would describe the events leading to heart disease in a different way. Contemporary theory — the one in most textbooks — explains that the initial damage to the intima (inner lining) of the vulnerable blood vessels is caused by, quite logically, the most actively reacting molecules in the body — the free radicals. These molecules, which I explained at some length in the previous chapter (see page 218), are unstable from the instant of their creation because they are electrically charged, by reason of the fact that they contain unpaired electrons. Just like patrons of a singles bar, these electrons seek instantly to be paired. The resultant electrochemical reaction is usually harmful to the area of the body attacked. So a *first* question is raised: How can we prevent free radical damage? (I'll answer the question in a minute; but first, read on.)

As soon as the blood vessel intima is attacked, the circulating blood platelets arrive to perform their function, which is to repair the damage. They clump, or agglutinate, over the injured spot, disturbing the smooth blood flow and liberating a platelet growth factor that attracts cells from the blood vessel intima (monoclonal cells). A *second* question, then, is: How can we prevent these platelets from clumping?

This platelet/intimal cell melange attracts fibrin, collagenous material, and cholesterol. One wonders where the cholesterol came from. Was it just there, or did it come because you ate a Western omelette, or did the body manufacture it and send it there, perhaps to achieve some beneficial purpose?

The process we have just described is atherosclerosis (waxy

hardening). In a later step, calcium comes along to play its healing/ scarring role. Calcium often reacts with a damaged area of the body, as it does when it walls off a tuberculous infection or calcifies a painful bursitis (as in, "Now I've got calcium deposits in my shoulder"). When it reacts with an atherosclerotic plaque, the result is arteriosclerosis (hard hardening). Since calcification is basically a one-way street, that raises a *third* interesting question: What can we do about the calcium?

The answer to the first of my questions is found in chapter 24, where I discuss antioxidant vitamins and minerals. The answer to the second is to take such platelet anticlumping substances as bromelain, EPA, GLA, and primrose oil. And the answer to the third question you already know from the chapter on chelation.

Implicating Cholesterol

We have just discussed the bottom line, which is that Complementary Medicine knows best how to deal with the damage caused by free radicals. But what about cholesterol? We know that it does play a part in plaque formation and that high cholesterol does correlate with a high rate of heart disease.

Some recent studies have confirmed this. In the 1987 Helsinki study, cholesterol levels were suppressed in a number of patients by the use of the drug gemfibrozil and their health course was then compared with a group of patients not given the drug.[2] There were significantly fewer cardiac events in the group that received the cholesterol suppressant.

Interestingly, the overall death rate in the two groups was found to be virtually the same. The control group suffered more deaths from coronary problems, but the gemfibrozil group made up the difference. How? They had more deaths from violence, accidents, and intercranial hemorrhages![*] What that second statistic means neither the Finns nor anybody else has been able to figure out.

Nonetheless, the results are significant with regard to heart disease events correlated with lowering of cholesterol. Although it is possible that gemfibrozil was affecting some other aspect of cardio-

---

[*] Since the same finding was noted in a cholestyramine study, it must be considered a significant fact that requires explanation.[3]

vascular disease as well as affecting cholesterol, we have no reason for thinking that. Therefore, the Helsinki study does suggest that blood cholesterol is not simply a marker but to some degree a cause of heart disease.

Cholesterol to the Rescue?

And yet the mystery of cholesterol remains. Not only is it an essential substance in the body and not only does the body produce it whether we have it in our diet or not, but there's reason to think cholesterol can act as a "good guy."

Dr. Elmer Cranton, president of the American Holistic Medicine Association and author of *Bypassing Bypass,* was the first to propose a theory that has influenced my thinking considerably. He suggests that perhaps the role of cholesterol is to help protect the body from free radical oxidation, that cholesterol is one of the body's antioxidants.[4] That would mean it is manufactured by the body as protection against oxidative damage by free radicals and that in the process of providing that protection cholesterol is converted into its oxidized form, which is harmful to the blood vessels (angiotoxic).

Dr. Harry Demopoulos points out that *oxidized* cholesterol is bound to low-density lipoproteins (LDLs) while *unoxidized* cholesterol is bound to high-density lipoproteins (HDLs).[5] This would explain why HDL is protective, and why LDL correlates more with heart disease than does total cholesterol.

What this could mean is that elevated serum cholesterol may be indicative not of a high intake of dietary cholesterol but of the metabolic and oxidative stress the body is under. If the body is suffering a high rate of free radical damage and is getting an insufficient quantity of effective antioxidants — such as selenium, vitamins E, C, and A, cysteine, and glutathione — it responds by manufacturing large quantities of cholesterol, which, having done battle with the free radicals, is converted into the harmful oxidized cholesterol, LDL cholesterol.

But the conclusion we will draw from this is not that cholesterol is the enemy; high serum cholesterol is probably just the result of the body's imbalance. The enemy is, of course, the oxidative stress the body is under, and reducing that stress solves the problem at its root. Once again we catch orthodox medicine treating a symptom, or in this case a potentially harmful indicator, when it should be treating the cause — stress and damage to the body caused by an inadequate supply of essential nutrients. The complementary approach is to simultaneously lower the LDL levels of serum cholesterol and protect the body against the metabolic stresses that cause heart disease by providing natural antioxidants and an appropriate diet.

With that under our belts, let's consider the rather wild-eyed hysteria that orthodoxy has shown in its assault on eggs and saturated fats.

The Attack on the Egg

The myth that eggs are somehow linked with heart disease received its impetus fifty years ago when research sponsored by the Cereal Institute (please *do* notice the sponsor) demonstrated that feeding eggs to animals and humans would raise their serum cholesterol level.

Recently, Bruce Taylor, M.D., of Albany Medical College, pointed out that all the compelling research of the early years was done by feeding dried egg yolk powder, not fried or poached eggs, as eggs are usually eaten. Then he proved that the dried yolk powder is an oxidized form that is toxic to the blood vessels. By rights, all the early powdered egg yolk studies would have to be thrown out as invalid. But Dr. Taylor's warning was not heeded, and cholesterol was still seen as the enemy of the heart.[6]

The Egg and Cholesterol

I treat many patients who come to me with a high serum cholesterol level, and I generally allow them all the eggs they want. Predictably, they ask: "How can you allow me eggs if my problem is cholesterol?" I answer: "The way you will eat them, eggs don't raise the cholesterol level. Almost all recent studies confirm that now."

The results of the powdered egg yolk studies in the middle part of the century,[7] have not been borne out in later studies done in the 1970s and 1980s.[8] There are now close to a dozen published studies showing very little, if any, cholesterol elevation from eating eggs. The most recent chapter in the egg saga was written by Professor Donald J. McNamara of the University of Arizona. He studied fifty men who spent six weeks on a diet containing half the typical American dietary cholesterol level, and then six weeks on a diet containing double the typical level — a fourfold increase. Two out of three of these subjects failed to show any increase in serum cholesterol when the dietary cholesterol was raised.[9]

What's Good About Eggs?

Could the cholesterol content of eggs be offset by their considerable content of lecithin, itself a very good cholesterol-lowering agent? An important nutritional axiom is that germinative foods are the most nutritious. Eggs, along with roe, plant seeds, and sprouts, fit into this category. These germinative foods, by nature's design, contain all the essentials for the growth of an organism. Further, the egg is considered the ideal protein source, containing the amino acids in the closest thing to a perfect ratio. Eggs are especially high in the sulfur-containing amino acids (cysteine, methionine, taurine), which are among the most clinically useful nutrients.

How to Judge a Nutritionist

As a matter of fact, if you want a quick test to judge whether a doctor is a good nutritionist, ask him what he thinks of eggs. If he insists that you must restrict your egg consumption, he's a poor nutritionist. If he says you must always make sure to include eggs in your diet, he's a good nutritionist. And if he says you should always include eggs in your diet unless you have a specific intolerance to them, he's an even better nutritionist.

How Bad Are Saturated Fats?

That brings us to saturated fats, for I'm convinced that in the not-too-distant future, the establishment will realize the egg scare has fallen by the wayside. At that point, even more stress will be placed on the evils of saturated fats as found in red meat, butter, and so on. If the orthodoxists attempt to show from this that a low-carbohydrate diet isn't healthy, I have an answer for them. Their statement about the dangers of animal fats is based on studies that compare two *high*-carbohydrate diets, one with beef and one without; but data from such studies *cannot* be extrapolated so as to become a criticism of a *low*-carbohydrate diet with beef. After all, in a low-carbohydrate diet, stored fat serves as the principal body fuel; in such a diet, the significance of the so-called excess intake of dietary fat is dwarfed by the effects of the body burning its own fat.*

If a study were made of the effects of a low-carbohydrate ketogenic diet (a diet in which the body goes into ketosis, i.e., burns its own fat) with and without animal fat, then I would respect its conclusions. The fact is that with the low-carbohydrate diet alone, I produced a small cholesterol lowering in my early patients. That was before I knew of the nutrients that would help me to lower cholesterol consistently — *and significantly.*

As for saturated fats, although I've produced plenty of evidence that on a low-carbohydrate diet they're not a critical issue, I do encourage my patients to consume them at a proportionally lower level than other fats. A diet high in fish, and thus high in polyunsaturated fatty acids that contain omega 3, is tremendously beneficial. Unsaturated fats such as linseed oil (also very high in omega 3) and walnut, soybean, sesame, sunflower, and safflower oils are also nutritionally valuable. Since fats are stored in the body much as we consume them, a favorable ratio of those fats to such saturated fats as beef, lamb, and butter is certainly to be recommended.

Good Results

In order to show what can be done when a low-carbohydrate diet is combined with cholesterol-lowering nutrients, I have devised a

---

*A recent study in the medical literature confirms the results I've been getting for two decades. Dr. H. L. Newbold put seven high-cholesterol patients on a low-carbohydrate diet high in beef and animal fats. The follow-up lasted from three to eighteen months, and the patients' average cholesterol readings dropped from 263 to 189. Their triglycerides dropped from 113 to 74. See "Reducing the Serum Cholesterol Level with a Diet High in Animal Fats," *Southern Medical Journal* 81 (January 1988).

tabular study on cholesterol, triglyceride, and HDL levels in one hundred patients of the Atkins Center. In order not to be accused of "stacking the deck," I have taken the cases consecutively. With the exception of patients upon whom no follow-up blood work was obtained, no one was left out.

Readers of my last book will note that a similar study was included in that volume as well. The reason I do this each time is that there is too broad a section of the population already brainwashed into an "it-can't-be" attitude concerning the lowering of lipid levels (lipids are fats, including cholesterol, found in the blood stream) with an unrestricted fat diet.

These are the results:

Results of One Hundred Consecutive Cases, All Patients
(1987 study)

	Mean Initial Reading	Mean Follow-up Reading
cholesterol	256.4	217.6
triglycerides	166.5	97.2
HDL	56.0	59.8
LDL	167.9	126.1

Mean interval between readings = 11.2 weeks.

These one hundred patients had all sorts of maladies. Some were on various medications, most were not. All were given one of the two diets listed in Appendices A and B, plus extra nutrients that I deemed appropriate to their condition. This is a retrospectively analyzed study; neither I nor the patients had any inkling they would be the ones used in the study. But there can be no sampling error, because there was no sampling; all were taken. Any patient whose initial cholesterol was over 175 and who generally followed the protocol was included.

When we did a similar study in 1980, the results were not as spectacular. In that group the cholesterol levels fell from 227.4 to 212.7 and the triglycerides from 133.6 to 84.9.

I attribute the more dramatic results in the 1987 study to the following factors: (a) The initial readings were much higher (we excluded those with low initial readings), and it is easier to lower a high reading than a "normal" one; (b) some patients had been on drugs with cholesterol-elevating effects (diuretics, beta-blockers, etc.), and the protocol enabled us to discontinue them; (c) the nutritional supplements, including the omega-3 and omega-6 oils, pantethine, and lecithin, are much more effective than the 1980 package.

Not all patients did well. There were five patients whose cholesterol went up. Conversely, there were several who dropped over 100 points. To keep things on a more personalized basis, let me tell you the story of one of these patients, an "anecdotal" instance that is just one part of the whole study.

Lou Ditizio

"I was running about twenty miles a week and I decided I needed a stress test because of my age (fifty-five) and it was summertime. After I took the test the physicians were ready to admit me into the hospital the very next day for an angiogram. They also gave me a prescription for nitroglycerine in case I started having chest pains. They scared the hell out of me! I left the hospital shaking but resolved that I was not going to have tubes stuck in my chest and arteries. That's what brought me to you, Dr. Atkins."

Lou told me that prior to the stress test, his physician had told him his cholesterol was too high.

When Lou came to see me on August 19, 1986, his blood work indicated a cholesterol level of 405 (confirming his previous readings), triglycerides 146, HDL 45, and LDL 330. His weight was in the normal range; his diet was free of red meat, heavy in fish, garlic, and olive oil, with plenty of grains, pastas, and fresh vegetables; and he exercised aerobically. He could not understand why he couldn't "break 400." In reviewing his family history, I noted that his mother, and maternal side of the family, always had high cholesterol levels, in the 350-to-400 range.

We put Lou on a generous low-carbohydrate diet (plenty of vegetables); when he reached his ideal weight, we would then add some grains. In addition to garlic and fish oils, he was given niacin, coenzyme Q_{10}, and some of the other cholesterol-lowering nutrients mentioned below.

When he returned just four weeks later, his blood test results surprised even me. Lou's cholesterol level was 181; his triglycerides reading was 105, HDL 36, LDL 124. Said Lou:

> *"I'm stunned at the results. I've done a lot of reading about cholesterol and I've never come across results like this."*

How Do You Do It, with Mirrors?

The success we get in improving our patients' lipid profiles is certainly not the result of pharmaceuticals. Because of my concern over possible adverse "other" effects, I am loath to prescribe them. Our success is strictly nutritional, and it is all the more gratifying since it flies in the face of the prevailing sentiment.

The low-carbohydrate diet must be assumed to play an important role in the cholesterol lowering, but the mechanism can only be speculated upon. Apparently, sugar has a worse effect on lipid levels than does cholesterol or animal fats.

There Are Valuable Nutritional Supplements

Several nutritional supplements have proven themselves effective. I think there is ample evidence of the lipid-lowering effect of lecithin, GLA nutrients (primrose or black currant seed oils), niacin,[10] and especially of EPA, a marine lipid, when an effective dose is given.[11] By effective dose I mean 8 or 9 grams of the marine lipid, providing nearly 3 grams of eicosapentaenoic acid (EPA) and 1600 milligrams of docosahexaenoic acid (DHA). One recent *New England Journal of Medicine* study proved the value of fish oils — the omega-3 fatty acids — in lowering coronary heart disease mortality risk.[12] It is quite logical to expect that the antioxidant nutrients will tend to improve the HDL/LDL ratio by relieving cholesterol of some of the antioxidant burden.

Other nutrients that may be of value are vitamin C,[13] most of the B complex, pantethine,[14] L-carnitine,[15] chromium,[16] guar gum,[17] pectin,[18] carageenan, glucomannoan, activated charcoal,[19] garlic,[20] mucopolysaccharides,[21] plant sterols such as sitosterol,[22] and a host of others. I am currently studying the cholesterol-lowering effects of a molecular compound including magnesium, pyridoxal-5 phosphate, and glutamic acid. It was quite effective in European studies.

All the published studies showing a nutrient-cholesterol connection have led me to the conclusion that *cholesterol elevation is more a sign of nutritional imbalance from a variety of causes than a sign of dietary cholesterol excess.*

16
· · ·

CONGESTIVE HEART DISEASE
A Complementary Approach

Allow me to pick up the threads I left dangling before I launched into my discussion of coronary heart disease, its prevention and treatment. There are three other types of heart problems that I, as a nutrition-cardiologist, am eternally grateful can be alleviated by the low-carbohydrate diet. They are heart failure, heart rhythm disturbance, and hypertension.

Remember when I said medicine can be a religion and is so for most doctors? Well, what I have learned over more than twenty years of treating heart patients turns out to be heresy to the "I place my faith in the Almighty orthodoxy" crowd. Since heretics do not endear themselves to religious fanatics, I will simply gather my facts and state my case.

Let's Start with Congestive Heart Failure

This condition, known in the previous century as dropsy, was the most prevalent of all forms of heart disease before the very modern epidemic of coronary disease, which had its beginnings less than fourscore years ago.

Congestive heart failure refers to a condition in which the heart fails to achieve its major purpose, to pump blood, allowing collections of fluid to escape from the blood stream, congesting certain vital organs.

There are two types of heart failure, left-sided and right-sided.

In the former, the heart's left compartment, or ventricle, whose job it is to pump blood from the lungs through the aorta to the body as a whole, does not do as good a job as the right ventricle, which has the task of propelling the blood through the pulmonary blood supply to the lungs, where it picks up its oxygen. Blood thus accumulates in the veins leading from the lungs and the lungs become congested. The terms *pulmonary edema, fluid in the lungs*, and *rales at the bases* all refer to this left-sided congestive failure. Its major symptom is shortness of breath, especially on exertion, but often in the middle of the night. Another symptom is inability to breathe while lying flat, thus having to sit up to breathe comfortably (orthopnea). When the pulmonary edema is acute, it is often fatal. As an intern, resident, and emergency physician, I spent more hours treating this complication — with the heroic, emergency measures that orthodox medicine excels at — than any other condition.

Right-sided Failure

When the right chamber does not keep up with the left, blood accumulates in the vessels leading to the heart from other parts of the body; excess fluid accumulated in the body, usually in the most dependent (closest to the ground) parts — the feet, ankles, and lower legs. The medical term for this finding is *peripheral edema*.

More often than not, both types of heart failure coexist. The causes of congestive heart failure (CHF) can be just about anything that affects the heart — congenital and rheumatic valve disease, cardiomyopathies (heart muscle diseases), grossly inefficient rhythms, pericarditis, drug toxicity, and the like.

The orthodox medical treatment involves treating for the underlying cause when possible, as well as salt restriction and a variety of drugs. The most widely prescribed drugs are the diuretics, which lower the workload of the heart by getting fluid out of the system. They do this by selectively poisoning the kidneys so that they no longer can conserve either fluid or a host of nutritionally essential trace minerals. A second group of drugs are called inotropic agents (drugs that cause the heart muscle to contract more forcefully), which include the digitalis derivatives. Several new agents, such as amrinone, shunt the surplus away from the blood circuit under greatest jeopardy.

I must admit that congestive heart failure is one area where some of the pharmaceuticals promoted by orthodoxy are very useful. I have prescribed inotropic agents in a number of cases and been thankful for them. Which raises an interesting general point: The drugs on which orthodox doctors place so much reliance are not bad things in themselves; indeed, many of them are splendid discoveries. What's bad is their use and overuse when there are better and safer methods of treatment provided by alternative medicine.

In the case of congestive heart failure, some of these drugs have proven to be a godsend, but here, too, nutrition therapy has a definite role to play.

The Low-Carbohydrate Diet

The low-carbohydrate diet doesn't do much for the underlying causes of heart failure, but it sure has a powerful diuretic effect. The academic research proof of this point is so well established that I won't try to annotate it. Suffice it to say that the AMA hatchetmen used this fact in their attempts to denigrate the diet, when they stated that most of the weight lost on the Atkins Diet was water loss, due to its diuretic effect. A diuretic diet, in sharp contrast to diuretic drugs, does not poison the kidneys, raise creatinine, uric acid, cholesterol, or triglyceride levels, or cause depletion of potassium, magnesium, zinc, or other trace minerals.

Encompassed in the entire field of Complementary Medicine are numerous nutritional substances that may be beneficial to the underlying condition. Add them to the low-carbohydrate diet and you have an extremely helpful regimen.

A Complementary Approach

In short, congestive heart failure provides an excellent showcase for Complementary Medicine. On the orthodox side, the pharmaceuticals — from the old standby digitalis to the new ones that are currently proving their mettle — seem to have a favorable effect (and when congestive heart failure is present we sure need emergency measures). At the same time, the advantage of carbohydrate restriction is clear, and diuretic nutrients such as B_6 and taurine and heart-strengthening nutrients such as coenzyme Q_{10} and carnitine are also proving themselves worthy of being part of the treatment protocol.

17
...

HEART RHYTHM DISTURBANCES
The Drugless Approach

One of the great categories of moneymaking pharmaceuticals is listed as anti-arrhythmics. There are about a dozen major choices in this category, and all are poisons.

In my opinion, most of the sales profit from these drugs is contrived. It is based on the combination of the interventiveness of scientific medicine and the refusal to see a nutritional, or dietary, connection in disturbances of heart rhythm.

Rhythm Disturbances

Most variations in heart rhythm are quite benign — even rather healthy people have occasional premature hearts, skipped beats, or other abnormalities. A very small percentage of them can be fatal — ventricular fibrillation is the best example of that.

There are about as many different kinds of heart rhythm as there are cardiologists. But, since we're interested in a succinct discussion, let me divide them into two groups, fixed and unstable.

As to the fixed rhythm disturbances — those which are not about to change — I do not have a great quarrel with the orthodox offerings. I find myself recommending a pacemaker implant for a complete heart block or prescribing digitalis for chronic fibrillation. My main concern is with the treatment of unstable rhythms, those which come and go, or vary in intensity. It is their very changeability that renders them treacherous.

Modern-day medical management of suspected unstable arrhythmia patients centers around a recording made over a twenty-four-hour period by a monitoring device called the Holter monitor. Because of the readings so obtained, patients who would otherwise be left alone are now on constant anti-arrhythmic medication.

The Worst-Possible-Case-Scenario Intervention Theory

Let's see how this works. Medical orthodoxy, feeling it can improve upon nature simply by applying the scientific method, loves to intervene in matters of health wherever possible. But interventive action of the type that has risks in and of itself needs justification. Medicine has solved the justification problem with a ploy I'm sure it is not aware of. It's called Worst-Possible-Case-Scenario logic.

With this logic, one can do any sort of intervention one chooses, as long as it prevents the Worst Possible Case. Now one can remove gallbladders of symptom-free patients ("It might obstruct"); one can do tonsillectomies on everyone ("They could become chronically infected"); one can perform hysterectomies on all fibroid patients or thyroidectomies on all thyroid nodules ("They could turn malignant"); or one can inoculate an entire nation against swine flu ("There could be a case, one day"). In this specific instance, the Worst-Possible-Case Scenario is that a patient who shows a run of consecutive ventricular beats (premature contractions) could go into fatal ventricular tachycardia — a not very *likely* outcome, but possible. So, to prevent this Worst Possible Case, even the innocent have to take anti-arrhythmia medicine.

The Atkins Arrhythmia Theory

For the past twenty years, I have had a theory about the cause and management of episodic arrhythmias. I have never seen a study on the subject, so I can't give you any references. But I do know that I cannot recall a single patient with unstable arrhythmia who didn't benefit to some extent from the dietary therapy appropriate to this theory.

The theory is this: Most arrhythmias are aggravated by an out-pouring of adrenaline, the quick-acting fear response hormone. This same adrenaline is a counterregulatory hormone for blood glucose, spewing forth whenever blood sugar falls too rapidly. The Atkins sugarless diets, all of which are designed to stabilize blood glucose, avoid any need for an adrenaline response, and all will have the profound effect of avoiding the arrhythmia.

Let me show you how this theory worked in one young man's case and saved him from lots of medical problems.

Michael Shepard: The Drugging of the Kid Next Door

"The doctor had me in tears. He actually told me I couldn't do anything. He told me I could walk and breathe."

Michael is the typical adolescent, and you might say he looks just like the kid next door. I first met Michael in May of 1985. He came into my office with a hospital record about a hundred pages long. His problem began with fainting spells at the age of fourteen. The first time, he was rushed to the hospital; a CT scan and EEG (electroencephalogram) were done, and they showed nothing wrong with him. He was sent back home and continued his ordinary activities, including "eating everything put in front of me, including junk food and a high-sugar diet," noted Michael.

The second time Michael passed out, he was again rushed to the hospital. The same tests were done and this time Michael was fitted with a Holter monitor, which showed a brief but definite string of ventricular beats, which was diagnosed as ventricular tachycardia. So began Michael's odyssey into the world of drug therapy. He was placed on propranolol, a beta-blocker. Shortly after, he began to complain he had no stamina and tired a lot.

"I would fall asleep during basketball practice, and I was labeled by the coaches as the kid with the heart problem. I really think the medicine affected me. I'd come home exhausted and had several incidents where I hallucinated."

Michael was not given any dietary advice, just propranolol. When he did complain of the effects of the medication, he was asked to read a medical journal article. It discussed the truths and consequences of the drug therapy and left him with the idea he would have to accept the symptoms.

When Michael came to see me he asked for an alternative to his medication and said he wanted to feel energetic again. Although a battery of tests and CT scans had been done at the hospital, a glucose tolerance test had *not* been given. When we saw him at the center he had a perfectly normal standard blood screen. But we also administered a glucose tolerance test, as we always do in these cases; Michael's blood sugar went from 82 to 176 in the first hour, but over the next two hours dropped to 31! He definitely had a blood sugar problem.

What We Did for Michael

It was pretty clear that Michael was another of hundreds of examples I've seen of rhythm disorders due to low blood sugar. I explained to Michael and his father what I proposed to do and told them that it would not be without risk, since we would be decreasing the dose of what might prove to be heart rhythm stabilizing medicine. They both agreed to go ahead. We were to cut his beta-blocker in half for a week, and then we would cut it altogether, provided he would be letter perfect in following the Meat and Millet Diet. We supplemented the Basic Formula with magnesium orotate (a recent *Lancet* study indicates its ability to reduce arrythmia[1]), L-glutamine (to stabilize blood sugar), and additional vitamin B constituents (B_1, B_6, and folic acid). Two weeks later, when Michael complained he had a problem swallowing, all except Basic Formula and magnesium were stopped. By July 1985, less than seven weeks after starting our program, we looked at a new Holter monitor readout. This time his rhythm was perfect, except for three isolated premature contractions, over the twenty-four-hour span! We saw him again in December 1985, and no evidence of any rhythm problem ever reappeared. Michael is normal, healthy, drug-free, and still on a sugarless diet. "If we hadn't gone to see Dr. Atkins I don't think hypoglycemia would ever have been brought up," noted Michael. Chris Shepard, Michael's father, reports that his cardiologist feels his son is doing well and has to see him only once a year now.

In Michael's case we again see the heroics of medicine misapplied. The Worst-Possible-Case Scenario was combined with arrogant disregard of a simple diet connection. Look at what orthodoxy prescribes.

The Orthodox Position

Orthodox medicine offers typical blocking agents, drugs that suppress the excitability of various areas of the heart, such as quinidine, propranolol, or procainamide. All of these blocking drugs act by depressing, or in truth, by poisoning an area of the heart from which an abnormal rhythm might arise. In a recent review of medical literature, reports have indicated that the beta-blockers have an effect on the central nervous system.[2] Some of the symptoms that have been noted are malaise, depression, drowsiness, and hallucinations. This is in many ways orthodox medicine at its worst. Substituting one disorder for another may cause symptoms that require more drug therapy and may even be fatal to the patient. Usage of such agents has never been challenged, because these drugs have been successful in teaching hospitals, where emergency medicine must be practiced and where most medicine is learned. However, because of this heroic approach, physicians have failed to consider even more fundamental questions, such as, What causes a person to have a rhythm disturbance? and What can be done about it?

The Nutritional Approach

It is here that nutritional medicine shines. The medical nutritionist cares about the *cause* of the arrhythmia. By stabilizing the cause, he can prevent the irregular rhythm without at the same time poisoning the heart. My experience would lead me to postulate that the biochemical upset initiated by changing blood sugar and the body's effort to compensate by releasing adrenaline-like substances is one of the mechanisms that is at work in well over 50 percent of unstable arrhythmia cases. As I mentioned previously, we don't know why some individuals fibrillate and others have premature contractions. But there is ample evidence that a rapid outpouring of adrenaline occurs when blood sugar is falling fast and that persons with rhythm disturbance do excrete higher amounts of adrenaline by-products. Besides helping to restore blood glucose to normal, adrenaline makes the heart beat faster.[3] My theory, then, is that adrenaline can cause the heart to beat so rapidly that whatever underlying instability exists within the individual will be emphasized, thus causing fibrillation, palpitations, tachycardia, or some other disturbance.

Can We Prove Our Point?

The proof of this is indirect. The proof, in fact, is nothing more than one significant bottom-line observation. That is that just about everyone with an episodic rhythm disturbance will improve clinically if placed on a diet that stabilizes blood sugar. This phenomenon is reproducible and at the Atkins Center we have observed it for over twenty years. It is not at all uncommon for a patient to say, "I did not have a single irregularity in my heart until Thanksgiving, when I cheated on my diet." I have observed this since 1964, but it is a fact that has been rarely discussed in the medical literature. Tinsley Harrison wrote about it in 1943, yet there has not been one study done to look into this striking phenomenon.[4] There *is* a recently published study describing the rhythm-disturbing effects of caffeine, a substance notorious for producing low blood sugar. It is not clear whether the effect is mediated through the glucose mechanism or is a direct, druglike effect of caffeine.[5]

Not only is there very little written information about the sugar trigger of rhythm disorders, but there is very little about any nutritional treatment in these disorders. All that exists is the logic that episodic rhythm disturbances must reflect more the influences acting upon the heart than a defect in the heart itself.

Enough Holter monitors have been performed that all cardiologists recognize the time-locked nature of waxing and waning rhythm disturbances (that is, they recur at the same, or similar, time of day). If they can be awakened to the possibilities, they will see that, along with physical and emotional stress, the daily vicissitudes of blood sugar mechanics can be observed in virtually every patient with an unstable heart rhythm.

I have often stated that the territory Complementary Medicine claims is the vast frontier between consistent observations of efficacy and medically acceptable documented proof. According to this understanding, rhythm disorders will be better managed by complementarists for many years to come. No one has even started to research this connection; no one is in the wings to prove this point.

Lessons Taught Us by Mitral Valve Prolapse

Mitral valve prolapse (MVP) is a common condition in which there is a physiologic change in the valve separating the left atrium from the left ventricle. The mitral valve is not anatomically deformed, but it does billow out, like a sail flapping in the breeze, into the left atrium. This phenomenon may be detected in as many as one out of every ten people, but only a small percentage of them have symptoms, usually chest pain and irregular heart rhythm.

When doctors began to ask, "What causes the symptoms when there is mitral valve prolapse?" the result was a little unexpected. They found that a significantly higher percentage of those with symptomatic MVP had detectable irregularities in sugar and adrenaline metabolism, two findings which strongly support the position that much of the symptomatology of MVP is, in reality, the symptomatology of low blood sugar.[6]

All too often the diagnosis of MVP leads to semiautomatic prescribing of beta-blockers, and to prescribing routine antibiotic usage during dental procedures to avoid possible bacterial endocarditis (a bacterial inflammation of heart tissue that disseminates bacteria throughout the body). Both interventive actions seem unwarranted, as both involve drugs with frequent, severe "side effects." (I use the words *side effects* in quotation marks because they are, as I've said earlier, direct effects of the drugs, not side issues. Doctors tend to dismiss these unwanted direct effects as something that might go away if given a name that implies inappropriateness.)

Our experience with the numerous cases of MVP we have treated clearly indicates that it is a benign condition whose symptoms go away when the underlying hypoglycemia is corrected nutritionally. The incidence of endocarditis on such valves is exceedingly rare.

Nutritional Pharmacology of Rhythm Problems

Every nutritional protocol we employ takes into account the dietary management and the nutritional pharmacology. In management of rhythm disorders, there is not much information from other nutritionally oriented physicians, so I call upon my own experience, which centers around the minerals magnesium and potassium, both of which have been mentioned frequently in scientific papers as being essential for a stable heart rhythm.

For example, Dr. Robert Lude and his team of investigators at the University of Southern California examined more than one hundred coronary care unit admissions and found that over half of them had deficient magnesium levels.[7] And a study of 130 patients with heart attacks (acute myocardial infarctions) was done with the sacred double-blind protocol in Copenhagen by Dr. H. S. Rasmussen and his associates. By giving magnesium (as magnesium chloride) by intravenous drip for only the first forty-eight hours after admission, the Danish cardiologists were able to reduce the number of patients who needed treatment for arrhythmias by 55 percent and the overall death rate by 63 percent. Think of the success they might have achieved had they continued the magnesium for the entire hospital stay (and thereafter). This certainly confirms the value of treatment practices of complementarists, who have been using magnesium for twenty years.

The most recent development in this story is that there are currently being conducted, in several medical centers, studies showing the benefit of giving magnesium salts to patients with mitral value prolapse. The improvement has taken place so consistently that magnesium administration has to be considered a must in MVP.[8]

The uniquely complementary aspect of administering these minerals centers around the use of orotates, the salts of orotic acid.

Magnesium Orotate Is My Number-One Treatment

Orotates were introduced into nutritional medicine by the brilliant West German physician Dr. Hans Nieper as an example of a "mineral transporter." Mineral transporters enhance a mineral's ability to penetrate cell walls; the concept implies that the minerals in question are transported as intact molecules, rather than as loose ions in the serum, to the cell wall, where the exchange of ions (between calcium and magnesium, or potassium and sodium, for example) actually takes place. I am not 100 percent certain that this mechanism bestows a therapeutic superiority on the orotates, but I have been pleased with their effect.

Other nutrients are also employed at the center in our heart rhythm control protocol. Some are beginning to be documented in published medical studies. They are potassium (we prefer the orotate),[9] L-carnitine,[10] coenzyme Q_{10},[11] and taurine.[12] We believe we have also found additional benefits in the use of octacosanol and in the herb from the hawthorne berry (crataegus).

Compare this with the orthodox medical practice of employing anti-arrhythmic drugs, whose capacity for treachery was brought to the profession's attention in a 1986 study published in the *Journal of the American Medical Association*.[13] The authors studied 123 consecutive patients with a history of ventricular tachycardia or ventricular fibrillation who had received anti-arrhythmic agents. Of these patients, 95 had side effects, and 36 of this group had major reactions. In the group studied, 23 died and at least one of these deaths was directly attributed to the anti-arrhythmic drug.

18
· · ·

HYPERTENSION
The Great Pharmaceutical Rip-off

Forgive the militant title this chapter has, but there is no subject about which my clinical experience makes me more certain. Over the two decades I have been treating patients nutritionally, at least 15 percent of them were hypertensive when they came to me. Since our patient roster has now reached thirty-five thousand names, it is fair to say we have treated more than five thousand such cases.

A review of three different patient inventories, or tabular studies, clearly indicates an improved status in more than 90 percent of those who have followed the regimen prescribed for them, and nearly 80 percent of those on medications have succeeded in getting off all medications.

The successful outcome of the nutritional management of high blood pressure has been observed so consistently that I am now in a position to safely begin to wean the patients from their medications from the very first day. In other words, I no longer have to wait to see if the protocol works; the results of frequent replication virtually assure that it will.

For Orthodoxists, Treatment Means Drug Treatment

Now that I have introduced you to the fact that there is an extremely well replicated nondrug treatment for hypertension, I invite you to leaf through any of the hundreds of recent medical journal articles informing our doctors how best to treat this condition. Virtually without exception, all treatment protocols are pharmaceutical. The treatment possibilities begin and end with the prescription pad.

Do you realize what that means in dollars and cents? According to 1987 figures of the National Heart, Lung, and Blood Association, 10 percent of the American population, or 25 million people are taking prescription drugs for the treatment of hypertension. This enriches the coffers of the pharmaceutical industry by 4 billion dollars a year.

If I'm right, and according to contemporary principles of statistical analysis, the chance that I am wrong is one in 100 million, then most of that money is made by one big society-wide rip-off.

What the Rip-off Is Not

It does not represent a deliberate attempt of doctors to defraud the public. The likelihood that elevated blood pressure readings, even though they usually cause no distressing symptoms, constitute a real threat to future health has been so well proven that I cannot imagine the most rabid anti-establishment mentality refusing to accept it. In tracking down the risks of blood pressure elevation and in making the public aware of the urgency of dealing with it, the profession has mixed its techniques of scientific analysis with the concept of prevention in an extremely admirable way. The assiduous efforts to prevent strokes and heart complications by controlling the blood pressure *before* it induces them is one of the crowning achievements of twentieth-century medicine.

It's just that the control can be achieved without resorting to drugs.

Drugs Make Their Presence Known

Millions of those on drugs seem to be doing "just fine," tolerating their medications well and having normal blood pressure readings. But many millions are achieving their blood pressure control at a price. The price is not just the cost of the medications, but the discomfort of having symptoms that weren't there before the treatment.

Depending on the drug used, the symptoms center around fatigue, depression, impotence, lightheadedness, and many more, and the "side effects" can be serious. In the case of the most widely prescribed category of drugs, the diuretics, the adverse consequences may be insidious changes, rather than symptoms that can serve as a warning to doctor and patient that a change must be made. Losses of nutritionally essential trace minerals such as magnesium, zinc, copper, manganese, and chromium are logical consequences of a drug that impairs the kidneys' ability to hold on to minerals. Diuretics are also known to disturb sugar metabolism, raise uric acid, cholesterol, and triglyceride levels, and subject patients to heart rhythm disturbances.

And the beta-blockers, currently the alternate number-one choice, cause so much depression that a recent computer survey of Medicare patients revealed that one in every four patients prescribed beta-blockers is also prescribed antidepressants.

Now I want to show you how the management of hypertension spotlights many of orthodoxy's glaring weaknesses.

Why You're Being Ripped Off

To understand the shortcomings of the existing hierarchy in medicine, you have only to find answers to this question: Why is the Atkins system not in widespread use? Certainly, it should be. It's drugless, it works better, the lab results are better, patients feel better, and it avoids side effects.

The following defects in establishment medicine contribute to the failure to adopt the better system:

▪ Medicine has, for the most part, equated "treatment" with "drug treatment."
▪ When orthodoxy uses nutrition, it refuses to use it for a pharmacologic purpose, to accomplish a therapeutic goal.
▪ Very few in orthodoxy recognize the insidious infiltration that pharmaceutical propaganda has made in their consciousness. They are sincerely unaware that alternatives exist.
▪ Orthodoxy accepts only reports in peer-reviewed journals.

Large blocks of patient data of the type I have amassed have no reality for them.

- The "religion" within medicine can accept no heretical ideas.
- The idea of a nutritional treatment was never sponsored by one of the avowed experts in hypertension, and the medical mainstream accepts ideas only from within the established hierarchy.
- The proof I offer is tabular; it is not double-blind.

What Constitutes Proof for Me

First of all, it's nearly impossible for the average person in everyday life to see something happen over and over again without being absolutely certain that the same phenomenon will continue to happen again and again. That's why a horse who wins every race will be made an overwhelming favorite by the bettors when it races again. If something happens often enough, we all come to expect it.

Well, I see blood pressure drop on my nutrition protocol as consistently as I see my office light up when I flip the light switch. I have come to expect both.

Now, with Dr. David Seegal's words echoing in my ears — "A doctor's duty is to *convince*" — I want very much for the medical profession to see the untold havoc they are wreaking with their down-with-the-blood-pressure-the-patient-be-damned attitude. In an effort to convince the obstinate of the obvious, I have completed the records of one hundred consecutive patients with hypertension to present the only kind of study that has a place in the evaluation of real medicine: a tabulation of results.

I know this effort will not convince the purists; it was not designed to be a scientific study in *their* sense. I merely hope it will convince you that there is ample justification for thinking that the nutritional approach we have been using at the Atkins Center will work for virtually everyone with a blood pressure problem,* to the extent that it should be a part of the management of every case.

---

* Blood pressure is measured in millimeters of mercury — that is, every unit of blood pressure represents the force required to lift a column of mercury one millimeter. A typical blood pressure reading for a healthy young adult would be 120/80. The first, higher, num-

We analyzed two groups of patients. Those in the first group (39 patients) were not on medication at the time of their first visit to the center. The initial mean blood pressure reading for this group was 164/102; after three to four months of their following the nutritional protocol, the mean blood pressure reading had dropped markedly, to 145/89.

The second group (61 patients), who were on medication to begin with, could not be analyzed in the same fashion, since the medication masked their hypertension. However, over the same time span (three to four months), we were able to achieve the same or better blood pressure control while in most instances removing or greatly reducing their medication. Thirty-three patients were able to discontinue drug therapy altogether; 12 patients were taking only 10 to 50 percent of their original dosage; and 6 patients were taking 50 to 90 percent of their original dosage. Ten patients continued to take the same amount of medication or more, but they nonetheless experienced a further blood pressure drop (from 165/104 to 147/93) as a result of our program.

What These Results Mean

From the extraordinarily high percentage of patients who achieved satisfactory blood pressure control following our program, I believe the proper conclusion is that the first line of defense against hypertension should always be a nutritional program similar to the ones my patients receive.

Now, I want you to pay special attention to the group who came to me already on hypertensive medications. Eighty-four percent of them were manageable on less medication and 54 percent were able to get off all medications. There are three possible explanations for this. One is that hypertension is a condition that is self-correcting. But we know that this is not so; hypertension, untreated, is more likely to worsen than to improve. Another possible explanation is that the patients' original doctors had prescribed drugs

---

ber records the highest pressure reached during forceful contraction of the heart muscle; this is called the systolic pressure. The diastolic pressure is the lower number and is the pressure recorded when the heart is at rest between beats. Both numbers are significant, but the diastolic is generally a more crucial indicator of hypertension. A diastolic reading above 95 is usually considered cause for concern.

incorrectly. But remember, my patients come from the New York City area, a city with more medical schools, hospital beds, and professors of medicine than any other city in the world. My patients' previous doctors were, by orthodox standards, no slouches. I believe the patients in the study group had been treated, for the most part, in accordance with the standards of the mainstream medical community. The third possibility, then, is that my treatment program works. *This is what I've been trying to tell you all along.*

I have a stock comment that I like to offer to my patients after it becomes obvious that their blood pressure is going to be just fine without medication. I say: "You see, you never had a blood pressure problem; you merely had a dietary problem." This is my way of emphasizing that if a condition has a nutritional correction, it must have had a nutritional cause.

What Is the Best Diet for Hypertension?

Would you believe, I don't *know* the answer to that question. I certainly *think* I know. But then, I've only studied two diets for high blood pressure. There is a third diet generally espoused for controlling blood pressure by orthodox medicine and a large segment of the alternative community as well — one based on the principle of sodium (salt) restriction. Salt restriction has had a very modest success except when the restriction is severe, in which case it works quite effectively, though it can limit the flavor of food and is sometimes associated with weakness characteristic of the low-sodium syndrome.

A low-salt diet can be made pleasant enough mainly because there are so many wonderful herbs and seasonings that don't contain sodium. But only a small percentage of patients can use salt restriction to get off medications.[1] Most of my hypertensive patients still requiring medications were already on salt restriction when they came to me. The belief in low-salt dieting is, in fact, doing our society a disservice. Too often the doctor prescribes it for a month or two, and when his patient returns with the same blood pressure, he immediately thinks: "See, nutrition doesn't work. Now where's my prescription pad?"

The Atkins Sugarless Diets to the Rescue?

My experience has been with the low-total-carbohydrate diet (Atkins Diet) and with the low-sugar diet (Meat and Millet). Of these, the low-carbohydrate diet is the more effective; on its own it solves the blood pressure problems of about half the patients who follow it. The second diet, which allows complex carbohydrates as well as proteins, is only moderately effective. The lower carbohydrate diet is the better one because there is a major diuretic effect associated with the switchover from a carbohydrate metabolism to a stored-fat-burning one.

The problem is that only overweight persons should be on the lower carbohydrate diet;[2] slim hypertensives have to rely on the somewhat less effective sugarless diet, plus some very effective nutritional supplements (more about them in a minute). I'll bet you overweight hypertensives didn't know how lucky you are; all you have to do is restrict carbohydrates, and your problem will just about vanish.

The fact that consuming sugar can induce hypertension was confirmed by R. A. Ahrens and his associates in both rats and humans, in whom he was able to raise the average diastolic blood pressure 5 points in just five weeks.[3] The hypertensive effect of alcohol has been confirmed in numerous studies.[4]

If you are hypertensive and have been "doctoring" for it, your doctor almost certainly did not place you on a sugarless diet, even though it does and will work far better than whatever you were probably told to follow. The fact that he didn't is just another consequence of the pharmacologic brainwashing all doctors are subjected to. In this case, it is not for lack of a scientifically established rationale to support such a diet.

The key concept here is that a significant proportion of cases of hypertension are cases of hyperinsulinism. Four major studies published in the "big" journals since 1985 have made that an "established medical fact."[5] These people also have glucose intolerance (diabetic tendency), insulin resistance (creating a vicious circle leading to more diabetes and higher insulin levels), and high levels of triglycerides.[6] None of this is obscure knowledge, since Stanford's eminent professor Gerald M. Reaven has been elaborating on these points for over two decades.*

* Those of you who find it necessary to convince your personal cardiologist should tell him

Now let's extend that logic toward a therapeutic diet for high blood pressure. Question: What diet completely bypasses the need to provide insulin? Answer: The lower carbohydrate diet. And that's just what we see: The vicious carbohydrate-insulin-hypertension circle is broken with the Atkins Diet.

What Else Works?

When I wrote my previous book, *Dr. Atkins' Nutrition Breakthrough,* I enthused about the protocol built around diet, garlic, magnesium orotate, and B_6. True, indeed, that protocol worked. But there have been some recent developments that have improved our results quite dramatically and have contributed greatly to the successful figures I just presented to you.

First and foremost, I can't say enough about the effect the marine lipids EPA and DHA have on blood pressure. The key to their successful use is to take enough. One needs 4000 milligrams of the two constituents combined, and many people take more, with further benefit. Medical studies worldwide are just beginning to appear, to confirm the antihypertensive effect of EPA.[7] The mechanism seems to center around providing a nutritional precursor for a prostaglandin series that has only members which dilate (open up) blood vessels and none which constrict them. (Following our usual diet, the prostaglandins generally derive from arachidonic acid, which gives rise to both effects.)

The same mechanism applies to the unopposed prostaglandin E_1, which we get in sufficient amounts only if we take in a source of GLA. That means that nutrients such as the seed oils of the evening primrose, or black currants, or borage can also contribute greatly to blood pressure control. And the evidence for this point is beginning to appear.[8]

Taurine for High Blood Pressure

The clinical value of this sulfur-containing amino acid is just now beginning to be discovered by the scientific community. It is currently being used as a preventive for convulsive seizures (epi-

about Dr. Reaven's important essay in *Lancet*, August 22, 1987, page 435, and get him to read it.

lepsy) — for which I have used it in about fifty patients, with good results — and for congestive heart failure.[9] In doses of 3 grams and up it has a definite blood-pressure-reducing effect. Presumably all these benefits derive from its ability to remove sodium from cells.

Magnesium and the Other Nutrients

I had been totally convinced of the powerful effect that magnesium salts have in the treatment of hypertension long before the doctors working with Dr. John Laragh's New York Hospital hypertension group demonstrated the consistent low level of magnesium in the red blood cells of their untreated patients[10] as well as their ability to lower their pressures by giving them magnesium.[11] The major ongoing decision centers around which magnesium preparation to use. T. Dyckner and O. Wester lowered blood pressure in nineteen out of twenty subjects using magnesium aspartate.[12] I have always favored magnesium orotate, because of my long experience with it. Basic research indicates that the orotate (as well as aspartate) molecule transports the magnesium to a position at the cell membrane where it can be most effective. I have recently supplemented the orotate with salts such as magnesium oxide in order to increase the total magnesium intake and blood levels. (Caution: Just a small amount of the oxide can induce diarrhea in susceptible individuals. It should always be started at a low dose and built gradually up to bowel tolerance.)

Minerals and Blood Pressure

In the medical journals, the mineral story is a fascinating one. Currently, there is a great deal of interest in the blood-pressure-lowering effect of calcium, which apparently has been reproduced in study after study.[13] Calcium and magnesium, as we have seen earlier, interrelate very closely. In the serum (blood), the ionized calcium *parallels* the magnesium; thus, one can raise the calcium level by giving magnesium. At the level of cell wall interchange, they are *competitors*. It is magnesium that relaxes the blood vessels by displacing calcium. Based on that logic and my own impressive (to me) clinical experience, I predict that future studies will confirm that magnesium (the transported kind) will prove to have the more powerful blood-pressure-lowering effect.

And Don't Forget Potassium

Potassium parallels the magnesium effect. Its competitor at the cell membranes is sodium. Sodium is thought to be one of the villains in hypertension, and many studies bear that out. It should come as no surprise, then, that potassium supplementation lowers the blood pressure. The first study was done on normal subjects. Soon, I presume, researchers will begin to find potassium useful in hypertensives. At the Atkins Center, we have known this for some time.

CoQ$_{10}$ — The Newest Kid on the Hypertension Block

Our success rate recently went up a few more notches, to the point where our doctors are perhaps too arrogant and self-confident in predicting success with blood pressure patients, with the recent availability of a nutrient that had been getting rave reviews in Japan. I'm speaking of coenzyme Q$_{10}$.

In one study, more than half of a group of hypertensives had a greater than 10 percent decrease in blood pressure when 60 milligrams of CoQ$_{10}$ were given daily.[14] We seem to be getting the same degree of success, but in our case, it is added to a program that has been lowering blood pressure for decades.

Our Old Standbys

Garlic — I don't know whether to classify it as a nutrient, herb, or drug, but it sure has a beneficial effect on the blood pressure. The current controversy over whether it is better to include or exclude garlic's powerful sulfur-containing constituent, allicin, is replete with lawsuits between the leading purveyors of each type of garlic supplement. Testimony has revealed that the "allicin-free" product in fact contains allicin. Both work very well in lowering the blood pressure. Please bear in mind, though, that for garlic's antibiotic, antifungal action, the allicin is the most important constituent.[15]

Another important nutrient is used for the same reason that diuretics are so popular in orthodoxy; anything that decreases the total volume of blood that circulates will lower the blood pressure. In addition to the diuretic effect of carbohydrate restriction, and of taurine, the best nutritional supplement for this purpose is pyridoxine (vitamin B_6). I have been prescribing B_6 in the range of 200 to 600 milligrams daily; this dose is enough for diuretic effectiveness while avoiding the potential toxicity of megadoses (too much can cause a reversible peripheral neuropathy, which can be seen when doses over 1000 milligrams are given without providing adequate amounts of the rest of the B complex). Instead of pyridoxine, I often administer the active form of B_6, pyridoxal-5-phosphate, in doses approximately 25 percent that of pyridoxine. This seems to avoid the small risk of neuropathy.

Rounding out the list of helpful nutrients are the sedating nutrients, such as inositol, pantothenic acid, tryptophan, and niacinamide. Of this group, I prefer inositol because of its consistently good response. The rationale for sedating nutrients should be obvious. Many hypertensives are "hypertense," meaning keyed-up, excessively hard-driving, type A personalities. Providing nutrients that neutralize these inner tensions or anxieties can help lower blood pressure when emotions are playing a role. It may be of more than passing interest that two of the best sedating nutrients are the aforementioned minerals calcium and magnesium.

It's Time for a Case History

I'd like to show you how all of the above works in concert to change a person's life. How do you pick whose case to use when you have five thousand successes to choose from? You pick the next one to walk into the office on the day this chapter is coming due. Nominated thus is Mary Campbell, and this is her story.

Mary Campbell

Mary Campbell first visited the Atkins Center on May 22, 1987. She had been on medication for high blood pressure for almost six years. Since Mary's blood pressure had always been high, she had been keeping to a salt-free diet for the previous thirty years.

Now, at the age of sixty-nine, this brisk, active homemaker was finding her physical troubles becoming almost unbearable. A month before she first saw me, she had had a hypertensive crisis with blood pressure of 200/110 and had been hospitalized for ten days. While in the hospital, she was also diagnosed as having congestive heart failure and a mitral valve prolapse. When she returned home, she found that her medications, which now included Inderal (a beta-blocker), Procardia (a calcium channel blocker), plus diuretics and tranquilizers, were keeping her condition in check, but at the expense of her being exhausted and short of breath on climbing less than one flight of stairs. She developed a sleep problem in which she would awaken after one or two hours and not be able to get back to sleep.

This prompted Mary to seek our help one month after her discharge from the hospital. On her first visit, we found her blood pressure to be controlled well enough at 140/90, and her physical examination showed her to be five feet two, 154 pounds, and *not* in congestive heart failure. Her lab tests showed the effects of her medication: Her potassium and chloride levels were quite low, she had an abnormally high alkali content in the blood, as shown by a high CO_2 level, and her cholesterol and uric acid levels were elevated. Her blood sugar findings, after glucose, showed a peak of 211 with a drop to 79. All these abnormalities were consistent with the effect of the diuretic she was taking.

I generally speak out against "routine" treatments using a fixed protocol, but in the case of any overweight hypertensive, especially one with a sugar/insulin disorder, there is a program so time-tested we do use it rather automatically. Accordingly, I placed Mary on a low-carbohydrate diet and a list of nutritional supplements to be taken daily which read: 4 Basic Formula capsules, 6 Antihypertensive Formula capsules, 6 L-taurine 500 milligrams, 6 mega-EPA, 6 oil of evening primrose capsules, 3000 milligrams magnesium orotate, 500 milligrams B_6, and 1000 milligrams calcium orotate. I immediately stopped the diuretic.

The battle was over as soon as it was begun. From the opening bell it was obvious that the blood pressure would succumb to the nutritional regimen. Visit by visit, drugs were discontinued and Mary felt better. In six weeks, she was off all medications. All blood pressure readings were below 130/84. After ten weeks she reported that she was able to climb three flights of stairs without stopping and that her walking on a level was unlimited. All her lab values went back to normal, too. Her cholesterol went from 262 to 219, triglycerides from 131 to 94, LDL from 181 to 130, and uric acid from 8.6 to 3.8.

"A few months before I came to you I had my grandson with me for a week. During that whole time I never slept, and when I took him out for a walk, people in the neighborhood, and I've lived in this neighborhood for more than thirty years, didn't even recognize me. They thought I was an old woman of ninety. Since I've been on the diet and gone off medications, I'm myself again."

Mary has been a good example of the utter simplicity of treating hypertension with a low-carbohydrate diet and the time-tested nutritional supplements we use. The fact that we began to lower her medication level before we observed a blood pressure drop indicated the confidence we had in her response to our program. The most gratifying aspect was that Mary, like most of our patients, noticed that she felt better with each reduction of medication. To me, this is the hidden benefit of not having to take medications that orthodoxy insists "you'll just have to put up with."

To Sum Up

I've just run you through what seem to me to be the advantages of being a cardiovascular patient of a complementarist. It means that if you're willing to take charge of your own health, you will probably be able to avoid a lot of surgery and medications. And for most of you, it won't be too late to start.

There is another major aspect of medical care in which the complementary system, almost by definition, can accomplish what orthodoxy is only beginning to deal with. And that's what I'd like to show you next.

PART III

...

Immune Disorders

19

...

IMMUNE DISORDERS
A Complementary Outlook

Where do you suppose a medicine based on heroics and on a treatment system requiring toxic chemicals would have its greatest difficulty? Of course, it would be in chronic degenerative conditions. Heroic measures and foreign drugs just don't get the job done. That's why the next group of conditions we will be dealing with all have such a discouraging prognosis, according to the dominant medicine. Yet with all of them, Complementary Medicine has had a notable success.

Everyone nowadays is becoming increasingly aware of the role that our immune systems play in safeguarding our health. When I went to medical school, the principle that we must "build up our immune systems," was, as now, very well accepted. The problem was, as I look back, that we didn't have very many facts to base our knowledge upon. Most of the understanding of the roles that our immune systems play in our patterns of illness has developed in the last two decades.

We now can study an impressive variety of specific elements conferring "cellular" or "humoral" immunity, along with an equally impressive array of laboratory tests which can identify and follow specific disorders. And then, no sooner was this technology in place than we *had* to use it, to follow and understand a new and frightening epidemic called AIDS (acquired immune deficiency syndrome).

The net result is that we all know that our health depends in large part upon the quality of our immune systems.

Autoimmune Disorders

Amidst all of this conversation, we occasionally hear the term *autoimmune disorder,* and judging from the many times I've had to explain this to patients, most of you probably need some help in understanding this concept. We are talking about illnesses that come about when our wonderful immune systems, for some reason still unclear, turn their wrath on some element of our own bodies, and begin to protect us from ourselves, or parts of us. The result is a chronic degenerative disease, that disease being the body's cell-by-cell destruction of itself. When I was a medical student, there were only a handful of illnesses that were accepted as bona fide examples of autoimmune illness. Good examples were lupus erythematosus and other collagen disorders, thyroiditis, some forms of pneumonitis, and other relatively rare conditions. But now that the technology for quantitating auto-antibodies against specific organs is being developed, there are more and more conditions in which autoimmunity is thought to play a causative role, and they are some very prevalent conditions.

I have picked some examples of illnesses that are now being looked at as probable autoimmune disorders, and we will go into detail about three of them. They are multiple sclerosis, irritable bowel syndrome, and arthritis. Add to this one we have already dealt with, diabetes, and you see that this type of illness accounts for a lot of visits to doctors' offices.

Degeneration and Regeneration

Orthodox medicine, in its own mind, is comfortable with autoimmune disorders. They do represent, after all, a disease process. Orthodoxists fight it in their familiar idiom with natural immune suppressants such as prednisone or synthetic ones such as Imuran. They feel they are helping if the harm wrought by the medication is less than that of the illness. But remember, degeneration is not as well handled by *opposing degeneration* as by *offering regeneration*.

Orthodox medicine has not dealt in regeneration. The consensus is simply that it is not possible. But Complementary Medicine *may be* dealing with the possibility of regeneration.

This could happen in two possible ways. One is by providing optimal nutrition. The other is through a healing art I have little discussed to this point: biologic medicine.

The term *biologic medicine* means *to treat with living cells or substances derived from them.* Historically, when the concept of biologic medicine began, it was focused on the area of providing live cells representing specific organs of the fetuses of other species. Sheep cells were the ones mainly used by the pioneers of this science, of whom Dr. Paul Niehans is the best known. Now there are dozens of derivatives, using peptides, sera, RNA material, freeze-dried and lyophilized organs plus numerous fractions derived from them.

Biologic medicine produces some profound beneficial effects. That it works clinically can be proven. What remains to be proven is whether real regeneration of tissue has taken place.

I mention this now not because I shall be telling you about our successes with biologic medicine. Our experience in this area is too short, and we have to see what the future will bring. But I want to mention that regeneration techniques, when they arrive on the scene, will be a part of Complementary Medicine, not of orthodoxy.

Let us now see how Complementary Medicine handles several diverse autoimmune disorders, and then let us see how it can support our entire immune system and contribute to the management of cancer.

20
...

MULTIPLE SCLEROSIS
It Can Be Halted

Of the three illnesses I am offering as examples of autoimmune disorders, the one most widely accepted as such is an increasingly prevalent neurological condition called multiple sclerosis (MS). It will serve to show you the difference between the old and the new medicines in treating these disorders.

But first, let me tell you a little about this illness.

The Effects of Multiple Sclerosis

Multiple sclerosis is an illness prevalent in industrial areas in temperate climates, affecting comparatively more women than men, usually beginning between ages twenty and forty. In the United States it is the most significant crippler and debilitator of those between fifteen and fifty years of age. The effect on the 250,000 Americans afflicted with multiple sclerosis varies but it ranges from minor to difficult to almost unbearable.

Multiple sclerosis can affect any part of the body, from the feet to the eyes. The disease causes scarring or destruction of the myelin sheath, the outer covering that protects the nerves. This myelin destruction affects the signals sent from the brain through the nervous system, causing anything from partial blindness, tremors, weakness, tingling sensation, jerky movements, or atrophy to a complete paralysis of the muscle involved.

The illness runs its course over a rather protracted time span —

approximately thirty years — usually waxing and waning at first, as if responding to some inner therapy. But in most cases, the neurological deficits become permanent and patients tend eventually to end up in a wheelchair, often with poor bowel and bladder control. Multiple sclerosis probably does not shorten the lifespan by much, but there are some exceptionally rapid downhill courses.

Causation: Who Knows It?

Although no one is certain of the cause of MS, there is ample evidence that the myelin destruction really begins as an autoimmune reaction. I have my own way of understanding the causation of this illness. It is just as speculative, and just as plausible, as anyone else's. To me, the autoimmune reaction directed against the myelin is the final common pathway of untoward reactions, no matter what the cause. There is not much else nerve cells can do, when in trouble, except demyelinate. The cause could be a chemical sensitivity (as to a pesticide or industrial chemical), a heavy metal poisoning (as by mercury,[1] lead,[2] or aluminum), a food intolerance (as to dairy products), or a reaction to a previous viral illness or to a parasite. The autoimmune reaction could even be triggered by abnormal electromagnetic fields in the patient's home environment. More than likely, the disorder is the result of a variety of the above. This understanding of the illness may not be provable, but it is pragmatic. It is what leads me to the success we get in treating this condition.

But I do have some information to pass on to you that's not in any textbook, medical journal, or even underground publication. I am certain that no one has ever collected as large a series as I have of glucose tolerance tests performed on MS patients. In its own quiet way, without publicity or fanfare, the Atkins Center has studied 140 patients this way. And friends, this I can tell you: There is an unusually high incidence of glycopathies, especially reactive hypoglycemia, among them. If we include tests with borderline low blood sugar findings, the figure approaches 70 percent of the entire group. We've also done a large number of cytotoxic tests, and here the reactions are considerably more numerous than the general run of our patient population. (The range of "allergic" foods usually resembles that of a candida patient.)

Further, we have studied a large group of our patients homeopathically with the Interro computer. This computer measures the electrical potential differences transmitted through acupuncture points on the hands and feet. These points reflect the condition of various internal organs. When the measurements indicate problems, the problems can be dealt with over time, either by doing away with substances to which the body has shown itself to be intolerant or by choosing proper homeopathic remedies. (The effect of these remedies can then be measured through the acupuncture points and any necessary fine-tuning can be carried out.) The MS patients present far more abnormal readings on the Interro than do other patients who are actually sicker. As we work with them, it soon becomes apparent that they are exquisitely sensitive to homeopathic remedies.

My conclusion from all this is that multiple sclerosis must be an illness that develops in individuals who are unusually sensitive ecologically.

What About the Treatment?

Sorry I had to do all the explaining first, but *there is no condition we have discussed, or will discuss, in which the difference between orthodox medicine and Complementary Medicine is so vast, or the superiority of the alternative approaches so patently obvious.*

Inflammatory language, you say? Arrogantly self-serving, you say? Well, I'm certain about this one, because (are you ready for this?) *orthodox medicine has no treatment.* And *complementarists do.*

Is There No Orthodox Treatment?

We often hear it said: "Give a neurologist an hour and he'll spend fifty-nine minutes on diagnosis. He has no treatment to offer." He has, for MS, a few symptomatic remedies, such as drugs to improve bladder control. Occasionally there are patients who respond to cortisone-like drugs or ACTH (adrenocorticotropic hormone), particularly during exacerbations (flare-ups). Heroic treatments such as immunosuppressive agents or blood exchange techniques are tried in research settings, but have never been adopted by the mainstream. In short, orthodoxy does not know what causes this illness or how to treat it. Within this paradigm, it is perfectly appropriate for a neurology professor to state to a patient: "There is nothing that can be done to help you overcome your illness; you'll have to learn to live with it. Let me know when you need a wheelchair."

The sad fact is that the professor can devastate his patient by uttering such an egregious lie without even knowing he is telling an untruth! The truth is that there is *plenty* that can be done to overcome the illness. We do it every working day with great success.

Want an Example?

My closest childhood friend became a neurologist in a major Great Lakes city (which is the very part of the country where MS is in its most epidemic concentration). One day, five years ago, he called me: "I understand from one of my patients that you have a treatment for MS. Could you see him for me?" I said, "Of course," and I waxed enthusiastic about the "breakthroughs" we were achieving in this illness with our nutritional techniques, expecting that he would ask me how we did it. But to this day, that question has never come. I wonder how many patients over that same time span he has informed that there was no treatment.

The Results We Get

Let me re-emphasize that we have treated approximately 140 multiple sclerosis patients over the last five years. Now, the condition is rather common, but it's not *that* common. Since we were in no way soliciting this type of patient, it is obvious there were lots of word-of-mouth referrals. Could this be because we had an effective treatment, or even because we offered *any* treatment?

The tabulation of our results is more frustrating in this instance than in any other illness we have studied. The follow-up percentage is too low to qualify as a good tabular study. The reason for this is that our program is based on frequent intravenous injections of an unapproved, unreimbursed, moderately expensive nutrient. And this is with a group of patients who have great difficulty getting around. Any one of these patients who experienced only modest benefit was inclined to drop out of the program.

Nonetheless, certain facts have emerged from the study. Almost all patients on our program, which I'm about to describe to you — even those who got no neurological benefit — reported a remarkable clearing of the nearly universal symptom of fatigue. And some 66 percent of those we followed reported improvement in neurologic parameters, ranging from modest to dramatic. What this often meant in practice was improved balance and better walking. Most also reported being more hopeful and optimistic about their illness, and much more able to lead a productive life.

The disquieting feature is that a few of the responders subsequently showed some flare-ups. Our data, because of the large group we were unable to follow up, do not give us a clear indication of how often this happened, but it appeared to be a minority of total cases.

What Is the Treatment System?

First, let me say that I am not one to make medical discoveries. My research terrain is in the medical library or at conferences, where I learn of other people's discoveries, and at my medical office, where I try them out.

The Atkins Center protocol for MS has two major parts. One part is the application of the principles we apply to any and all patients: *Find out what the patient needs and provide it; find out what harms the patient and remove it.* The other part is our adaptation of the time-tested, twenty-year, fifteen-hundred-patient experience of the extremely innovative German physician Dr. Hans Nieper.

The Nieper Contribution

The literature of alternative medicine is replete with articles by and about Dr. Nieper's discoveries and clinical results. Because he developed both the concept and the products involved in a series of compounds called mineral transporters, his discoveries found use in treating heart disease and cancer as well as multiple sclerosis. So, in the summer of 1981, I decided to pay a visit to Hannover to learn what I could. Dr. Nieper was very gracious and took me with him on his rounds at the Paracelsus-Silbersee Hospital and his private "praxis," as he called it.

There I learned that the key mineral transporter is the calcium salt of colamine phosphate, also called phosphoethanolamine, also called EAP. I saw patients improving on the calcium-EAP therapy and I heard their stories. It seemed to me that I was observing the first substance ever discovered to be therapeutically effective in the majority of cases of multiple sclerosis. Dr. Nieper informed me he had treated over a thousand cases (the number now exceeds fifteen hundred) and that the majority of them had come from the United States, most from the urban belt on the south shore of Lake Erie. He felt his records indicated that the progressive nature of the illness had been halted in almost all of his patients.

I Replicate Nieper's Work

I managed to locate an American cache of the German mineral transporters and began to use Dr. Nieper's program on my own patients. At the same time, I included other nutrients that American complementarists had been using with good success, especially octacosanol and a source of GLA. The diet recommendations fell into place naturally after the glucose tolerance test and food intolerance tests told me what foods my patients had to avoid. In addition, most were asked to heed Dr. Nieper's special warning to avoid dairy products.

The results were immediately gratifying. I had never before, as a physician, had the experience of inducing a remission in this condition. It was one of the most rewarding medical experiences of my life. Shortly after this, more and more patients came to my office and our learning process proceeded. Today, our treatment program seems to be far more effective than it was in the beginning, thanks to our learning how to use homeopathic computer diagnosis to locate the specific intolerances to certain substances that seem typical of patients with MS.

If ever the axiom "Health is balance, disease is imbalance" held true, it is in the management of MS. We are constantly striving to find all the causes of imbalance in our patients' very sensitive constitutions. It is a never-ending struggle, but it is rewarding.

I will now tell you about three of these patients. One is an early case, one of our first; the other two are more recent patients at our center. Perhaps the similarities and differences in their treatment may be informative.

Jason Savage: A Homegrown Response

Jason Savage, a thirty-five-year-old man, six feet five inches tall, weighing 202 pounds, entered my office showing a loss of some motor power and skill to his right side and a noticeable limp stemming from what appeared to be an atrophy of his right leg muscles. Jason had been diagnosed as suffering from multiple sclerosis some fifteen years earlier.

His symptoms began when he was in the Marine Corps and grew worse over the years. He described numbness in his right hand, burning bladder, general weakness, lethargy, and fatigue. It became increasingly difficult for him to work at his regular occupation as a house painter.

During these years, Jason had seen the best-known doctors working in traditional medicine and multiple sclerosis. He was treated at veterans hospitals, and in 1981, Jason went to Albert Einstein, a New York City teaching hospital, where a prominent doctor told him: "There is no cure. There is nothing that can be done for you. I can't help you. Go home, put your feet up, and rest in an air-conditioned room and sip lemonade."

As Jason stated in this first interview:

> "I had lost all confidence in doctors, and became extremely depressed. My multiple sclerosis was getting worse, and all of the doctors were telling me there was no hope, only continued deterioration."

The most significant findings of his initial testing were a high level of the toxic mineral aluminum, and hypoglycemia.

OUR TREATMENT PROGRAM

Jason was given a multipronged regimen: an elimination diet emphasizing the no-sugar rule to control his hypoglycemia; nutritional supplementation consisting of the EAP salts of calcium, potassium, and magnesium, plus calcium and magnesium orotates (all of these constitute the Nieper mineral transporter regimen); plus my own favorite therapies — primrose oil,* octacosanol, lecithin, and pantothenic acid, as well as extra vitamins A and C. We gave him an ampule containing 10 milliliters of calcium-EAP solution by rapid intravenous administration. I told him he would have to give himself an ampule every second day, by vein, which he agreed to do.

JASON'S RESPONSE

Within one week Jason indicated that he felt better. By the end of the second week, he noted that his depression and mental tiredness were gone, his energy was returning, the tingling in his right hand was less, and his bladder pain was markedly reduced.

By the end of the third week, Jason had no further dizziness or headaches and strength was returning to his right side. By the fourth week, he indicated that he felt like he had years earlier, with the exception of the foreshortening of his right leg and right hand, which had atrophied beyond natural correction.

THE MS SOCIETY "RESCUES" JASON FROM CHARLATANISM

During his fifth week, Jason went to visit a local chapter of the Multiple Sclerosis Society to tell them of his good fortune. There, the staff intimidated him by telling him that possibly all he was going through was the "placebo effect," feeling better because he wanted to believe so badly, and soon all of his symptoms might return. He was also told that many who had used EAP had developed kidney stones. (Not true at all, by the way.) Remembering the pains of his burning bladder, he decided to stop taking his EAP, but continued the rest of his regimen.

* Nieper states that GLA sources interfere with the role of calcium-EAP. If so, this is the first example of an antagonism of two nutrients, each valuable independently. My experience suggests that these *can* be used together with success.

In the four days Jason went without EAP, every symptom that had disappeared over the previous five weeks returned — headaches, weakness, and lethargy.

> *"I made a decision, kidney stones could not be worse than what began happening again, and now I knew that it was the regimen that was making me better."*

After six days of returning to his regimen, Jason felt better, and after another six weeks he stated:

> *"I am bouncing out of bed refreshed again. I can now work longer than I have for years. I feel like my old self again. I now have a life with my family."*

Even though Jason was one of my early successes, the follow-up is not so terrific. Somewhere along the line, Jason went off the regimen (he said it was for financial reasons), and he fell back to square one. There is no reason to assume he will not respond to the calcium-EAP injections once again, if he decides to resume treatment.

Patricia Lyle

> *"I have that sparkle back in my eyes, love being with my husband again, and feel ten years younger."*

Patricia first came to the Atkins Center in June 1984, leaning heavily on a cane. She was five feet four inches tall and weighed 236 pounds. Patricia had been diagnosed as having multiple sclerosis in 1978 after a skiing accident.

> *"Dr. Atkins, I am not going to kid you. I am here because I have no alternative and am scared to death. Recently while I was in my office my left leg gave way and I fell partially through the window, cutting my forehead and face. Over the last few weeks I have fallen at least a dozen times. No one has been able to help me. I am simply told*

*that I will have to live with my condition and should re-
duce my activities. This is totally unacceptable to me! I
talked with a close friend and she told me about your
book* Nutrition Breakthrough. *I read part of it, and here
I am."*

Patricia indicated that just six months previously, she had had a
heart attack and had had adverse reactions to the drugs she was
treated with. She now had additional symptoms: a bladder problem, which resulted in her often being incontinent; her sex drive
had "evaporated"; she had developed a twitching in her left eye
(nystagmus), which prevented her from driving; and her hair was
falling out.

Patricia received our regular battery of tests, including cytotoxic
testing. Her glucose tolerance test indicated a borderline glycopathy. She also had a slight abnormality of liver function. Her hair
analysis revealed a high mercury content and indicated she was low
in selenium, calcium, and magnesium.

PATRICIA'S PROGRAM

I began slowly to wean Patricia off her medications and placed
her on a low-carbohydrate diet for weight loss. All of the following
constituted her nutritional program: a calcium-EAP injection, calcium and magnesium orotates, the EAP salts, octacosanol, pantothenic acid, oil of evening primrose, extra folic acid, B_6, and B_{12}.
She also received our Antioxidant Formula and our Acute Infection
Formula.

By Patricia's next visit, four weeks later, she had lost six pounds
and reported that she was feeling stronger. In another two weeks,
she recounted:

*"I am using my cane less and lean on it less heavily. My
hair is no longer falling out. My eye condition has improved, and my bladder is back to normal."*

On the next visit, she told me: "I feel wonderful." She was continuing to lose weight, her nystagmus had completely corrected
itself, her hair was growing back healthier. By this time, Patricia
had received only three EAP injections. She also had been com-

pletely removed from her medications. When Patricia saw me on October 16, she was down to 200 pounds. She walked without the use of the cane and there was no limp. She said she felt as though her left side was as strong as her right. She noted that all of the conditions that had brought her to me were gone.

Diana Vargas

Diana Vargas walked rather slowly and gingerly into my office one morning in May 1986. She was putting on a brave front, but I could see her underlying fatigue and depression.

Diana had first noticed numbness in her trunk and limbs in 1979, and by the next year MS was diagnosed after a lumbar puncture. Since then the disease had followed its typical downhill course, with particularly severe exacerbations in 1983 and 1984. In the summer of 1985, Diana was hospitalized because of weakness.

> *"I was so tired that, even in between flare-ups, I had difficulty holding my job, and when I went home at night, I just collapsed."*

Diana's medications were furosemide for premenstrual fluid retention and prednisone, a steroid given to suppress the immune system, from which she had just completed weaning herself. She felt that her condition was gradually worsening. She walked with difficulty, the numbness in her limbs was increasing, and she had considerable pain and stiffness in her knees and fingers. For Diana, as for most MS patients, fatigue was nearly overwhelming.

Her lab values were typical in that she had moderate hypoglycemia, low levels of folate and B_{12}, and a pattern of food intolerances on the cytotoxic test. Her reactions were to milk and to all yeasts and molds tested — these are common in MS — plus vanilla, cashews, lima beans, and pepper.

I began treatment by putting her on the Meat and Millet Diet with no yeast or dairy products or the other reactive items. We then began intravenous injections of calcium-EAP, first one ampule three times a week, then two at a time. (Her husband learned to give these injections.) For the first month she showed no progress; in fact, she was going downhill. But with perseverance the progress began.

> *"I always felt it was the calcium-EAP that made the difference. It seemed to me I could feel the effects of those injections almost immediately, especially if I was having a bad day. Before I came to the center, I walked around feeling like my spine was made of glass. Within a few weeks, it didn't feel as if it might break. Let me tell you, that was a relief."*

With continued administration of calcium-EAP, Diana did show marked improvement. Equally important was her vitamin regimen, which consisted of EAP and orotate salts of calcium and magnesium, plus octacosanol, antioxidants, primrose oil and EPA (our basic protocol), plus extra pantethine, folate, B_{12}, and CoQ_{10}.

While the nutritional changes and calcium-EAP were operating, the third aspect of our protocol was also proceeding. My physician assistant, Dan Dunphy, was, visit by visit, using the Interro and making discoveries of intolerances to a variety of influences, such as mercury, giardia, and gonococcus. I personally am convinced that the results effected by homeopathics selected by the Interro have been responsible for a lot of our success.

Three months after I first saw Diana, her numbness was less than half what it had been, and her joint stiffness was gone. She also had an unexpected bonus: Her eyesight had improved so much, she needed a new prescription. Diana looked radiant as she told me about the changes she had experienced.

> *"You can't imagine what it's like, Dr. Atkins, to be able to walk again, to be able to do things. My husband and I go out together, and I walk as much as I want, which I haven't been able to do for years. And I'm no longer exhausted when I get home in the evening."*

Diana began to proselytize for calcium-EAP, and, at a meeting of the MS Society, she told the members about her treatments. She was surprised at the response.

"They were not at all receptive. They said people often have remissions and told me that calcium-EAP was not recognized by the FDA."

Diana decided, however, that she knew more than the FDA, and so far, like most of the other patients on calcium-EAP, she has been right. As time went on, what impressed her most was her body's reactions when MS reminded her that it was still there. Formerly, when she had a flare-up, she found herself confined to bed for two or three weeks, and she was generally unable to end the exacerbation except by taking steroids. Eventually they would end the attack, but the price she paid was an overwhelming exhaustion. Now she usually found that a flare-up could be quieted if she rested for two days. "My body gets back on course on its own now."

Diana's course has not been entirely smooth. In the summer of 1987, she got an ear infection and, in the aftermath of that, went through the worst flare-up of MS she had experienced since coming to the center, with return of considerable numbness and great fatigue. Even on this occasion, however, her recovery was quicker than it had been in the past.

"It was so good to hear somebody say there are alternatives. And everything you told me came true. The treatments changed my life. I still have MS, but I'm one hundred percent better than I was a year and a half ago."

Talk about mixed feelings! Every successful multiple sclerosis patient I have treated — and there are many more like the three I have just presented — fills me with professional satisfaction and with intense chagrin. If you are beginning to know me a little from the words on these pages, you will easily understand the satisfaction I feel. The chagrin? Well, that comes from the realization that only a handful of the victims of this illness will ever be treated in this or any other similarly effective way.

The Ca-EAP Story

Let me tell you a little about calcium-EAP. It is unequivocally the best treatment available today for multiple sclerosis, and it is effective in all autoimmune disorders. I have used it in a variety of conditions: rheumatoid arthritis, irritable bowel syndrome, peptic ulcer, nephritis, polymyalgia rheumatica, polymyositis, and lupus, as well as several other demyelinating disorders, such as amyotrophic lateral sclerosis (ALS, Lou Gehrig's disease). By giving it in greater than usual doses (two ampules daily), I have witnessed day-to-day improvement in ALS, the first time I have ever seen such a response. It is completely safe. It has been tested and found so. I have supervised the administration of hundreds of ampules intravenously and have never seen an individual who did not tolerate it reasonably well.

It is difficult to classify the transporting half of the molecule, the EAP, colamine phosphate. Colamine phosphate is one of our body's own substances, perhaps a neurotransmitter, although no role for it has ever been discovered. For Dr. Nieper, it is a cell membrane protector that inhibits autoimmune response. Perhaps it is *the* mechanism our bodies depend on so that we won't turn our immunity on ourselves. So we can consider it to be an intermediary metabolite, a nutritional substance. But to the U.S. government, it is a drug, and an unapproved one at that.

And that's the problem. For nearly a thousand of Dr. Nieper's American patients, shipments of calcium-EAP provide a lifeline protecting them against progressive multiple sclerosis. In Germany, calcium-EAP is produced by a legitimate medium-size pharmaceutical firm, the F. Kohler Company, and its approved package insert has for twenty years stated that a proper "indication" is in multiple sclerosis.

In this country, it has not been approved simply because the approval process takes millions of dollars. A lay group of Dr. Nieper's patients is trying the unprecedented maneuver of getting the substance approved by the FDA without the necessary financial investment.

The Compassionate Use of EAP

Perhaps the patient group can get the substance approved for use under the FDA provision for the "compassionate use" of unapproved drugs. The trouble is that the FDA is itself totally without compassion. All the while this dialogue has been going on, the FDA has been halting the import of shipments of calcium-EAP to the individual patients who are dependent on it.

And the bureaucrats have issued bulletins accusing Dr. Nieper of "promoting" these (you guessed it) "unproven treatments" and of "encouraging Americans to visit his clinic." I'm in pretty close contact with Dr. Nieper and I can assure you he needs to do no "promoting." With a six-month waiting list, he would prefer to slow the tide of American MS victims who are not content to "live with it."

In the December 12, 1986, issue of the *Journal of the American Medical Association,* Dr. Stuart Nightingale, the FDA's associate commissioner for health affairs, compassionately explained the FDA's compassionate position: "The FDA is concerned not only that these unproven remedies may be unsafe, but that they will deter patients from undergoing potentially beneficial — and even lifesaving — accepted treatments."[3]

I do wish Dr. Nightingale would be compassionate enough to tell the rest of the profession just what those beneficial accepted treatments are: They don't seem to know any.

But think about it. Can't you just imagine this dinner table conversation between one of the FDA's policymakers and his wife?

"Did you have a good day at the office, dear?"

"Super! Why, today alone our agents kept a hundred and ten multiple sclerosis victims away from their unproven lifesaving medications!"

What Else Helps?

The mineral transporter system, which should belong in mainstream medicine, works; but it is not the whole story.

The prostaglandin protocol, meaning the provision of either omega-3 fatty acids[4] (salmon oil, EPA, marine lipids) or gamma-linolenic acid[5] (primrose or black currant oils), can be very protective of the delicate immune systems that MS patients seem to have.

The wheat germ oil concentrate octacosanol is an incredibly valuable nutrient for the central nervous system. Dr. Carlton Fredericks used or recommended it in his protocol for patients in coma. There have been hundreds of examples, nationwide, where this nutrient has brought comatose patients back to consciousness. If calcium-EAP is the number-one nutrient for MS, then octacosanol is surely number two.

The Avoidance System

There certainly is more to do than administer "wonder nutrients." The real nitty-gritty in managing these cases lies in finding the trouble spots. Basically, MS patients are clinical ecology patients. This means they have numerous food and chemical sensitivities in response to a variety of environmental problem sources. Here our system of searching for causation comes into play.

Since the glucose tolerance response is usually abnormal, I start by eliminating sugar and sugarlike foods from the diet. Then I do a cytotoxic test and follow the leads it provides me. I look especially for yeast-related foods (the fermented ones, including anything with vinegar in it), dairy products, grains, and spices. But I always try to find intolerances that are real, that are confirmed by real-life reactions. I use hair analysis to look for any accumulation of heavy metals — dental mercury, or cadmium, aluminum, or lead. If I find it, I try to remove it by antioxidant nutrients, homeopathic concentrations of the metal(s) found, or chelation therapy.

I ask my assistant to study my patients' responses on the Interro machine and very gingerly use the homeopathic remedies indicated by the testing. In short, the patient is studied, visit by visit, until more and more adverse elements are uncovered and removed. It is a painstaking, careful, complicated system of medicine. It is not the superficial, nonpersonalized, statistical system we learned in medical school. It is work, but it is rewarding.

21

IRRITABLE BOWEL SYNDROME AND THE MANY WAYS TO HEAL IT

The more complementary physicians I meet, the more I learn about their emphasis on bowel function. It is fitting, then, that our next example for comparing the two medicines should be the illness centering around disturbances in these functions.

There is a certain commonality to these bowel disturbances, and this fact is reflected in the nomenclature that the experts offer for categorizing them. I will use the term *irritable bowel syndrome* (IBS) as an all-encompassing one, characterized by the symptoms that result when the colon (large intestine) is dysfunctional, *for whatever reason*. Symptoms are spasms, cramps, blood and mucus in the stool, frequent bowel movements, dyspepsia (disturbed digestion, usually attended with lack of gastric acidity), rectal bleeding, anemia, weight loss, signs of intestinal obstruction, and even ulceration with bleeding.[1]

Because of the increasing frequency with which the mucous membranes of the colon are being studied (by colonoscopy, sigmoidoscopy, and the like), it is possible to be more accurate in the diagnosis, and doctors can readily distinguish between a functional disturbance with few or no anatomical changes and a variety of illnesses that cause inflammatory changes. To classify the latter group, the terminologists spun off a very important subcategory and named it *inflammatory bowel disease* (IBD). Ulcerative colitis, ileitis, Crohn's disease, and others fall into this category.

As we proceed in this chapter, I will maintain this distinction when it is appropriate, but when it is not, I will stick with the term IBS. To me it seems that in many cases there is a natural progression from IBS to an inflammatory condition.

Bowel disease producing IBS is the most common complaint treated by American gastroenterologists. The probability that many types of it, especially IBD, are really autoimmune disorders is becoming more widely accepted in academic medicine.[2]

Even though IBD is a "modern" disease in terms of its increasing frequency, it has been around for centuries. There are reports of it as far back as 1769. Medical studies in 1912 are written in terms of "chronic interstitial enteritis" (chronic inflammation of the intestines). In 1932 Dr. Burrill Crohn and his associates discovered a new location of the disease. This form, Crohn's disease, was named after Dr. Crohn.[3] In this instance, IBD is found at the lower portion of the small intestine, between the ileum and the ileocecal valve, which closes off the small intestine from the "blind pouch" at the beginning of the large intestine, the cecum. When the disease is found anyplace along this route from the ileum to the ileocecal valve, it is called Crohn's disease. Crohn's disease, therefore, appeared to have an origin different from IBD in the colon, or large intestine, but does it?

My Awakening

My on-the-job education started me questioning a taught belief that the bowel illness originates in the part of the intestinal tract where the pathology is found. Instead, I came to believe that wherever the site of the illness, it may have its origin *in the upper part of the gastrointestinal (GI) tract*, especially the stomach. Actually, my awakening was brought about through the use of two uncomplicated diagnostic techniques designed by orthodox physicians but, unfortunately, never picked up by orthodoxy — the Indican (Overmeyer) and Heidelberg tests.

The Indican test evaluates the amount of a substance called indole in the urine. When food is properly digested, there is an absence of indole in the urine; thus, its presence indicates improper food assimilation. Using this "alternative" diagnostic test and finding it positive in most IBS cases, I began to suspect that the problem of IBS began when the large intestine was given the job of processing substances that were incompletely digested as they left the upper part of the GI tract.

The second clue that led me to finally believe that IBS might be a digestion problem was the Heidelberg test, or gastrogram. In IBS patients, the test often demonstrated low hydrochloric acid (HCl) production.

When I found low HCl production in an irritable bowel syndrome case I gave HCl pills (in the form of betaine-HCl) to replace the missing stomach acid. Usually the patient's condition improved. In approximately 70 percent of the cases in which low HCl was found *and* the Indican test was positive, the betaine-HCl regimen improved the condition (if a large enough dose was given). When these individuals were tested for food sensitivities (cytotoxic test) and the foods so identified were eliminated from the diet, recovery generally followed, regardless of the site of irritation. Now, scores of successful cases later, what was once a theory has become the basis for a regimen that I have found works in the vast majority of IBS cases.

The Food Allergy Connection Is More Than Proven

The food allergy approach is fully ready for acceptance into mainstream gastroenterology, except that it has not been accepted. Mainstream specialists don't do food-allergy testing. But if replicated studies in peer-review journals are what the foot-draggers demand to accept a new idea, then let them try this one on for size.

There have been, since 1982, at least eight different experimental studies published in peer-review journals such as *Lancet* and the *Annals of Allergy*. All of them consistently suggest that two of three cases of IBS or IBD will respond dramatically to the elimination of food intolerances.[4] The greatest offender, by the way, is wheat, followed by corn, dairy products, and yeast.

The Causes of IBS

No one is absolutely sure why IBS occurs at certain age periods, disappears, and then often returns. Is it a disease that is triggered by food intolerances? Is it an autoimmune disease? Is it psychosomatic? Is it some combination of all of these? Or is it that IBS is not a single entity, but rather a common response to a variety of causes?

Orthodoxists and Complementarists Treat IBS Alike?

Since the causes of IBS may be as varied as autoimmunity, yeast infection, parasitic infestation, improper diet and nutrition, and food intolerances and sensitivities, the keys to successful treatment must also be varied. *Both orthodoxists and complementarists treat IBS based on what works best.* However, there are differences in the methods of treatment, and perhaps the rate of success. Complementarists do not pigeonhole patients into a diagnostic category so that a standard treatment can be given. Their search for unique features may be leading to an understanding that, in approximately 60 to 70 percent of IBS cases, there probably is an overgrowth of *Candida albicans.* At the Atkins Center, when candida is found to be highly positive on cytotoxic testing and we treat the patient with an anticandida regimen, the IBS improves as the candida is brought under control. When candida seems not to be the problem, our basic protocol may be sufficient. In all cases, an elimination diet is employed.

Let me show you the complementary approach in action.

Christine Stevenson: The Chronicity of IBS

Christine Stevenson, a five-foot-four-inch, 92-pound eighteen-year-old, first came to see me in September 1983. She came with the diagnosis of irritable bowel syndrome fully established.

When I asked why she had come to the center at this time, she indicated that she had been suffering from IBS for the last six years and although she had seen many traditional doctors and gastroenterologists, none of them had been able to help her.

> *"I am constantly in pain. I have spasms that double me up, and the prednisone and other antibiotics that the doctors have given me don't seem to help at all."*

Her other symptom was an overwhelming fatigue. Christine was carrying approximately a straight-A average and was determined to get into medical school.

I asked Christine if she ever noticed that her condition worsened under any set of circumstances, and she said:

"The one thing I have noticed is that when I have exams my condition is impossible."

OUR EVALUATION AND TREATMENT

Christine's glucose tolerance test revealed, as I suspected, that she was hypoglycemic. Christine's blood sugar hit 120, then dropped to 60 in the third hour. This is a fairly common finding in patients with IBS. She was also anemic, another fairly common finding.

I placed Christine on a diet low in refined carbohydrates (but with plenty of unrefined ones) and began her withdrawal from prednisone and antibiotics. Her vitamin and mineral supplements included extra pantothenic acid and injections of extra vitamin C, calcium, zinc, and iron.

The following week Christine returned feeling better, commenting that her diarrhea had started to decrease and that she had more energy.

In October, Christine began seeing our acupuncturist. Acupuncture is one of the healing arts that make up Complementary Medicine. It depends on an "anatomy" and bioelectric physiology that doctors don't learn in medical school, an energy flow through meridians that represent the various organs. In Western terms, acupuncture is very useful in balancing the autonomic nervous system. Since this is the nerve pathway controlling the intestinal function, including the colon, acupuncture treatment has been consistently helpful in IBS. Christine received a total of ten treatments. After the third, her spasms stopped, her pains became less, and her diarrhea decreased moderately in frequency. My assistant complemented the acupuncture with a freeze-dried Chinese herbal combination of peonia and cinnamon.

After her seventh treatment, Christine returned to me for an evaluation. She smiled from ear to ear as she told me how very much better she felt.

"Dr. Atkins, you can't imagine what is happening to me. Although my diarrhea is there, it is so much better. I actually now have a stool rather than just water, and the pain has subsided almost completely and I rarely get spasms. I'm just feeling a great deal better."

By Christine's tenth acupuncture treatment, she no longer had spasms, pain, or diarrhea — except when taking examinations.

"When I'm studying for the exams I'm fine, and I know that I know the work. I'm even fine the night before, but when I get up in the morning and I go to class to take them, that's when it really begins to hit me."

That's the good news. The bad news is that Christine is not cured. Christine comes back to see us from time to time and has her share of setbacks. All setbacks are related to her going off regimen. Would you like to know which deviation from the regimen does it to her? Well, it's the times she has *sugar* — one more example of how we learn the major causation of most modern illnesses.

Margaret Corrigan: She Saw All the "Best" Doctors

"My life is miserable. I cannot eat. I can't plan. I have no social life. I am ready to jump off the edge of a cliff if you can't help me."

Margaret Corrigan first visited the center on January 22, 1985. For ten years she had been diagnosed and treated by clinicians at Columbia Presbyterian Hospital for ileitis, or Crohn's disease. Margaret came to me, she said, because her symptoms had gotten so much worse that she had to try something else.

She indicated that in the previous six months she had had an "unbelievable" flare-up: cramps, diarrhea, sweats, blood and mucus in the stool, nausea, general weakness, depression, headaches, and pains in her back and joints.

For the past ten years her physicians had always prescribed

medications for her condition. When she arrived at the center, she was taking 15 milligrams of prednisone daily, along with 6 Azulfidine pills.

Margaret was five feet five inches tall and weighed 110 pounds. The side effects of her medication were painfully apparent: moon face, skin infections (blotches on her face and hands), and conjunctivitis.

In 1973, according to her file, Margaret had had an appendectomy and received large doses of antibiotics. The following year she developed food allergies, particularly to cocoa, citrus fruits, and green vegetables. In 1975, at the age of twenty-two, she had her first ileitis attack. These attacks never let up. I wondered whether she had not been treated as though the symptom, IBS, was the cause of her illness.

It was obvious to me that the antibiotics related to allergies and finally to her irritable bowel syndrome. I strongly suspected that Margaret was suffering from *Candida albicans* imbalance with irritable bowel syndrome as the major symptom. I immediately withdrew Margaret from Azulfidine and gradually, over the next six months, removed her from prednisone.

On her first visit, the Indican test was positive, revealing that she was not fully assimilating her food. The cytotoxic evaluation indicated a classic candida profile: high sensitivity to brewer's yeast and all fermented foods (e.g., mushrooms, vinegar, mustard), as well as wheat and other grains, not to mention *Candida albicans* itself. She had a flat glucose tolerance curve, which suggested why she was constantly depressed. Her folic acid was low and her red blood cell count was marginally low, perhaps indicating that she was showing the adverse effects of her Azulfidine. Folic acid is the most consistently found nutritional deficiency in ileitis patients.[5] The hair analysis showed low selenium, chromium, and zinc but high copper.

TREATMENT

Margaret's system had to be buoyed while we addressed both the irritable bowel disease and the *Candida albicans* overgrowth. I prescribed the Antioxidant Formula, oil of evening primrose, zinc, manganese, magnesium, calcium, 400 units of vitamin E, bioflavonoids, vitamin C, B_{12}, B_{15}, and folic acid. I placed Margaret on a low-refined-carbohydrate rotational diet. (A rotational diet is one in which no food is repeated in any four-day period, thus making it easier to determine which foods a patient is sensitive to. Of course, we excluded foods to which we already knew Margaret was allergic.)

ACUPUNCTURE TREATMENT

On February 12, she first saw the acupuncturist. For the next five months she had acupuncture treatments once a week and continued her diet and nutritional supplement regimen. To stop her diarrhea, the acupuncturist gave her a non-milk-based acidophilus culture (milk for Margaret acted as a laxative), and a Chinese herbal combination. By the end of April, Margaret was much stronger and had more energy, and all of her symptoms were markedly reduced.

ANTICANDIDA REGIMEN

In June we started Margaret on our anticandida program, with the Chinese herbs ginseng and tang kuei, then a homeopathic candida program, and finally caprylic acid. When Margaret returned to me for a re-evaluation, she was radiant.

> *"My headaches are gone. I no longer have cramps. My periods don't even bother me the way they used to, and I don't have diarrhea. Only when I go off my diet do I get attacks."*

I indicated to Margaret that this was the proof of her improvement and that from now on she was responsible for her condition.

We continued treating Margaret for candida through August, at which time she said:

> *"I feel fantastic. Now, I always have a ravenous appetite. I eat three meals a day and I'm snacking all the time. I have gained ten pounds. I am so happy! I even have a social life again. Just getting me off that prednisone has made me see that I really am an attractive woman and*

*not that blotchy, moon-faced, bloated creature that first
came in here."*

What These Two Cases Show

Margaret and Christine are but two typical examples from my IBS
files. According to our tabular studies, our treatment regimen has
yielded an 80 percent improvement rate in a population made up
primarily of treatment failures of other physicians. This means that
both the diagnoses and treatment regimens are falling into a predictable response pattern.

Diagnosis

Our diagnostic approach begins with glucose testing, Indican and
Heidelberg tests, and especially the cytotoxic test. The cytotoxic
test identifies the nonallergic aspects of food intolerance and the
degree to which the sensitivity to certain foods can break down the
leukocytes. It is invaluable in making dietary guidelines for any
patient. In Margaret's case it not only told us what foods her body
was reacting to, but the pattern of results tended to confirm our
diagnosis that Margaret had a yeast problem, probably caused by
her frequent exposure to antibiotics.

For any patient with possible IBS, the diagnostic understanding
starts with the stomach. Complementary Medicine is always concerned with causes; in the case of IBS, the lesions are in the intestine, but the cause may be elsewhere. Suppose that one of
the causes of intestinal malfunction is that improperly digested
food particles are entering the GI tract; to find the underlying
cause you would look at the stomach. That's where we begin our
search, employing either or both the Heidelberg and Indican
tests. The Heidelberg test, you'll recall, measures the level of
hydrochloric acid production. The Indican test, which for both
Christine and Margaret was positive, detects the presence of
indole in the urine, which is an indication of improper food assimilation.

Treatment

Because of its varied causes, irritable bowel syndrome can sometimes be difficult to treat. Highly creditable orthodox institutions
and doctors treated both Margaret and Christine for six to ten years
with limited, if any success. The orthodox physician has a problem
in treating IBS because by choice (he rejects alternative approaches) he has a limited range of therapeutic options. Further,
there are other diseases that look like IBS but are not; parasitic
disease, for example, can readily pass for irritable bowel syndrome.
This confusion is further compounded by the fact that when a direct swabbing of the rectal mucous membranes rather than the
standard stool specimen is used, parasites, particularly *Endamoeba
histolytica* and *Giardia lamblia,* are found in approximately half of
those IBS cases already complicated by candida. Therefore, one is
never 100 percent sure what combination of factors causes the colon
to "go wild."

A Six-Part Regimen

There are many possible causes of IBS; therefore, there are various
aspects to our IBS treatment regimen. The basic treatment is a six-
part regimen: (1) where necessary, withdrawal from pharmaceuticals; (2) withdrawal from foods to which the patient is sensitive; (3)
a diet appropriate for blood sugar control; (4) bowel cleansing; (5)
nutritional supplementation; and (6) a "curative" regimen directed
against the pathological organisms.

Pharmaceutical Withdrawal

Unless you began this book with this chapter, you know by now
that my number-one therapy is getting people off medications
whenever possible. In the case of IBS, this may involve the gradual
tapering down and, if the program works properly, elimination of
prednisone or other steroid drugs. The risk of these drugs is so
universal that all doctors, orthodox and otherwise, agree on the
advisability of this. A commonly prescribed drug for IBS is sulfasalazine (Azulfidine), which in addition to its own list of adverse

effects is known to antagonize the effects of folic acid.[6] Folic acid, in turn, is a remarkable treatment for chronic diarrhea (see The Folate Story, p. 294). Antibiotics, another possible drug approach, may even be contraindicated in that majority of patients in whom a yeast overgrowth is contributing to the syndrome, as in Margaret's case.

Dietary Changes

I hope by now you are ready to accept the notion that the irritable bowel syndromes are indeed diet-related disorders. The food-allergy aspect is clearly the most well-researched clinical connection.

The Atkins Center's orientation to most patient care always includes an evaluation of the blood sugar and its management with a sugarless diet. It is no coincidence that both the case examples in this chapter showed evidence of glycopathy, for that is true in the majority of IBS cases. Moreover, the dietary indiscretion most likely to cause a flare-up is not so often a violation of the food-intolerance rules as it is the intake of sugar, as in Christine's case.

I was supported in my antisugar conviction by an article by D. S. Grimes, writing in *Lancet* in 1976, who opined that high-refined-carbohydrate diets helped cause IBS through the mechanism of smooth muscle spasm, which he, in turn, attributed to the reduced bulk of the fecal material in refined diets.[7] Crohn's disease patients are more likely to be sugar consumers than are the other types.[8] Perhaps that's why German researchers in a randomized controlled study were able to show symptomatic relief in 80 percent of Crohn's patients on a diet low in total carbohydrate and permitting no refined sugar.[9]

The Low-Carbohydrate Diet and Bowel Movements

Suppose you go beyond sugarless to low total carbohydrates? The advantage of the low-carbohydrate diet for IBS patients is that it slows bowel motility. In some instances, this can be its weakness. The reduction of frequency of bowel movements can be a godsend for those who have diarrhea, yet for persons with constipation, this can be disadvantageous and adequate fiber or other bulking agents must be used.

Colon Cleansing — Does It Help?

Bowel cleansing derives from a long tradition of "natural healers" who saw the accumulation of toxins in the colon as the cause of most disease. Unfortunately, this has not been an area to which orthodoxy has given much credence. Orthodoxy usually pooh-poohs the idea of bowel cleansing. I was taught in medical school that "if you have one bowel movement a week that's fine, there's no problem." Meanwhile, complementary physicians have consistently maintained that the hygiene of the bowel is vital to health. For years, colon therapists have used natural ingredients to cleanse the bowel in the belief that systemic toxins arise with the accumulation of nitrogenous putrefying waste material in the bowel.

Methods such as coffee enemas, juice fasts, large and/or steady oral doses of psyllium seed husks and adsorbent clays such as bentonite have all been used to accomplish this "gut detoxification."

Most of my IBS patients are given psyllium husks and bentonite either separately or as ingredients in commercial preparations called bowel cleansers, which in addition may contain prune concentrate, aloe vera, comfrey powder, sodium alginate, celery powder, acidophilus (lactobacillus), papain, flaxseeds, golden seal, alfalfa, vitamin C, or garlic.

Nutritional Supplements for IBS

Every patient I see at the center gets a set of diet instructions which includes nutritional supplement prescriptions. For IBS patients, after I provide for the basic needs with our Basic Formula and for any vitamin and mineral undersupply that our intake testing uncovers, I then add certain nutrients specifically for the IBS.

My pen first turns to the line imprinted "pantothenic acid/pantethine." I may give 600 to 900 milligrams of each. Pantothenic acid is the chief supporting nutrient for adrenal cortical insufficiency and can help take the place of prednisone, which does have a profound effect in relieving this condition. Pantethine is the precursor of coenzyme A, which is markedly decreased in the mucous membranes of colitis patients, even when pantothenic acid levels are normal.[10]

The Folate Story

Then I write for folic acid. Ever since L. B. Carruthers's what-should-have-been-a-landmark article in 1946, in which he told about collecting eight patients with chronic diarrhea and being able to normalize their bowel function at will by giving or withholding folic acid in a 40-to-60-milligram dose, doctors might have known that folic acid was "worth a try."[11] Certainly, the majority of IBS patients have low folic acid levels,[12] especially if they have been taking sulfasalazine. Remember the dosage problem created by the archaic and grossly inappropriate FDA regulation that limited over-the-counter dosing of folic acid to 0.8 milligrams. This means that IBS patients who do not work with a physician enlightened enough to *prescribe* the effective dose would have to take a bottle a day to get Carruthers's effective dose.

More Nutritional Tips

I will also prescribe vitamin A, because it helps protect mucosal surfaces. Research has shown that colitis patients do not absorb or assimilate oral vitamin A as well as do normals[13] and that Crohn's patients have lower vitamin A serum levels than do normals.[14]

Minerals that have been found to be deficient in IBD worldwide are zinc,[15] especially, plus magnesium,[16] calcium,[17] and selenium.[18] Zinc is a critical factor in hydrochloric acid production, which is often involved in IBS.* I usually try to see that these minerals are included in the supplement program.

---

*Remember we found that there was poor food assimilation in Margaret Corrigan's case? Generally, this means low hydrochloric acid production. The stomach's parietal cells produce HCl, which requires carbonic anhydrase, which utilizes zinc as the metalloenzyme.

The Autoimmune Aspects of IBS

I have concluded that IBS has so many causes that we don't know *the* cause of this condition, but a lot of attention is being paid to the concept that autoimmunity is involved in the causation. In the previous chapter, I described the value of the nutritional compound calcium-EAP as a protector of this autoimmune response. Accordingly, we often give this compound to IBS patients in the same dosage schedule as in multiple sclerosis.

Acupuncture and Herbal Treatment

We employ acupuncture and Chinese herbal medicine in tandem. Their purpose is to help balance the various systems that are out of balance and causing disease. In both the cases I described, the acupuncture points that my assistant stimulated related to acidic flow, neuromuscular reaction, and intestinal balance.

The Implication of Acupuncture

The success of acupuncture in this condition in many ways completes the profile of Complementary Medicine. Before I elaborate, I must tell you of our success rate, as tabular studies demonstrate. More than 80 percent of our IBS and ileitis patients have improved, many to the extent that Christine and Margaret did, to the point where they no longer "need" our services. But I must confess that we could not have achieved this result without the services of my physician assistant, Dan Dunphy, who developed his acupuncture skills to the point that acupuncture, more than diet and supplements, was the effective therapy.

Look at what this means. My axiom "A good physician will not do anything for you; he will teach you what you can do for yourself" is certainly not applicable here. The role of physician as healer, as a hands-on therapist, is in this instance the curative force. Complementary Medicine thus clearly provides for the dual role of doctor-as-teacher *and* doctor-as-healer. I trust that sensitive physicians, even those in hospital settings, will recognize that as the ideal of medicine, and will shudder a little at the role that orthodoxy expects of us: doctor-as-impartial-scientist.

Now Prove It

Suppose, just suppose, that Dan Dunphy was even more skilled than he is now and was getting a 100 percent cure rate. No matter how severe or how chronic the case, patients would walk away after a few treatment sessions as normal as anyone else. How could I prove to the profession, and the world, that the treatment worked and should be adopted by the mainstream of medicine?

There is nothing in the currently accepted criteria for proof that provides for the interaction between a skilled healer and his patient. One cannot in any way create a double-blind experimental protocol to test our hypothesis. Orthodoxy sometimes tries by substituting an inept, unconvinced administrator of the protocol and gets negative results, which may be widely publicized when it is politically expedient to squelch the alternative treatment. Two examples of this are the infamous cancer studies, headed by Dr. Charles Moertel, "proving" that Laetrile and vitamin C were ineffective. All they really proved was that there is nothing quite so easy to achieve as failure.

And so, orthodox medicine can continue to dismiss successes of this type as "unproven therapies," and continue to prescribe prednisone, Azulfidine, and antispasmodics, and to perform colostomies.

If the public cannot see that this indifference to the effectiveness of treatments not yet sanctified by double-blind proof is the single greatest weakness in orthodox medicine, then I will simply retire to writing another book about how to lose weight.

22

...

ARTHRITIS
The Great Proving Ground

If there is one single condition that can best be used to evaluate a system of medicine, that condition most certainly is arthritis. Arthritis provides enough chronicity and confusion to frustrate any attempt at healing.

Arthritis, which really is a term for a number of pathological conditions affecting the joints,* is a perfect proving ground for therapy-testing. It has features in common with most conditions we have been treating. It is widespread, chronic, has elements of allergy, autoimmunity, microorganism, and free radical involvement; it is related to diet, nutrition, and environmental influences. It is a discomforting, disabling, discouraging, degenerative disease.

Arthritis even has the politico-economic protection of its own special interest group, the Arthritis Foundation, more determined than any of its counterparts to insure its own continued existence by hammering home the Big Lie that all treatments which are non-pharmaceutical are quackery.

For all these reasons, you would do well to understand that whatever works in treating arthritis would work for most illnesses.

---

*I have discussed the types of arthritis and its nutritional treatment in my book *Nutrition Breakthrough*. Some of the discussion will not be repeated here.

Why I Think Complementary Medicine Is Better

Almost every patient who is on some orthodox treatment protocol for arthritis when he or she comes to see me shows some degree of improvement on the complementary program. You cannot get results like that in a crossover situation unless the second treatment plan is better. (*Crossover* refers to a testing system in which a patient is evaluated first on one treatment plan, then another.) The tabular study that we conducted on a recent series of arthritic patients gives you some idea of our success rate. There were 50 patients who received our program in this time span. Of these, 38 showed definite improvement of 20 percent or more (less pain or less medication required), 8 showed slight (less than 20 percent) improvement or had a variable course, and in 4 cases, the course was essentially unchanged. None got worse. To orthodox medicine, this proves nothing. With arthritis in particular, it is virtually impossible to prove anything, but I hope our results do indicate that our system is worth trying insofar as it does not have the capacity to produce adverse effects, as most of the "recommended" arthritis therapy does.

Let's look at two cases from our study group just to show you that there is still much to be learned from a case history.

Maria Diamante

"I try not to look back, but I wonder what I would be like if I had seen you in the beginning instead of those other doctors."

Maria Diamante, a fifty-five-year-old woman, came to the center in October 1983, a victim of rheumatoid arthritis. As she entered my office, it was obvious that she was in great pain, and that she could barely walk. At five feet one inch and 152 pounds, she presented that overblown look that overtreated rheumatoid victims have.

PREVIOUS MEDICAL HISTORY

Years earlier, following two operations (one for gallbladder, one for thyroid), she began having the symptoms of bursitis in her shoulders, for which she was given cortisone injections. Shortly afterward she complained of arthritis pain in all of her joints. Doctors then prescribed Indocin, gold injections, and Motrin. All medical treatments failed, and soon Maria was recommended for surgery.

In 1978 surgeons performed a bilateral hip replacement and four years later, both of Maria's knees were also replaced. Still, this was not enough. Maria continued to be in pain. The next surgery was on the big toes and then the right wrist.

This "radical intervention" (as surgery is called in medical circles) did not succeed in slowing the progress of Maria's arthritis, so her doctor returned her to a pharmaceutical routine. On the day she came to my office, Maria was on aspirin, Naprosyn (a nonsteroid anti-inflammatory drug, or NSAID), and prednisone, as well as hydrochlorothiazide, a diuretic given to offset the side effects of the NSAID and prednisone.

ATKINS CENTER'S EVALUATION

Maria's medical evaluation demonstrated the expected high sedimentation rate (the laboratory sign of chronic inflammation), as well as elevations of other rheumatoid factors in the blood. We found, as had her previous doctors, that Maria was anemic, and that her alkaline phosphatase (a bone-related serum enzyme) level was high. We gave Maria a glucose tolerance test. Her blood sugar levels went through violent swings, starting at 76, soaring to 215 at the end of the first hour, and then dropping to 43 at the fourth hour, at which point the test was discontinued because she became weak and dizzy. The confirmation of Maria's hypoglycemia, along with high insulin level, told me that Maria's carbohydrate metabolism was awry. Further, Maria's hair analysis confirmed an iron deficiency.

HER TREATMENT AT OUR CENTER

Immediately, I started Maria on a treatment regimen. We began by having Maria stop taking aspirin and hydrochlorothiazide. I also removed nightshades (tomatoes, potatoes, paprika, eggplant, green pepper, tobacco) from her diet, since foods in this family are known to aggravate arthritis. Beyond this dietary prohibition, Maria followed the center's routine low-carbohydrate diet, which also served to eliminate some widely implicated food intolerances.

NUTRITIONAL SUPPLEMENTS

Maria was placed on our Anti-arthritic Formula, to which I added superoxide dismutase (SOD) and pantothenic acid. In the second month, she received a series of intravenous vitamin drips of vitamin C (40 grams), plus 5 cubic centimeters each of vitamin B complex, vitamin B_6, folic acid, zinc, manganese, and magnesium. By mouth she was also taking bromelain, one teaspoon of vitamin C crystals three times a day, and niacin at bedtime. By the third month, Maria had received six vitamin drips. She felt stronger and was more active.

PHARMACEUTICAL WITHDRAWAL

I felt that Maria's condition would improve more rapidly if I could remove her from all of her medications, but in order to prevent trauma to her system this would have to be done gradually. As I continued her withdrawal from Naprosyn and prednisone, her rate of improvement accelerated. By February, her complaints were limited to some numbness and tingling in her joints; the pain had gone.

NUTRITIONAL SUCCESS

By March you would not have recognized her. Her ankles and wrists were virtually free of pain. The nonsurgical wrist was far more mobile and painless, and she had lost twenty pounds. On each successive visit, Maria showed improvement. In 1984 she told me:

> "When I first came to you, I could hardly walk. Now I don't think about it, I just walk without pain. I can even lift and use my right arm. I really feel good. Last month I broke my shoulder, so I had to go the hospital, and not one doctor could believe what he saw. I was seen as a

miracle. They couldn't believe how well and free of pain
I am."

Subjectively, Maria felt and looked better. What I like best is that Maria has kept up her visits to the center at regular intervals, such that five years after her first visit, her improvement has continued. Compare that to the course of her illness before she visited us, where the only relief was obtained through surgery.

Robert Kelley

"I can walk two miles a day and cycle wherever I want,
and without any pain whatsoever."

Bob Kelley was one of the more challenging patients I have treated, because he had been a patient of a highly competent alternative physician. Bob, a sixty-six-year-old retired engineer, was having severe shooting pains in both his knees.

PREVIOUS MEDICAL HISTORY

He was already on a rather satisfactory diet and he had been receiving intravenous vitamin-and-mineral therapy from his alternative clinician, so his overall health was fine. But his medical past revealed some pretty serious problems. In 1959 he had had a heart attack and in 1976 he had had coronary bypass surgery. It was his desire to recover as completely as possible from the bypass surgery that led Bob to consult with a nutrition-oriented doctor.

Although Bob was suffering from arthritis, his main concern had been his heart and overall health. He had been told that exercise was vital to his maintaining good health after his heart operation. His major source of exercise became walking. He walked two miles each day. Now walking had become very painful. Bob was frightened that a lack of exercise would adversely affect his heart. This fear caused additional stress, which itself had an effect on his cardiovascular system.

Unfortunately, the regimen of his alternative clinician was not working and so he had turned to the Atkins Center.

THE ATKINS CENTER INTERVENES

Bob received our standard evaluation, including a glucose tolerance test, which revealed that he was slightly hypoglycemic; but there was little need to change Bob's basic diet, which was a good one. I concentrated instead on the cytotoxic analysis. Here I discovered that Bob was sensitive to nightshades, yeast, cheese, wheat, mushrooms, broccoli, carrots, oranges, and vinegar.

TREATMENT

I started him on our anti-arthritic nutritional supplement formula, adding only vitamin C, extra vitamin E, and cod-liver oil. We took Bob off the foods to which he was sensitive but asked him to test his food sensitivities by eating small quantities of the suspected food at intervals over the following weeks.

One week after the allergies had been identified, and Bob had eliminated the implicated foods from his diet, he was walking with only mild discomfort. From his testing, he found that, indeed, eating the suspected foods regularly resulted in pains in his knees. By the second week of staying away from these foods, the pains disappeared. They have not returned.

The last time Bob had an appointment with me, he came bounding into my office.

*"I am free of worry because I can now exercise regularly
and I know my arteries won't close."*

He was not only walking long distances, but he added bicycling and gardening to his exercise routine. If you didn't know that Bob had undergone serious cardiac surgery, you would probably guess he was a good ten to fifteen years younger than his sixty-six years. I can't honestly say now whether what I've done for Bob constituted a cure or a remission, but he is still well.

Patterns of Success

These two cases are examples of the consistent pattern of at least partial success we have achieved. No two were treated the same and yet all were treated the same. *They were all treated as individ-*

uals with specific individual regimens. It is this emphasis on finding the breakthrough for each individual that has led to Complementary Medicine's high success rate. Yet, in spite of our successes, there probably is no single modality used at the Atkins Center that would pass muster when subjected to orthodoxy's double-blind analysis, for there is no *one* standard treatment modality that would help a majority of arthritics. The flaw in the logic is pigeonholing. The idea of reducing a multifaceted disorder into a single category will not work with arthritis, and many other illnesses, for that matter. To practice medicine well we should understand causation, not diagnosis. As these two cases illustrate, the diagnosis may be the same, but the causation — and thus the key to treatment — is different.

The Complementary Approach to Arthritis

If you have followed my exposition carefully to this point, you may be getting the impression that the treatments we use for patients with conditions as diverse as bowel disorders, headache, or arthritis have much in common. If so, you have grasped the point I have to make. The complementary approach concerns finding and correcting causation, and the same causation can cause different problems in different people. We soon learn that most causation centers around our twentieth-century diet and twentieth-century environmental factors.

In the case of arthritic patients, as in so many others as well, we look for food intolerances, sugar disorders, heavy metal accumulations, yeast or parasitic overgrowth, and autoimmune reactivity. Once the causative factors have been identified, the "hand plays itself." Remove the cause of the imbalance and the patient gets better.

The Orthodox Way

How different this approach is compared to the total sympton-relieving system of orthodoxy. Orthodoxy rarely digs deeper into causation than to recognize that arthritis (especially the rheumatoid variety) is caused by inflammation. This leads to the use of anti-inflammatory agents, which admittedly are one step deeper into dealing with causation than are simple painkillers. *But what causes the inflammation?*

If you are concerned enough to seek an answer to that question, you are not orthodox; in fact, you are a quack. And if you use agents that protect against this type of causation, you are using quackery. That is, if you can believe the organization that speaks for orthodox rheumatologists, the Arthritis Foundation. This powerful entity is really worth scrutinizing, for it, more than any other, save perhaps the American Cancer Society, shows you exactly what is wrong with American medicine.

What Is the Arthritis Foundation?

The Arthritis Foundation is a typical example of a large, extremely influential, private, nonprofit foundation. Headquartered in Atlanta (as is the Coca-Cola Company, one of its benefactors), the foundation has seventy-one chapters and over 150 offices nationwide. It publishes newsletters and numerous free pamphets and booklets for the general public, as well as the medical journal *Arthritis and Rheumatism,* the bible for most American rheumatologists. The Arthritis Foundation's activities serve to illustrate a point I made earlier, when I voiced my concern over the role that financial considerations play in the control of a medicine that is deeply rooted in establishment economics.

The Arthritis Foundation has grown large with charitable contributions from a naive public, all of whom give willingly in the unselfish belief that their bequests will somehow benefit victims of arthritis. The sad fact is, these dollars have contributed more to the perpetuation of arthritis than its eradication.

My Evidence Speaks for Itself

All you have to do is study some of the many documents the Arthritis Foundation has released in its vigorous campaign to "educate" the public as to how arthritic patients should be treated. Let's start with its published statement of purpose. In addition to finding "the cause and cure for the many forms of arthritis" and to providing services to patients, the foundation's purpose is to create public understanding of these diseases and to "combat unproven remedies." Well, the foundation is quite up front about this, and for that I give them *credit*. If someone else is foolish enough to give them *money*, then we're all in trouble.

Who Benefits When Unproven Remedies Are Combated?

Unless you started the book with this chapter, you must, by now, absolutely know for an unchallenged fact that many of *today's unproven remedies are tomorrow's established therapies*. Who but an utter misanthrope would lock himself in *combat* with these promising leads to relief from this disabling condition? Somebody who was "raking it in" with the present system, that's who. The Arthritis Foundation, for one.

And combat the fledgling therapies they do. They fight them with vigor, venom, virulence, and a vast volume of vocal, vicious, and vengeful vilification and vituperation. (Sorry, gang, just showing off.)

The Pamphlets Speak

One pamphlet, entitled "Arthritis, Unproven Remedies," urges its readers to "be wary" and "be suspicious of" a roster of treatments that looks to me, speaking now as a physician who has been busting his gut for twenty years seeking ways to help my arthritic patients, to read like a *Who's Who in Effective Treatment for Arthritis*.[1] On the list of quack remedies are the allergy elimination diet, nonightshade diet, vitamins, cod-liver oil, homeopathy, acupuncture, herbs and botanicals — all the basics that no compassionate doctor who wants to help his patients would dare be without.

The Foundation's Idea of Real Medicine

Lest you think the Arthritis Foundation does not have a therapeutic suggestion, let me assure you that nothing could be further from the truth. In the pamphlet "Arthritis, Basic Facts and Answers to

Your Questions,"[2] you see what the Arthritis Foundation considers to be good, proven medicine. The entire gamut of therapy runs from toxic drug A clear through to toxic drug Z, with a little surgery in between.

Without exception, every drug on the Arthritis Foundation's "recommended" list has great potential for toxicity, not as "side effects," but as direct harmful effects explainable on the basis of the known action of the drug. That's why so much treatment of arthritic patients must be handled by experienced rheumatologists. By my definition, a rheumatologist is a joint disease specialist so skillful that he is able to simultaneously administer six different extremely toxic drugs in such a way that his patients remain breathing.

Complementary Techniques in Arthritis

This concludes our accentuation of the negatives, so that we can briefly review our therapeutic protocol. There are dozens of types of arthritis and millions of cases. Since our treatment is individualized, there is a potential for millions of treatment outlines. But there are certain basic principles.

The Arthritis Foundation's position statement that diet has no role in arthritis notwithstanding, the first principle *is* an avoidance diet. Avoid sugar, avoid nightshades, avoid whatever you are addicted to, and avoid the foods indicated to be problem areas in food-intolerance testing. Second, there *are* anti-arthritic foods — central among which are the oils which lead to omega-3 fatty acids (salmon or cod-liver oils or linseed oil) or to PGE_1 (primrose, black currant oils).

There Is a Diet-Arthritis Connection, Admit It

The last decade has witnessed the beginnings of what promises to be a long series of studies confirming the value of intolerance-elimination diets. In 1979 Scandinavian researchers were able to effect an improvement of a majority of rheumatoid arthritis (RA) patients who require NSAIDs (nonsteroid anti-inflammatory drugs) with a seven-to-ten-day juice fast.[3]

Then, J. A. Hicklin produced "objective improvement" in 20 out of 22 RA patients within eighteen days on an allergic-exclusion diet (after testing for allergies).[4] More recently, a really significant study by L. G. Darlington was published in *Lancet*. In this blind, placebo-controlled study, improvement was effected in 33 out of 45 RA patients simply by eliminating the allergenic foods. I have located three other studies that help prove the point that diet and arthritis *are* connected.[5] Meanwhile, the NSAIDs, the most widely prescribed *drug* category, have been shown to increase intestinal permeability to food antigens, the very mechanism thought to underlie nonallergic food intolerances.[6] How can the Arthritis Foundation ignore these findings?

Nutritional Supplements in Arthritis

In *Dr. Atkins' Nutrition Breakthrough* I described how I used library research on nutrients for arthritis, plus a belief in the teamwork of nutrients, to come up with a formula combining vitamins B$_6$, niacinamide, pantothenic acid, PABA, vitamin C and bioflavonoids, and vitamin E, plus zinc and copper to produce a single tablet that the arthritic patients at the center could take.*

In terms of rate of clinical response, this formula was more successful than any other formula we use at the center and contributed greatly to our 92 percent improvement rate. Maria and Bob both received this as foundation therapy. I believe that the updated formula, which you will see in Appendix C, by adding selenium and L-cysteine and doubling the manganese content, will provide even greater success.

Reviewing the Medical Studies

Supportive studies in the medical literature are still spotty, largely because, I believe, of the organized opposition to nutrition. But Dr. E. C. Barton-Wright's studies about the value of pantothenic acid were eventually picked up by the General Practitioners Research Group in the United Kingdom. They reported on a double-

---

*I later updated this formula (see Appendix C), adding certain nutrients and at the same time taking out others that were included in our updated Basic Formula.

blind study in rheumatoid arthritis in which pantothenic acid alone, in doses of 500 to 2000 milligrams, produced significant reduction in morning stiffness, pain severity, and degree of disability.[7]

There have also been studies on the decrease of vitamin C levels in rheumatoid arthritis patients, and the mechanism of its action has been elucidated; but still more research needs to be done to show with absolute clarity vitamin C's rather obvious (to me) beneficial effect.[8]

The Copper-FDA Saga

Meanwhile, research into the anti-inflammatory, anti-arthritic effect of copper has proceeded in a most impressive manner under the guidance of John R. L. Sorensen of Little Rock, Arkansas. The salicylate form seems still to be the most effective.[9] You'll *know* it is good when I tell you this: The FDA has made the sale of copper salicylate illegal. As a card-carrying FDA watcher, I find time and again that the FDA has an unerring record of acting only on nutrients that *work*. This is not as much of an exaggeration as it seems, for the FDA is interested in protecting its jurisdiction over drugs (which it defines as anything used in the treatment of illness). When a nutritional agent is proven to work, the FDA feels compelled to remove it from commerce as an untested new drug. Nothing that cures disease can be administered without its permission. Ineffective nutrients, on the other hand, it almost never deigns to notice. What, after all, would be the point?

In all fairness to the FDA, I must point out that it has taken the position that copper salicylate is a drug and must be submitted for study as such. In all fairness to arthritics, that simply is not going to happen. This is a nontoxic, extremely effective, proven substance that could help millions of people. Does anyone in Washington care?

The Fatty Acids, Once More

The real breakthrough of the 1980s is the ongoing work with the EPA-containing fish oils (omega-3 fatty acids) and the gamma omega-6 fatty acids (primrose oil). It is already clear from the studies that *both* have a favorable effect on rheumatoid arthritis.[10] In one Scandinavian study, the researchers did a controlled study minus the immorality or unethicality of a placebo study. One half of the group got standard NSAID therapy (so they received an acceptable standard treatment); the other half got primrose oil, combined with the cofactors zinc, vitamin C, niacin, and B_6 (all favorites of ours). The two groups did equally well with the arthritis, but the nutritionally treated group was not subject to the NSAID side effects![11]

Our Program

All of this discussion leads to our supplementing the Anti-arthritic Formula with 6 capsules or so of primrose oil, EPA and/or linseed oil, antioxidants, more copper, superoxide dismutase,[12] L-histidine,[13] quercetin, or more zinc or selenium.

Our basic approach for arthritis patients runs like this. We begin with the appropriate avoidance diet and nutritional supplements I just outlined. But I tell my patients that we are holding a trump card, the opportunity of giving an injectable program. Among the biologic substances available for injectable programs are high doses of vitamin C (intravenous) with the key minerals and B vitamins, calcium-EAP (see chapter 20), the penetrating carrier molecule DMSO,* ozone therapy,† and a series of biologicals that derive from fetal synovial (joint) cells.

As you can see from this list, complementarists can choose from a wide range of nontoxic therapies, and our European counterparts have another dozen or so time- and experience-tested biological therapies to call upon.

My Conclusions

I know of no condition for which there are more effective treatments that obviously work but whose success is greeted with more

---

*DMSO is an industrial chemical with remarkable properties of penetrating biologic cell membranes. It recently received FDA approval for the treatment of interstitial cystitis. Its therapeutic potential extends far beyond that, according to Dr. Stanley Jacob, its leading proponent.

†The administration of ozone also has widespread clinical applications. It is virucidal and bacteriocidal, yet seems to have a supportive effect on the immune system.

across-the-board denial by the establishment propagandists than the various forms of arthritis.

Any arthritic who can overcome the brainwashing we've all been exposed to can get significant relief from arthritis, and even more significant relief from the unpleasant drugs used to treat arthritis. I realize this statement qualifies me on several counts to be a quack according to the Arthritis Foundation's self-serving definition. But let me serve notice that this is one quack who (a) has the arthritic patients' best interests at heart and (b) has the documented results to back up his statement.

23

. . .

CANCER THERAPY
Orthodoxy's Most Willful Negligence

Sometimes the difference between an entrenched medical system and my nominee for the incoming new system is merely the superiority of one technique over the other. But at other times, it can be a matter of life or death.

There is no better example of the weaknesses of our dominant medicine than its clearly ineffective War on Cancer. There is no better example of the superiority of a complementary approach than in the management of this dread disease.

As much as this book concerns the issue of whether the old orthodoxy must be replaced by a contemporary medicine whose scope grows exponentially when other healing arts are added to it, we are equally concerned about whether mainstream medicine's demand for proof works to maintain it at its current level of ineptitude.

Anecdotal Evidence Revisited

I have repeatedly claimed that one can glean really valuable information from case histories and that these case histories *can* be used to establish proof of a sufficient degree to change one's course of action. In a few moments I am going to ask you to do some serious soul-searching. I am going to ask you the following question: Could there be a *single* case history that could cause you to reject the advice strongly urged upon you by a cancer specialist and to pursue a course he did not approve? Form your answer carefully, because your conclusion may one day save — or cost — the life of a loved one, or your own.

Pauline Platten: Case in Point

"Logically, I knew I was going to die. But I didn't feel I was going to die. I was simply angry. I had read everything I could get my hands on about what alternatives I might have and came to ask you where to go. When I found you had been thinking about all of them, I felt this was the place for me."

Pauline Platten was a vigorous, active, sixty-two-year-old housewife and retired attorney when she and her husband, a prominent suburban dentist, went away for their Christmas 1985 vacation to Puerto Rico. Neither was alarmed when, after exposure to the tropical sun, her skin turned dark. On her return, she accompanied her husband on *his* visit to their family internist. Upon seeing Pauline, the doctor exclaimed: "My God, your eyes are *yellow*."

On January 12, 1986, Pauline was admitted to Winthrop University Hospital, a teaching institution affiliated with the Stony Brook College of Medicine. Hepatitis was quickly ruled out, obstructive jaundice was ruled in, and in a few days Pauline underwent surgery in which a shunting procedure was done to relieve her obstruction. The surgeon's worst suspicion was confirmed: an inoperable cancer in the head of the pancreas, and the biopsy confirmed it to be a typical pancreatic adenocarcinoma with extension to the lymph nodes.

WHAT DOES PANCREATIC CANCER MEAN?

In orthodox circles, a diagnosis of inoperable adenocarcinoma of the pancreas is as certain a death sentence as is a midair plane crash. Every year, twenty-five thousand Americans get this diagnosis and twenty-five thousand of them die. Official statistics claim a one-year survival rate of 2 percent. Those "lucky" five hundred consist principally of four groups: (a) cases in which there was a successful surgical resection, (b) cases of the less virulent islet cell carcinoma, (c) incorrect diagnoses, and (d) patients who received alternative therapy.

Notice that chemotherapy does not work here, not even a little bit. One recent study compared three different chemotherapy protocols with untreated controls — *all lived only three months*. And I can guarantee you that those who were subjected to the chemotherapy had a much *sicker* three months than those who were not.

CHEMOTHERAPY AS A FAIT ACCOMPLI

This did not stop Pauline's oncology consultant from (a) "giving" her four months to live and (b) recommending that she receive a course of chemotherapy. By this time, Pauline had already been reading up on the subject and she was not very enthused about being subjected to a course of powerful chemical agents with myriad unpleasant and debilitating "side effects." She said, politely, "I'll think about it. For now, I just want to go home."

Which was her way of saying, "No way, José, you're not selling *me* any one-way tickets."

This did not stop Pauline's oncologist (an oncologist is a tumor specialist) from writing the orders he sincerely thought were in her best interests. And three days later, a cheerful nurse arrived with the transport stretcher and announced, "It's time for your first chemotherapy treatment."

Pauline bolted out of bed into the hall, holding her intravenous bottle aloft like the Statue of Liberty holding her torch.

> *"I was livid. I said, 'I don't know who wrote those orders, but you strike them right now.'*
>
> *"Then I left the hospital to do some more reading on the subject. My first stop was to see you because you work with Dr. Carlton Fredericks, and he seems to know everything."*

OUR FIRST ENCOUNTER

I remember that first meeting with Pauline quite clearly. She appeared calm and intent on getting answers to a long list of questions, but her eyes presented the appearance of a frightened doe.

She asked me about the work of Emanuel Revici,[1] of Lawrence Burton, and of Stanislas Burszynski. I said, "Wait a minute. All of these doctors have made splendid contributions, and each of these is a perfectly valid healing system, but you left out a lot. There are a dozen or so other biologic treatments that have to be included as well."

Let me confess here and now that I was unabashedly making a pitch for Pauline to become my patient. I had by that time grown beyond my previous stance of steering clear of cancer patients, a self-protective device employed by nearly all alternative physicians, who soon learn that the cancer establishment is exceedingly protective of its domain to the point that it goes for the jugular — and for the "trespasser's" license to practice. Quite the contrary, cancer treatment was becoming an ever-increasing part of my professional career.

I told Pauline I had treated only one pancreatic cancer patient before her but that she had done surprisingly well. However, I continued, my German colleague Professor Friedrich Douwes reported over a dozen cures with his biologic therapy, and enzymologist Karl Ransberger had reported on thirty-eight cases of total remission (collected by no less an official than the Austrian minister of health) using his world-renowned Wobe-Mugos enzyme.[2] (Incidentally, Wobe-Mugos enzyme was "run out of the country" by the ever-compassionate FDA. Evidently the FDA felt that these European biologic treatments would keep the pancreas cancer victims away from the "definitive cures" that American medicine is famous for.) "So, you see, there is plenty of reason for optimism," I told her.

PAULINE AND I BOTH KNEW

As I said that, I could see the relief come over her face and I knew then and there that Pauline would do well and would be a curable *person*. (I have long known there are no incurable *diseases*.) Pauline had the two most valuable traits of all — fighting spirit and the emotional unwillingness to accept the idea of being sick. That very day, I was so enthused I told my family, "I've just met the perfect case for the cancer chapter."

Don't miss the point of all this. To overcome overwhelming odds, *both* the doctor and the patient must *believe* the treatment will work. *Without this collaboration, there can be no healing.* This is the point where orthodoxy fails. In the current approach used by oncologists, the doctor sees too much failure, too consistently, to be himself convinced, or convincing. In double-blind research, the problem is compounded; here even the optimistic doctor knows there is only a 50 percent chance his patient is getting the genuine treatment and not the placebo. A cancer patient can win only when confidence creates success and success has created confidence.

PAULINE STARTS HER TREATMENT

On February 24, 1986, just three weeks after her hospital discharge, Pauline returned for her first treatment. My game plan was "kitchen sink complementarism" — meaning I would use everything I could think of in the way of health enhancers, immune stimulants, and enabling agents. I was out to *build up the body, not to tear down the cancer.* To this end, I would throw in everything but the kitchen sink.

HOW I ARRIVED AT KITCHEN SINK COMPLEMENTARISM

Let me leave my narrative long enough to tell you how I arrived at this treatment philosophy.

Can you imagine how many ambitious mothers have told their gifted children: "Be a great success, find the cure for cancer"? Well, they got it wrong. The correct statement reads: "Want to lose your license and your credibility? Find a cure for cancer."

There have already been *many* cancer cures, and all have been ruthlessly and systematically suppressed with a Gestapo-like thoroughness by the cancer establishment. The cancer establishment is the not-too-shadowy association of the American Cancer Society, the leading cancer hospitals, the National Cancer Institute, and the FDA. The shadowy part is the fact that these respected institutions are very much dominated by members and friends of members of the pharmaceutical industry, which profits so incredibly much from our profession-wide obsession with chemotherapy.

I had evolved an idea of combining all the many bona fide yet suppressed, effective yet ignored, clinically tested yet dismissed, health-enhancing cancer therapies and *using them all* — or as many as I could fit in. The beauty of this system is the beauty of Complementary Medicine. If everything I use enhances health and none poses any danger, then the worst that can happen is that I may use a few agents that make very little contribution. But the best thing that may happen is that the body may find in my offerings something it can use to *achieve its own healing*. There is nothing I gave Pauline that I wouldn't take myself if I wanted to feel better and improve my resistance to disease.

I WRITE THE ORDERS FOR PAULINE'S CARE

First, we established the good news that Pauline's immune system was intact. (We always keep tabs on the precise quantification of cellular immunity by ordering the lab study called T and B subsets, the same tests doctors use to follow the progress of AIDS patients. Hospital oncology stubbornly refuses to do likewise, perhaps out of reluctance to chronicle the immune system's systematic destruction under chemotherapy.) Having also found that Pauline's tumor markers (immunologic blood tests) indicated no spread of the cancer, we sat down again while I wrote her orders.

I prescribed a diet that was not very different from diets I use regularly, the Meat and Millet type. I toyed with the idea of using a macrobiotic, low-animal-protein diet simply because Dr. Max Gerson and Dr. William Donald Kelley had obtained such gratifying success with it.[3] I opted for keeping her off sugar (increasingly, studies are connecting sugar consumption to various kinds of cancer[4]) and off chemical additives, and specified that she must include 16 ounces of freshly squeezed carrot juice every day and that 80 percent of her vegetables should be uncooked.

ENZYMES AND ANTIOXIDANTS

Pauline was to take 6 enzyme tablets (bromelain and pancreatic extracts) with each meal. My reading had taught me that enzyme therapy is particularly important in pancreatic disease. She was given 12 antioxidant capsules every day. Other nutrients included beta carotene, which with the antioxidant, totaled almost 200,000 units. Vitamin A is the best documented anticancer vitamin, and beta carotene is the precursor and the safest form to give it in.[5] It is also an important one-two punch when used with pancreatic enzymes. She was also to take vitamin C,[6] ascorbic acid, in crystalline form, totaling 3 teaspoons (15 grams), as well as lots of magnesium orotate,[7] plus copper and manganese.

The oral treatment also included primrose oil and squalene, a shark oil derivative, plus extracts of valerian root, the Venus-fly-trap *(dionaea)*, and a few other herbal immune boosters.

Over the next thirty-two days, Pauline received 13 intravenous drips containing 50 grams of sodium ascorbate, plus minerals and adrenal cortex extract. She also received ozone, thymus extract, and the hormone dehydroepiandrosterone (DHEA). Our understanding was that this would be the treatment until she could make it to a resort hospital in West Germany run by Dr. Douwes, for more intense biologic treatment.

THE TRIP TO GERMANY

Pauline was in quite good shape when she left for Germany and in wonderful shape when she returned three weeks later. Throughout these two months, she had regained all eighteen pounds she had lost in the hospital and was back at her lifelong weight of 118 pounds.

In Germany, Dr. Douwes gave her regular treatment with his biological therapies, organ-specific peptides derived from liver, spleen, and thymus. "A very important therapy," Dr. Douwes said, "is what German alternativists call Symbiose Lenkum, which means, balance the bacterial flora of the bowel."

On April 30, Pauline proudly proclaimed, "I feel better than ever," and proved it by continuing the program of speed walking she had started in Germany. The CT scans could no longer demonstrate a pancreatic tumor "with certainty." A more recent sonogram localized the site of the tumor, but noted that there was no sign of any enlarging of the head of the pancreas. The tumor markers stayed down, with one, the LASA test, dropping from a suspicious 21.4 to a normal 15.7; her liver tests remained normal and even improved, and her red cell count went from 3.8 million to 4.5 million.

Pauline remained sympton-free for over a year, until she developed problems secondary to nonmalignant obstruction at the site of the original surgery. When a second surgery was performed to correct that problem, the carcinoma in the head of the pancreas was no larger than it had been one and a half years before. Kitchen sink complementarism — and Pauline's spirit — had fought this killer to a stalemate. Pauline is now the third two-year survivor out of the six pancreatic adenocarcinoma patients we have managed. In standard circles, it requires three hundred admissions to find three such cases.

There are still a lot of items in our sink that Pauline has *not* received. Items with names like iridoides, tumosterone, ukrain, carciverein, mandelonitrile, carcalon, cesium chloride, germanium sesquioxide, Neoblastine, Immucothel, Regeneresen, urea, transfer factor, serrapeptase, and dozens more are all examples of therapeutic biologic substances that have had written documentation of excellent results. And this list does not include the systems of the aforementioned Dr. Burton, Dr. Revici, or Dr. Burszynski, nor of William Donald Kelley, nor Andrew Ivy, nor the countless others who have faded into obscurity because of cancer establishment suppression.

The suppression of a promising technique almost always takes the form of ignoring it or placing it on the American Cancer Society's (ACS) "unproven methods" list. The ACS quite pointedly presents this list as a tabulation of "cancer quackery," as modalities to be shunned, in a vein very similar to the Arthritis Foundation's "be suspicious" list, mentioned in the previous chapter. To the ACS, *unproven* is *disproven*.

But now just suppose that the American Cancer Society were more interested in cancer *patients* than in cancer *corporations* (which is probably the most far-fetched supposition I'll ever ask you to make). How would a philanthropic entity view a compendium of unproven cancer therapies? With great hope and enthusiasm, just as I have. By noting that proof is very hard to come by, by scouring the list for promising yet-to-be-proven therapies, and by offering to help test and ultimately prove their value.

Pauline Platten's good response was achieved exclusively with unproven therapies. If she had been intimidated enough to be treated by proven therapies, she would have been dead in four months, if we can accept the pronouncements of her previous physicians.

How I Got Started in This Field

My move into cancer management really came in stages. At first I entered the picture merely by providing nutritional support for patients already on some form of definitive cancer therapy. Nutrition seemed to have been an area totally abandoned by the oncologists serving as case managers. Yet logic, practice experience, and reviewing the nutrition "literature" all demonstrated that such a limitation simply shouldn't be.

Reports were beginning to appear on the cancer-preventing effects of beta carotene and/or vitamin A, selenium, vitamin C, and cysteine or glutathione. It should be noted that all of the above are antioxidant nutrients. Dr. Carlton Fredericks had suggested the use of antioxidants in cancer patients over his WOR radio program (which is now my responsibility). This produced a dramatic remission in the wife of a physician at New York's Peninsula Hospital. And this led to the beginning of a formal double-blind study on the effect of giving the entire system of nutritional antioxidants, which was showing promising results until the Compassionate Ones (the FDA, remember?) put a stop to it.

When it became apparent to me that the patients seemed to be benefiting more from the nutrition and the biologic treatments (referring to the enzymes, botanicals, and organ extracts) than from the chemotherapy, we began to suggest "holding off" on the chemotherapy unless it became clear that the safer treatments were not getting the job done. We felt we were thus following the Hippocratic dictum of *Primum, non nocere* by offering our treatments in the sequence of safest modalities first, most dangerous modalities last.

Many of the patients did very well on the nontoxic therapies alone. Chester Delmas is one example.

Chester Delmas

Chester Delmas is a sixty-five-year-old retired undertaker who has been a ray of sunshine in the lives of all the staff at the Atkins

Center. But on his first visit to us, on June 3, 1987, he didn't look so happy.

Chester was more than a little concerned about his health. Four years before I met him, Chester had been successfully operated on for colon cancer. He apparently did quite well until early in 1987, when a lung cancer was diagnosed. Chester went under the surgeon's knife in April, and a tumor the size of a golf ball was removed, along with the middle lobe of his right lung. The pathologist, noting that mucin was produced, diagnosed it as a metastatic lesion, that is, one that had probably begun in the original site, the colon. Chester's recovery was rapid. A few weeks after the operation, he went with his son, a practicing physician in Pennsylvania, to talk to his original surgeon about his prospects. The surgeon's recommendation was that Chester take some chemotherapy "as preventive medicine." He was about to mention the names of a few oncologists when Chester beat him to the punch by rattling off the names himself. The surgeon looked a bit surprised.

> *"I had to remind him that I was funeral director, and he looked a little queasy when I added: 'I know those names all right — they've signed more death certificates than Carter has liver pills.' "*

Chester was clear on one thing: He wasn't going to be taking chemotherapy. Since he had heard of our center, he decided to come see me. I explained to Chester that there are two ways to win a battle. One is to weaken the enemy; the other is to build the allied forces. When I told him we would give him only agents that would build him up, the apprehension left his face. I have never seen an unhappy look on Chester's face since.

Chester's lab tests looked like anything but those of a cancer patient. He had high cholesterol (326) (cancer patients often have very low cholesterol), and his blood sugars even had that high-low pattern, dropping from 196 to 51. His immune profile and tumor markers of all kinds were quite normal. His only medication was a beta-blocker, and he was moderately overweight. I really had to treat him more like a blood pressure patient. Accordingly, I put him on 12 antioxidant capsules a day, 2 teaspoons of vitamin C,

75,000 units of beta carotene, 4 primrose oil capsules, 450 milligrams of germanium sesquioxide, pancreatic enzymes, thymus and liver extracts, plus our usual antihypertensive protocol. And we stopped his beta-blocker. I started him on intravenous vitamin C, with ozone, peptides from liver and spleen, and a program of mistletoe. The intravenous "cocktail" contained vitamins, minerals, and some of the biologicals with the most successful track records among the European protocols. He took fifty of these treatments in the first month.

There is nothing else to say about Chester's subsequent course, except that it was, as we doctors say, uneventful. In Chester's case, this meant he would come in twice a week, rosy-cheeked, robust, and loquacious, raising the spirits of every patient in our center. Today, all tumor markers and immune profiles remain well within the normal range.

> *"I don't know what I'd do if I didn't come here. I look forward to these visits so."*

Pay careful attention to these words, because I believe this is the key to the success we've been having. If visits to the medical facility provide optimism, support, love, and the conviction that getting well is not only possible but probable, then the healing of a cancer patient can really take place.

And that's what we work at. The interaction between doctor and patient creates the success. Has scientific medicine forgotten that?

Chester's first seven months under our protocol have been letter perfect, but it doesn't *prove* anything. Intellectual purists (including me) can muse, with hindsight, "Who's to say the second surgery wasn't curative?" At the time when only foresight was available, the physicians managing Chester's case recommended a course of chemotherapy so powerful that the treatment alone would have been debilitating.

In case you're wondering why I haven't written a paper about our results, let me point out that no meaningful paper can be written when free-living patients come to a private medical facility for treatment. Virtually every one of the 150 cancer patients I have

treated has interrupted our intended protocol in some way by in-
terludes with other therapies, breaks in the treatment, underdos-
ing or overdosing, other complicating illnesses, and the like. Add
to this the fact that each has a different kind of cancer, that each
was discovered in a different stage of the illness, that each has had
different treatment before seeing us, and you can see that no one
can make an intelligible paper out of this hodgepodge of information.

It is no wonder that the greats in the field — Ivy,[8] Nieper,[9] Revici, and the like — cannot give meaningful answers when asked
to present statistical proof of their success.

But one thing we note. Our patients' life quality is improved.
And very few are in pain on our program.

In the past twelve months, according to my narcotics prescription blanks, I have written for only three narcotic painkillers in a
time span when I was responsible for a hundred patients with cancer. Not all of my patients made it, to be sure, but the interesting
phenomenon is that, more often than not, we could *predict*, from
the initial interview, who would and who would not survive. Survival was not based so much on the severity of the disease as on
attitude. The survivors almost invariably were those who (a) adopted
a very fundamental this-is-not-my-time-so-cancer-I'm-getting-rid-
of-you attitude *and* (b) had not succumbed to the intimidation of
destructive orthodox medicine.

As Pauline recounted so succinctly: "I've gotten to know about
two dozen of your patients and the ones who had gone through
chemotherapy before they saw you aren't here anymore."

Unfortunately, this *is* often the case. The damage done to the
body by an unsuccessful course of chemotherapy is often so great
that the patient's immune system never recovers sufficiently for
him to stand a fighting chance.

What About Chemotherapy?

This brings me to the most troubling decision in my professional
career and one I have to make almost every working day. Cancer
patients, having heard of the success of Complementary Medicine,
arrive after they have been exposed to orthodox oncology and have

been offered, and often have begun, a course of radiation and/or chemotherapy. Their question, more often than not, is: "What can you do to make chemotherapy more bearable?" My gut reaction, which I don't verbalize, is: "Get you to stop the chemotherapy." But the question is such an important one that it deserves a much more carefully considered answer.

One of the criticisms of every alternative method that has ever been proposed is that it "takes the patient away from lifesaving approved therapies." I would never want to be guilty of that mistake. Nor would I, on the other hand, ever want to be guilty of *not* taking the patient away from *life-destroying* proven therapies. The problem is that only God knows which is which.

How to Make the Chemotherapy Decision

One of the advantages that orthodox medicine has over complementarism is that its track record is well documented, while the alternative medicine sails mainly in uncharted waters. This fact helps me greatly in advising patients who seek my opinion. From this we know that there are roughly three types of tumors: those that respond to chemotherapy, those that do not respond, and an in-between group that responds only to an unsatisfactory extent.

Tumors of the pancreas, stomach, lung, and colon, and melanoma are in the group that do not respond. Here the decision is clear-cut. *Chemotherapy, when it has no chance, or only a remote chance, to work is at best stupid and at worst criminal.* It takes what's left of a cancer patient's life and immediately creates more sickness than existed before.

But what about lymphomas, Hodgkin's disease, ovarian cancer — tumors for which chemotherapy has shown that it works? Here the answer is different, and more difficult to give. It's hard to turn your back on treatments that are known to work. But these people run into the same problems all patients receiving chemotherapy do: the immediate toxic effects leading to hair loss, vomiting, blistering, debilitation, and much more, plus the more significant delayed effects of a markedly decreased immune function, which creates a vulnerability to simple infections (actually an AIDS-like immune system) and to more cancer. I've seen the end stage of these treatments — very gritty people who had nothing left to fight with. And there was nothing I could to to help them.

Why Turn Away from the Proven?

For complementary cancer therapy to work, the immune system must be relatively intact. The biologic therapies work *through* the immune system; they cannot create a new one. To the immune system, chemotherapy is a disaster and a half. The inescapable conclusion is that even when chemotherapy works, alternatives must be considered.

My second point is the one that convinces me. If a tumor is docile enough to shrink from chemotherapy, don't you think it would respond readily to the biologic and nutritional systems that can handle the deadly cancers? My experience has already taught me that the answer is a resounding yes!

The third group of cancers are those that respond on occasion, or partially, to chemotherapy, breast cancer being a good example of that. Essentially the same considerations apply.

Let Me Modify the Question

The question I hear every day is: Orthodox or alternative, alternative or orthodox? I must say I really don't like this question, because it calls for one of two very foolish answers. The question is tantamount to asking, "Which half of the deck do you want to play with?" My answer is: "As long as both halves are there, let's play with the whole deck."

But that's just what's going on. *Patients with cancer who seek either orthodox or alternative approaches are entrusting their lives to doctors who are playing with half a deck.*

The Full-Deck System

Soul-searching decisions as to whether, when, or how much to use chemotherapy cannot be made well, and should not be made at all, by doctors who have not studied the entire deck. My patients ask intelligent questions: "How can I get the therapeutic benefit of chemotherapy without hurting my immune system?" "Should we use the safer biologic therapies first and hold the chemo in reserve?" "Can I get by with less chemotherapy if we use biologic medicine simultaneously?" "Which combinations have the best chance for success?" Questions like these can be answered only by doctors who have had the experience of using both approaches and who have seen their problems and their successes. My German consultants, Dr. Nieper and Dr. Douwes, for example, have used considerable chemotherapy and have that experience. I, too, have used chemotherapy when working with an oncology consultant in a spirit of mutual respect.

Our Solution to the Problem

The solution at the Atkins Center is to gather as much data as possible on each patient and then to apply what I call the Hippocratic pecking order, which means do the safest of the effective things first and save the riskiest for last. The data-gathering is a very important step. We study the immune system in detail, looking at the T and B subsets, including the helper and suppressor and natural killer (NK) cell counts. We do tumor markers of every conceivable kind and sonographic or x-ray studies of anything that may pertain. The importance of all this is that we must see whether we are getting a response to our initial treatments, because we must know whether the riskier treatments are necessary.

This system, which precludes giving destructive chemotherapy or radiation unnecessarily, runs counter to the accepted teaching, which quite clearly is based on *statistical probability*. Ours is based on *individualized response* and *on-the-scene judgments*.

The Problem with Orthodoxy

Assuming that the individualized, flexible system appeals to a cancer patient, he will have a hard time finding an oncologist who has that "mutual respect" for an alternative, immunologically oriented practitioner. I have encountered very few oncologists who are at all interested in the immune system. Incredible as it may seem, most oncologists are willing to bring the immune system from normal to near zero without drawing a single immune profile (blood test). The simple white cell and platelet counts that they order just do not give adequate information. If you have a doctor who will give radiation therapy or chemotherapy without checking your immune system, you could be in for real trouble unnecessarily.

The problem is that orthodoxists don't even want to know that the other half of the deck exists. Thus their results are not very encouraging.

The prestigious *New England Journal of Medicine* (May 8, 1986) published an analysis of the "war on cancer" by Dr. John Bailar, associate professor of preventive medicine at the University of Iowa.[10] In analyzing the cancer death total of 450,000 Americans per year, Dr. Bailar wrote:

> These data, taken alone, provide no evidence that some 35 years of . . . efforts to improve the treatment of cancer have had much overall effect on the most fundamental measure of clinical outcome — death.

He concluded:

> There comes a time to cut your losses, to admit privately and then publicly that it hasn't worked and then do something else.

That something else is being done today, by complementarists in Europe and now in America. It is an individualized, flexible, biologic, and nutritional medicine, which utilizes the destructive therapies to the extent that the immune system is preserved. All that is missing is the "proof" that it works.

BOOK THREE

. . .

THE TREATMENTS

24

•••

THE CUTTING EDGE
OF COMPLEMENTARY
NUTRITION

I f it were my intention to write a two-volume book, volume two would begin here, and it would detail all the treatment modalities used in Complementary Medicine. As essential as it is that all this be written someday, it might divert your attention from the main thesis of this book, which is, in case you missed it: *There are, and long have been, two major approaches to health management, and you do have a choice between them.*

Nonetheless, I do want to provide some of this information, both because it's valuable in its own right and because it provides background support for a point that needs to be made.

The point concerns the answer to the question: *Where is the real frontier of contemporary medicine?* Is it located in the research departments of the highest-powered medical center hospitals or the development laboratories of the pharmaceutical industry? Or is it in the private medical offices of a handful of starry-eyed complementarists, ever seeking the "last word" in healing techniques?

My answer to this question about progress is "Both places." Most of the *research* leading to real breakthroughs does come from the for-profit think tanks. But, for all the reasons I have been discussing, the *clinical trials* of greatest significance are being done by complementarists. When it comes to the clinical use of discoveries as they come "hot off the press," Complementary Medicine is, on a broad scale, ahead of the competition.

Nutrition Is the Best Example

Let me show you what I mean. In writing this section of the book, I wanted to provide you with a scientific understanding of some of the nutritional tools we work with every day. And so I sent an editorial assistant out with the project: "Find out what you can about these twelve nutrients that we use routinely."

> nutritional antioxidants
> gamma-linolenic acid nutrients (primrose oil)
> omega-3 fatty acids (DHA, EPA)
> mineral transporters (orotates, aspartates, and EAP)
> taurine
> carnitine
> bromelain
> coenzyme Q_{10}
> quercetin
> pantethine
> caprylic acid
> octacosanol

She went to a 1986 edition[1] of the most comprehensive textbook of nutrition, which was then only a few months off the press, and this what she found:

- ▪ Six of the subjects were not mentioned.
- ▪ Four were mentioned but no clinical applications were suggested.
- ▪ One category (the antioxidants) was only sketchily represented.

And only one, the marine lipid EPA, contained a brief discussion of its possible clinical values.

Now I would like to tell you about these nutrients, to show you what complementarists must know in order to practice their medicine. The information is recent, but it is published in the world's medical literature. I present it for three reasons. First, as a small part of the proof that it is Complementary Medicine and not the headline-grabbing academic medicine that operates comfortably at the frontier of medical discovery. Second, I present it to show you that empirical medicine has matured into a medicine based on scientific discoveries, and "provable" by scientific studies, and is thus fully prepared for a merger with mainstream medicine. Finally, I want you to begin to acquire some background for understanding some of the nutrients that will be household words in the near future.

Nutritional Antioxidants

Most of the credible theories about the causes of aging and the degenerative diseases such as arteriosclerosis, cancer, and arthritis focus on the effect of environmentally induced stresses mediated by extremely reactive chemical fragments called free radicals. The body has several built-in mechanisms that serve to protect it from this free radical damage. Since free radicals generally harm by oxidizing the healthy body parts and biochemical constituents, the body will protect itself by providing certain substances that offer themselves for oxidation, thus precluding the possibility of the oxidizing radicals harming vital tissues such as the linings of our arteries, lungs, or joint structures. These substances are called antioxidants. You have already learned that the enzyme superoxide dismutase (SOD) is one of them, and that our friend/enemy cholesterol may also be one of them. The entire network that the body has to call upon, which is more an abstract concept than an integrated system, is referred to as the antioxidant system.

The Nutritional Needs to Replenish Our Antioxidant System

Many of our antioxidants are enzymes that nature designed for the purpose: SOD (which requires copper, zinc, or manganese), glutathione peroxidase (which requires cysteine and selenium), catalase, and many more. Some are themselves vitamins, as vitamins E, C, and A.

For the past decade, many of the more progressive companies in the nutritional formulations business have been offering to the public their own version of an antioxidant formula. Since the Atkins Center developed its own such combination five years ago, it has been our most widely prescribed formula except for the Basic Formula itself. This is because I believe that antioxidants are, not just in theory, but in actual fact, our most valuable nutrients, for prevention of illness and for management of existing illness.

To see how we have updated our formula, refer to Appendix C.

What Is a Good Antioxidant Formula?

To provide a good antioxidant formula, the most important nutrients are cysteine and glutathione,* selenium, vitamin E, vitamin C, and vitamin A or beta carotene (provitamin A). If you want real antioxidant protection, and you should, *make sure the dose is adequate.* (Appendix C will give you a good idea of what I regard as an adequate dose.) Don't be satisfied just to see the name on the label.

There are certain B-complex constituents that support the antioxidant system. Minerals such as zinc and manganese are valuable as well. There are two other elements that we find useful, as our formula indicates: bioflavonoids and methyl donors, such as N-N-dimethylglycine.

When you consider that the antioxidant nutrient system probably protects us from aging, cardiovascular disease, arthritis, cancer, Alzheimer's disease, diabetes, pulmonary disease, and just about everything else, you can see why it is so widely prescribed.

GLA: Gamma-Linolenic Acid

The next two items on my list refer to one of the most important scientific understandings of the last generation — our prostaglandins. Prostaglandins are hormonelike, messengerlike substances that give signals to various structures in the body, telling blood vessels, or bronchial passages, or the uterus, or the like, to expand or contract. There is generally a balance between two opposing types of

---

*Cysteine and glutathione are for the same purpose, support of the critically valuable enzyme glutathione peroxidase. Glutathione is the more valuable substance, but it is expensive and cysteine is inexpensive. The beauty of cysteine is that much of it will convert into glutathione.

effect. One (prostacyclin type) is a beneficial series that relaxes our blood vessels and bronchial muscles, protects our joints, and relieves inflammation. The other (thromboxane type) effect is just the opposite, a tightening or contracting, and is generally undesirable.

Prostaglandins are named and numbered according to — and their actions are determined by — the structure of the fatty acids incorporated in their molecular structure. The body is not able to do much shifting of essential fatty acids from one molecular structure to another, as it can with carbohydrate metabolites, for example. Thus, for the most part, *what you eat is what you get*. With a typical Western diet, what we eat gives us arachidonic acid, from which derives a series (series 2) in which the thromboxane is particularly destructive. We *can* avoid this problem by providing our bodies with the essential fatty acids for manufacture of prostaglandins that have no adverse counterbalance. The first example is gamma-linolenic acid (series 1) and the second is the series based on omega-3 fatty acids (series 3).

The Value of GLA

Gamma-linolenic acid is incredibly valuable to us because it converts to dihomogammalinolenic acid (DGLA) which, in turn, converts to the most ideal prostaglandin of all, prostaglandin E_1 (PGE_1). Normally, we can expect some linoleic acid to mutate to GLA, but it just doesn't happen enough to supply our needs. Accordingly, we must scurry around looking for a dietary source of GLA. When we were babies, we had it made. Mother's milk is an excellent source of GLA. Unfortunately, most of us have had to grow up.

You cannot eat a so-called healthy diet and get GLA. It is found too infrequently for that. The only significant sources of GLA anyone has told me about (and I sure asked) are in the seed oil of a beautiful yellow wildflower called the evening primrose, black currant seed oil, and an herb called borage. So you see, bean sprouts, brown rice, and miso alone just don't cut it.

Most of the work on the GLA-DGLA-PGE_1 nutritional system has been done on primrose oil. The studies were masterminded by Dr. David Horrobin, one of the most brilliant minds in Complementary Medicine. Horrobin has succeeded in publishing studies of the type that orthodoxy *must* accept — double-blind, controlled, statistically significant, done at English-speaking teaching hospitals. They *absolutely prove* that GLA is the most effective treatment yet for premenstrual syndrome,[2] atopic eczema[3] in children, and the dry eye (Sicca) syndrome, as well as the related Sjogren's syndrome.[4] They virtually prove its value in a variety of allergy and immune disorders,[5] in lowering blood pressure and cholesterol,[6] in aiding alcoholism,[7] in breast tenderness,[8] in Raynaud's syndrome,[9] in diabetic neuropathy,[10] in rheumatoid arthritis,[11] and in autoimmune disorders such as MS,[12] lupus,[13] and scleroderma.[14] It has also been tested and shown to have favorable results in hyperactive children, depression, schizophrenia, and Parkinsonism.[15] Animal studies have shown a possible benefit in treating cancer.[16]

Has Science Helped the Acceptance of GLA?

Now, with an impressive bibliography of excellent double-blind studies such as those amassed on behalf of primrose oil, would you not think orthodox medicine would grasp it to its bosom and use it to treat some of these rather serious conditions I just mentioned? If your answer to that question was yes, you get an F. Would you believe instead that the ever-compassionate FDA would act against a leading health food retailer and try to halt the sale of the product to the unfortunate victims of these very illnesses? If you answered that one yes, your score is an A+.

Eicosapentaenoic Acid: A Household Word

Contrast the nonacceptance of GLA with the acceptance of marine lipids — the prostaglandin series 3 precursors eicosapentaenoic acid (EPA) and docosahexaenoic acid (DHA) — which derive from the oils of coldwater fish such as salmon, shad, and mackerel.

Orthodoxy is in the process of accepting this nutrient although its use is not widespread. The rationale for its use (the mechanistic mind must be given a plausible story to explain a phenomenon or it won't buy the bottom-line results) is similar to that for GLA: Provide an alternative to series 2 prostaglandins. The same number of good double-blind studies have been performed on both, but the ones on EPA get published in more widely read journals.

EPA Deserves Its Success

EPA is so good it can single-handedly wipe out the lucrative antihypertensive market and the almost as profitable anticholesterol market. A flood of recent studies proves that point. The trick is to give a large enough dose. One recent study showed a *group* cholesterol level dropping from 370 to 204, unheard of for a nutritional agent, but the daily dose was 60 grams (that's 60 large capsules). This means you can have as low a cholesterol as you want; it's only a matter of how much fish oil you're willing to burp.

I find EPA invaluable in cancer, arthritis,[17] allergy,[18] MS,[19] and just about everything else I've written about. It is particularly valuable in lowering elevated triglyceride levels.[20]

Now that real pharmaceutical houses have jumped on the bandwagon to sell those products, I believe the concept of marine lipids will take hold firmly and will create a measurable improvement in our life span statistics. I only fear a global salmon shortage.

Why Is EPA Accepted and GLA Rejected?

I can't answer this question with certainty. I believe it's simply a matter of sponsorship. The salmon oil people had the right sponsors; the primrose oil people apparently did not. It is frightening to note that medicine is so structured that finding the cure for some "incurable" condition may not be enough. You must also find the right promoter, as well. Perhaps this is why the world has been introduced to a score of cancer cures, yet the mainstream doesn't know of any.

Let's Pause Here

Do you want to know how good the two systems I just told you about really are? I can only describe a hypothetical situation to show you. Suppose there were a doctor so inept he never got a single diagnosis correct, but he agreed to give every patient adequate amounts of antioxidants and of the alternative prostaglandin precursors, GLA and omega-3 oils, and to keep his patients off sugar. Well, this dummy would get clinical results that would run rings around those achieved by the best doctor in the state who didn't use these nutritional godsends.

Mineral Transporters

As I said earlier, Dr. Hans Nieper developed the concept of mineral transporters, of which he works with three — the orotates, aspartates, and the salts of colamine phosphate (EAP). Electron microscopic studies place each of them at a different locus in the cell wall, giving each a different purpose.

Orotates

Orotates are manufactured substances made by combining minerals with the metabolite orotic acid. Orotic acid was once classified as a vitamin, and was given the name vitamin B_{13}. It is a precursor of pyrimidines, which are important in the structure of our nucleic acids.

Orotates improve cell penetration without disturbing the electrical activity of the membrane. It is this quality rather than their limited mineral content that provides their value. By combining an orotate with magnesium, for example, magnesium can get into the cells faster and with less waste.[21]

Aspartates are similar compounds, but have some differences. American complementarists have ready access to aspartates. In fact, aspartic acid salts were once an approved pharmaceutical.[22] Orotate, which provides the best delivery system of the desired mineral I have yet seen, is still available in the United States in only a few places. As a cardiologist, I am unrestrainedly enthusiastic over magnesium orotate in just about any cardiovascular condition imaginable.

EAP (Colamine Phosphate)

I have described the action of calcium-EAP in the multiple sclerosis chapter. The intracellular destination of calcium when attached to colamine phosphate is different from when it is compounded with orotates and aspartates. By somehow sealing the free lipid pores off all membranes, calcium-EAP decreases the permeability of the membrane to antibodies. This serves to protect the cell against autoimmune reactions. In this manner, Ca-EAP works in illnesses that can be treated by the class of drugs known as immunosuppressive agents. There is just one difference: Calcium-EAP is perfectly safe, having virtually no side effects, whereas the immunosuppressive drugs are among the most dangerous in the entire medical profession.

I have also used EAP in cases of rheumatoid arthritis (for which it seems to be one of our very best therapies), plus most kidney disorders, other neurological conditions, ulcerative colitis, collagen disorders, lupus, polymyositis, and an assortment of other conditions.

Dr. Nieper, in his two widely read clinical studies published (in English) in the international medical journal *Agressologie* some twenty years ago, also described the value of calcium-EAP in juvenile diabetes, gastritis and ulcer, erythema nodosum, thyroiditis, myocarditis, sarcoid, and Hodgkin's disease.

I really wish the FDA would look into this godsend, especially for patients with MS and ALS (Lou Gehrig's disease), and give it the fair trial it truly deserves and that the victims of these illnesses deserve. Rather than looking to find a way to help people, the FDA persists in its adversarial position. Thus, it accuses Dr. Nieper, who has no financial interest in the product, of "promoting" unproven therapies. May I ask the holier-than-thou people at the FDA this question: *What should a caring physician do?* When such a doctor sees people being helped when not even a hope existed before, and reacts by wishing that every sufferer had the benefit of this experience, must he be thought of only as self-serving? Could it be that the "authorities" are themselves so saturated with misanthropy that they can see only base motives in others?

Two Special Amino Acids: Taurine and Carnitine

The new frontier of nutrition medicine currently centers around the many individual amino acids. For a practitioner of nutrition pharmacology, amino acids double the opportunities to help. The possibilities of amino acid therapy are outlined in the landmark book by Dr. Eric Braverman, *The Healing Nutrients Within*. The exciting fact is that the book is drawn from over thirteen hundred references, most of which represent studies on the therapeutic effect of individual amino acids.

Taurine

One such amino acid is taurine. Taurine, the most abundant amino acid in the heart, is a boon to cardiologists. It is a major contributor to lowering of blood pressure and to relieving congestive heart failure.[23] Probably because it facilitates the removal of sodium from the cells, it can function as a safe diuretic. It seems also to help control heart rhythm irregularities.[24]

The most clear-cut clinical use for taurine is in the treatment of epilepsy.[25] We have now used it in over forty patients with seizure disorder, and it seems to be universally beneficial. We have lowered the anticonvulsant drug requirement in 40 percent of our patients and have gotten another 40 percent completely off their medications. This is a very specific area where a nutrient deserves a therapeutic trial. This, too, may never happen, because taurine, like all nutritional agents, does not have a sponsor. Proof costs money and there's no money here.

Carnitine — The Heart Tonic

Dr. Braverman labels L-carnitine the "heart tonic," and it is in this context that I include it here. Carnitine seems to benefit cardiomyopathies[26] and stabilize heart rhythm,[27] but its greatest use is in coronary insufficiency.[28]

Carnitine is a carrier of fatty acid molecules into the cells composing the heart and skeletal muscle tissue. These fatty acids can then be utilized by the tissue cells as a source of energy. Without sufficient carnitine there is no ketosis (proper metabolization of fatty acids for this function), which adversely affects healthy heart tissue and blood flow. Carnitine also appears to enhance the effectiveness of vitamin E, vitamin C, and other antioxidants by transporting them more effectively into the mitochondria where free radicals are generated. When there is inadequate blood supply to the heart or when there are arrhythmias, a reduced or depleted amount of carnitine has also been found. When carnitine has been supplied to the patient, both conditions have improved. Carnitine has also been prescribed for preventing the occurrence of ventricular fibrillation.

Carnitine has been shown to decrease serum triglyceride, as well as cholesterol levels, and to increase HDL.[29] I use carnitine in cases of metabolic obesity, to help patients who have difficulty getting into ketosis.

Bromelain: The Pineapple Enzyme

Bromelains are the proleolytic enzymes obtained from the pineapple plant. (They are obtained from the middle third of the root, not from the seductive fruit that wreaks havoc on your blood sugar.) Since bromelain was introduced as a therapeutic agent in 1957, more than two hundred scientific papers on its application have been published, showing positive effects as a digestive aid, anti-inflammatory agent, and smooth muscle relaxer. It has been used for enhancement of antibiotic absorption, ulcer prevention, sinusitis relief, appetite inhibition, shortening of labor, and enhanced wound healing. It increases tissue levels of a variety of antibiotics and is even used as an antibiotic in treating certain infections, for example, pneumonia, perirectal abscess, cutaneous staphylococcus infection, and bronchitis. It is widely used in treating sports injuries; because of its "spreading" action, it clears up bruising, reduces knee joint inflammation, and reduces pain.

I present bromelain to you here, however, for a special reason. Bromelain, in sufficient strength, exerts a powerful cardiovascular effect. The aforementioned Dr. Nieper is the chief proponent of its use in cardiology, where he combines it with the orotates and carnitine.

Bromelain and the Heart

Bromelain has a number of cardiovascular effects: It prevents the clumping (or aggregation) of platelets to produce the effect much desired by preventive cardiologists, since platelet aggregation is a key step in the development of atheromatous plaques. Bromelain also has the ability to inhibit the biosynthesis of thromboxane, the pro-inflammatory prostaglandin. (This makes it valuable in treating rheumatoid arthritis, as well.)[30] And it may even have the ability to dissolve already existing blood clots. "Thus," as Dr. Nieper has written, by intensive, long-term "therapy with bromelain, it is possible to 'clean out' the coronary arteries from the inside."[31] This effect, which follows from the powerful enzymatic protein-digesting activity bromelain is known to have, places it in the same therapeutic classification as the exciting new development of heroic, emergency orthodox medicine, the thrombolytic (clot-dissolving) agents like streptokinase and TPA. The latter agents are currently used only at the time of an acute heart attack; bromelain is a useful long-term therapy. I believe bromelain is the perfect adjunct to EDTA chelation therapy. EDTA is designed to remove calcification from the blood vessels, while bromelain is designed to "digest" the decalcified plaque.

The "Trick" to the Use of Bromelain

There is a major caveat. You must use a powerful bromelain. The usual digestive strength bromelain tablets available at health food stores won't cut the mustard. (They probably won't even *digest* the mustard, for that matter.) One would need a daily minimum of 2000 GDUs (gelatin digestion units) to begin to expect a cardiovascular effect.

Coenzyme Q$_{10}$: For the Contemporary Cardiologist

I am literally hoping that my readers who are heart patients have read the foregoing and are asking themselves: "Why didn't my doctor recommend that?" That's the first sign you are grasping the reality that doctors don't know everything. They don't even know everything they should.

That's why they also are very unlikely to offer you coenzyme Q$_{10}$, another key nutrient whose principal clinical use is in cardiology.

Coenzyme Q$_{10}$, also known as ubiquinone, is an enzyme derivative of the B-complex family. It is a cofactor in the biochemical pathway in cellular respiration from which ATP (adenosine triphosphate, a compound involved in the storage and transfer of energy in cells) and metabolic energy are derived. Since cellular functions are dependent on availability of energy, CoQ_{10} is essential for proper functioning of the immune system. Where deficiencies of CoQ_{10} have been found, clinical conditions such as cardiovascular disease, hypertension, and periodontal disease have been noted.[32] Coenzyme Q_{10} is a critical substance utilized in heart metabolism. By maintaining a balance of CoQ_{10} in the system one can reduce heart attacks and/or their severity. Also, it has been found that injections of CoQ_{10} lower blood pressure[33] and reduce angina.[34] CoQ_{10} has been found to be deficient where diabetes mellitus exists,[35] and the condition has improved when CoQ_{10} is supplied.[36]

The effect of coenzyme Q_{10} on the heart muscle in cases of advanced congestive heart failure was so dramatic and consistent that S. A. Mortensen and associates labeled it "a major advance in the management of resistant myocardial failure." In their study, eight of twelve patients who were failures with digitalis and diuretics, after a month of a daily dose of 100 milligrams CoQ_{10} showed significant improvement in every clinical parameter measured.[37] Coenzyme Q_{10} has also been shown to be effective in rhythm disturbances[38] and in seventy-one of eighty patients with cardiomyopathy.[39]

Add CoQ_{10} to carnitine, taurine, EPA, GLA, magnesium orotate, bromelain, and garlic and you have a formidable yet safe nutritional background for the heart patient. It's no wonder I grin from ear to ear whenever I meet a new heart patient. Since I am armed to the teeth with a nontoxic nutritional package that's stronger than any heart drug on the market, it is extremely gratifying to observe those patients improve almost on a daily basis.

Quercetin: A Special Bioflavonoid

The rest of the complex centered around vitamin C is a group of natural substances called bioflavonoids. I have long used the natural substances derived from citrus and did not pay much heed to the individual bioflavonoids.

But one of my colleagues told me to pay special attention to quercetin, and in the short time I have used it, it has been outstanding enough to be noticed.

Quercetin, which is derived from blue-green algae, protects vitamin C from oxidation in the body. It is an antioxidant and antihistamine, the most effective nutritional antihistamine I have seen yet.* Quercetin benefits those with hypertension and has been found to reduce small strokes (transient ischemic attacks, or TIAs). Quercetin also reduces capillary permeability and capillary fragility.

Bioflavonoids Are Good but Quercetin Is Better

I include quercetin among my list of twelve contemporary nutritional breakthroughs because of my personal experience with it — both as a victim and as a physician.

I told you about my Chinese restaurant headaches; I didn't mention that there are *many* foods which give me mild toxic headaches and I haven't discovered them all (but red wine is one of them). Every time I would wake up with one it would run its course, usually lasting until late afternoon. Once I discovered quercetin, the headache would vanish about twenty minutes after I took two tablets.

Accordingly, I have prescribed quercetin for my many patients who have similar problems of food and chemical sensitivities. More often than not, quercetin has made me some sort of a household hero. It is one of the few nutrients ever shown to be of benefit in the treatment of varicose veins.[41]

Pantethine: Who Knew?

The "cutting edge" philosophy is as much a part of Complementary Medicine as is its devotion to safer alternatives. This means that the search for new ideas is always on, especially since the nutritional agents employed present no risk to the patient. When the

---

*Biochemical scholars may be interested to learn that the flavonoid quercetin reduces allergic processes through its ability to stabilize mast cells and basophils, inhibiting degranulation and subsequent releasing of histamine and other inflammatory mediators.[40]

worst thing that can happen is nothing, there is no reason not to try promising ideas.

So when one of my colleagues noticed a 1985 article in the obscure scientific literature suggesting that pantethine, an intermediary metabolite with no previous clinical use, could lower the acetaldehyde concentration in the blood and could thus be a successful adjunct in the treatment of drinking episodes, he recalled that acetaldehyde is not only implicated as the cause of alcohol toxicity, but that it had also been hypothesized to be responsible for many of the symptoms of candidiasis as well.[42]

There is a great need in my practice for nutritional substances that reduce untoward reactions to environmental chemicals, or foods, or allergies. Vitamin C and the other antioxidants helped, but not always. Pantothenic acid (vitamin B_5) helped. GLA and omega-3 oils helped further. Since pantethine is a derivative of pantothenic acid, I began to use it in a variety of allergic patients and am now convinced that its value extends beyond its use in alcoholism and candidiasis.

The other side of the pantethine coin is equally promising. Because it is also the immediate forerunner of coenzyme A, pantethine can be very beneficial in treating heart disease, especially in lowering the LDL, cholesterol, and triglycerides, while raising the HDL levels. Between 1983 and 1986, five experimental studies confirmed this effect.[43] One of the researchers, L. Cattin, suggested that, because it was without side effects, pantethine was "the therapy of choice" for people with high cholesterol levels.

And if you believe the suppression of platelet clumping prevents heart disease, you'll be interested to know that pantethine does that quite nicely, too.[44]

Caprylic Acid

Sometimes the cutting edge is really the trailing edge. One of my nutritional colleagues has an interesting approach. Dr. Robert DaPrato specializes in scouting the medical library for ideas that were offered as promising nontoxic agents and then, as is the case with sponsorless nonpharmaceuticals, got lost in the shuffle. One such example is caprylic acid.

Caprylic acid is a short-chain fatty acid that is created in our intestinal tract by our resident bacteria. In 1954, Dr. Irene Neuhauser wrote about three patients with candida overgrowth of the large intestine she had treated with caprylic acid. Rapid clinical improvement was accompanied by disappearance of the yeast organisms from the stool specimens. Thirty years later, Dr. DaPrato came upon this article and told a nutrition product manufacturing colleague; thus the caprylic acid "industry" was born.

The trick was to mix the caprylic acid with an ion-exchange complex so that it would be released in the colon, where the yeast overgrowth is, not in the stomach.

I use this product as the treatment of choice for candida, which translates into 25 percent of my practice. It works and has the advantage over nystatin, the main treatment orthodoxists would provide (in those rare cases where they think of the diagnosis), in that very few patients show allergic manifestations to it. Many candida patients show an allergy to molds, from which nystatin derives.

Octacosanol

Octacosanol is a valuable portion of a valuable nutrient that teaches us a lesson about the power of nutritional substances. It is present in very small amounts in wheat germ and other vegetable oils. It is a 28-carbon-atom-long alcohol.

Wheat germ oil was well studied in the 1930s and in the 1950s and 1960s. Professor Thomas Cureton of the University of Illinois conducted extensive research into the effects of wheat germ oil on stamina, reaction time, and cardiovascular responses. Cureton concluded that octacosanol was the critical unknown factor in wheat germ oil responsible for its success.[45]

Octacosanol was a cult item among athletes and body builders, but it was not a major part of nutritional medicine until Dr. Carlton Fredericks became aware that it was extremely valuable for brain function.

He began to recommend octacosanol for patients who were comatose for a variety of reasons (all serious, you can bet) and was gratified, and rather excited, when a significant number of them improved. This led to our use of octacosanol in all conditions in which impaired brain function is critical: memory deficit, Alzheimer's, Parkinson's,[46] seizure disorder, multiple sclerosis, children's attention deficit disorder, and the list goes on.

Octacosanol is one nutrient that works so well you notice it. It is the closest thing to a "universal tonic" I have discovered. Try it, at least 8 milligrams for an adult, and you'll see for yourself.

Give These Breakthroughs a Break!

These twelve items do not constitute all that is new in complementary nutrition, but they do provide the flavor of the science. The point to take home with you is that these agents work for me and for hundreds of my nutritionally oriented colleagues. To us, using them is second nature. When we consider our therapeutic options in case management, these nutrients, and others like them, come to mind first, simply because they are as effective as the orthodox offerings or more so, yet they are generally without risk.

The disturbing aspect is that, even though the beneficiaries are our patients, many with life-compromising illnesses, orthodoxy has not only failed to show interest, but has actively complained *against* these innocuous therapies.

The real criminals in all of this are our governmental agencies, which consistently adopt a prove-it-to-me attitude even though they should full well know that proof is not an economic possibility. When there are lives to be saved or reconstructed and there are no moneyed sponsors to underwrite the costs of proving the worth of these natural therapies, then the government must act to do so. There are national institutes for just about everything, and they are funded. Why should they not be given the responsibility of testing that which the "medical underground" has found successful?

25

. . .

SUPPOSE YOU WERE
MY PATIENT . . .

I certainly hope that what you have read has made you want to
know the details of how our patients converted themselves from
sufferers to successes, from being case histories to being anecdotal
evidence.

One of my pet peeves is authors who tell you of their wondrous
achievements but never quite tell you *how* they do it. Because of
the complexity of Complementary Medicine, this may happen here,
but it won't be for lack of trying. Let me do this by walking you
through the very steps my own Atkins Center patients take from
the time they make their commitment to "go complementary."

The Disadvantage of Complementary Medicine

I guess I have neglected, until now, to tell you the chief drawback
of Complementary Medicine. Since in the next few pages you are
going to discover it yourselves, I had better confess now. This new
medicine is not easy or simple, like instructions out of a cookbook.
It is complex, elaborate, and requires decision-making at every turn.
It is so individualized that no two people get exactly the same program. Its disadvantage, then, is that it is too difficult for ordinary
mortals to understand. How utterly unfortunate this would make
things if our physicians were ordinary mortals. But, happily, they
are not; just ask them.

Let's suppose you decided to be a patient of ours. What would
it be like?

The First Visit: The Complementarist's Workup

A week or two before your appointment with me, you would go to a relatively quiet workup center, physically separate from our main office (not by design but because of the limitations of Manhattan real estate). There you will be met by one of my staff physicians, usually a young doctor with aspirations of becoming a great complementary physician.

You will fill out some six pages of questionnaires about any symptoms you may have noticed, plus your past medical history, family history, medications and/or vitamins list, and a description of your chief complaints. The nurse will take a careful dietary history. (That is the first thing I look at, because it tells me how much room you have for improvement.) The doctor may then use all that written information as a jumping-off point to take his own history. We call it an intern's history, because of the century-old practice at teaching hospitals of having interns get everything on paper, leaving no stone unturned.

The Naked Truth

Then you will be ushered into the examining room, where the same doctor will perform a head-to-toe physical, which is supposed to include sticking a gloved finger in every orifice that will admit one. He will pay careful attention to the skin, hair, nails, tongue, teeth, and gums, for these are the parts of the body which give evidence of your nutritional state, which he is expected to evaluate.

Before you are reunited with your clothes, you will get an electrocardiogram, pulmonary function test, and photomotogram (a quick screening test of thyroid function). An x-ray of your chest (or other part) will be performed only if the doctor feels it is appropriate.

You may also have a visual screening battery performed by one of our nurses, employing the grid that screens for peripheral visual field defects. You may have a dental examination, which includes a mercury vapor test to see if your amalgams are actively releasing mercury vapor. Or you may undergo psychological testing with the Minnesota Multiphasic Inventory (MMPI), or even the Rorschach (inkblot) test.

Our Use of the Medical Laboratory

All the while, blood testing is proceeding concurrently. You will have arrived sans breakfast and will then get a single venipuncture, with a handful of test tubes being filled. (Don't be concerned; all the tubes can be filled with less than two ounces, total.) At this point, we will probably begin a glucose tolerance test, which is a pivotal study because it can demonstrate the relationship of your particular package of medical problems to the various sources of sugar in your diet. This means you will get a bottle of corn syrup cola beverage to drink and that further test tubes of venous blood will be collected every hour for five or six hours (plus some on the half hour), while you and my nurses take notes of any symptoms you may notice. If the symptoms you are worried about are reproduced during this test, that provides the strongest evidence that the symptoms are blood-sugar-related. We also collect urine specimens throughout the morning.

The blood is analyzed for the entire routine screening panel of blood counts and twenty "chemistries." Our routine also calls for thyroid testing, IgE (allergy) blood levels, vitamin levels, and a complete lipid profile. It is semiroutine for our doctors to order a study of cellular immunity, the T and B subsets, or our famous cytotoxic test. The latter enables me to do your dietary counseling on a very specific, personalized level. I will be able to tell you which foods need most to be eliminated, according to the severity of reaction when your white blood cells are incubated on a slide with various food antigens.

Information about essential trace minerals or the toxic heavy metals can be obtained either by way of a one-ounce snip of hair from the nape of your neck, or by a more expensive blood test called the RBC/plasma mineral analysis.

Then You and Your Chart Visit Me

A week or two later we meet, and your chart is full of medical information, compactly gathered together. Just as Complementary Medicine is orthodox medicine *and then some*, so is complementary diagnosis. Your chart contains all the information required for an academic doctor's evaluation, *plus* information about nutrition, your immunity, your food responses, and your metabolism. I am looking less to find out the name of your illness than to find out what may be *causing* illness in you.

Part of the reason a complementary workup is so detailed is that the combined medicine represents a movement toward holism, which calls for the unification of medical care into the hands of a single, comprehensively informed physician (or group), and away from the disjointed compartmentalizing by specialists, none of whom accepts the responsibility for *integrating* the treatment plan. Your personal physician, therefore, must know at least a little bit about everything that pertains to your health.

Then we talk

I ask you first what you perceive to be the main reasons you are seeking help. From that point on, I am disciplining myself to see the big picture and trying not to get stuck on the many details we now have that make up that picture. The first thing I try to learn about you is whether you intend to get really healthy, or whether you would really rather have someone take care of you. Do you recognize that the conversion to good health will be achieved by you and not by me? If you don't, the whole emphasis of our meeting shifts until you see quite clearly that I am unable to *do something for you*. I can only outline what you can *do for yourself*.

Then, after giving you my working hypothesis as to what, in your lifestyle, might be the cause of the medical problems you are having, I begin by outlining a nutritional program for you. This consists of nutritional supplements of the type I have been writing about, plus a diet tailor-made for you.

The Atkins Center Diets

Our diets are open-ended; they consist of rules to follow, not specific foods. Thus, no two people eat precisely the same foods, even when the diets are printed on the same forms.

One of the most difficult tasks I ever assigned to myself was to write a form that I could use for all patients but that would still allow me to outline different specific instructions for each individual. Actually, I came up with two forms. This is how I use them:

I use two basic diets and select between them principally on the criterion of whether or not the patient needs a diet to counter a weight-gainer's metabolism. People who need to lose weight receive the lower carbohydrate diet, the Atkins Diet, the direct descendant of the diet I found so useful in *Diet Revolution*. If the patient cannot tolerate weight loss, he is given the more liberal Meat and Millet Diet, the one that allows starch but not sugar.

That is only the first of several choices I have to make for each patient. I must also decide whether it is appropriate in individual cases (a) to eliminate yeast-containing or fermented foods, (b) to rotate the food choices, and if so how many days should elapse before repeating a food, (c) to restrict salt, or (d) to perform a cytotoxic test and restrict foods that the test indicates as "intolerant" and, if so, which of those foods.

Then I have to decide how much of the foods that are "borderline" choices to allow in each case. And finally, visit by visit, I add (most often) or subtract (rarely) items in an effort to make the diet painlessly livable yet still an effective avoidance diet that achieves the successful result.

I now refer you to Appendix A and Appendix B so that you may see the diets as they are actually used at the Atkins Center.

The Nutritional Supplement System

Welcome back from the appendices. If you have it clearly fixed in your mind how you are going to be eating from here on in and have the resolve to carry it out, you have already solved most of your problem. Nonetheless, I assume that most of you feel that the real key to nutritional medicine lies in knowing about vitamins, minerals, amino acids, and all the other nutritional "goodies" you can gobble down as supplements. I'm certainly not here to downplay the role that nutrients can have as a safe yet effective pharmacology, but I must re-emphasize that *no nutritional program can get results unless you avoid what you must avoid*. There are too many orthodox nutritionists and registered dietitians who fail to recognize the single most important principle of nutrition medicine: *The value of a diet is not so much the good nutrition it includes as the acquired intolerances it eliminates*.

How Many Vitamins Do We Need?

I hope you realize that the days of the multiple vitamin supplement that supplies the minimum daily requirements are over — except in extremely backward places, like hospital dietetic departments. As a matter of fact, I could easily prescribe 80 vitamin, mineral, and other essential nutrient capsules per person per day and still not prescribe a single overdose, according to the amounts *orthodox* medical literature finds necessary to be effective. For example, a healthy middle-aged woman who wants to prevent cancer, osteoporosis, and dysplasia of her cervix would have to take 25 folic acid tablets, 9 calcium gluconate tablets, 9 primrose oil capsules, 9 marine lipid capsules, and 9 standard antioxidant capsules just to provide the amounts of those nutrients deemed to be effective in recent medical studies. Then add to this the rest of the B complex, the optimal amount of vitamin C, the fat-soluble vitamins A, D, and E, the more than a dozen essential trace minerals, and some important intermediary metabolites and you see how the number can mount.

And This Is Not Megavitamin Therapy

The term *megavitamins* applies to the use of quantities that are huge multiples of the usual requirements. What I have outlined is nutrients given in the quantities necessary to be effective. For example, of the more than sixty double-blind studies done worldwide on the use of primrose oil in eczema, premenstrual syndrome, lipid disorders, and the like, the *minimum* quantity that produced an effect was six capsules. The large number of vitamins to choose from is a function of the *breadth* of the nutritional possibilities recognized once a greater knowledge is acquired.

The Problem with Numbers

The main difficulty in working out supplement programs is that the optimal number of vitamins* is not optimal — for the stomach.

* In this context, I may use the word *vitamins* to include all nutritional compounds.

What may be physiologically the perfect quantity of a variety of nutrients as each is considered singly will, when dealt with in the aggregate, almost invariably be more than anyone's stomach will want to handle. Suppose someone goes down a list of health food store possibilities asking, What is the right amount of bee pollen, of liver extract, of mucopolysaccharides, of calcium, of lecithin, of pancreatic enzymes, et cetera, et cetera? Were I to answer each question to the best of my ability, the patient would end up with a supplement program that is not only indigestible, but more expensive and inconvenient than it could possibly be worth.

The Inescapable Conclusion

In planning a supplement program, we must be *selective*. We must pick and choose what we, as individuals, need most. I have struggled with developing such programs for all those who have been patients at the center and have gradually evolved a system that works better than any other I have used to date.

The Building-Block System

The Atkins Center system of dietary supplements is based on using a series of unique building blocks — vitamin formulations created for specific purposes. Rather than use individual vitamins, we work with formulas created by the expedient of gathering together into a single capsule all the nutritional ingredients that I and other clinical nutritionists have found to be most useful in a common clinical situation.

Thus, you have read of some patients getting the Anti-arthritic Formula, the Antihypertensive Formula, the Osteoporosis Formula, or the like. So far, we have developed more than a dozen formulas, which are listed in Appendix C. Some of you will recall that I did the same thing in *Nutrition Breakthrough*. You will note that all the formulations are somewhat modified, reflecting the fact that we are constantly updating as new nutritional knowledge is acquired.

On our production line are formulas for hypoglycemics, dieters, potency in men, PMS and menopause in women, immune system support, candida, and memory (which I will order as soon as I remember what it was that helped so many of my patients).

How I Would Use the System for You

You will need a basic formula. This is still the single most important building block, for it provides the minimum necessary amount of a broad list of nutrients. (Since the last book, cysteine, vanadium, and molybdenum have been added, and iron and iodine have been removed, not because they are not important, but because a few patients react to these minerals.) I usually start every adult on the Basic Formula with the idea that six tablets a day, two after each meal, is the usual dose. (For those taking no other vitamins, nine tablets a day may be the better dose.) There is a second basic formula, which I use for women who must lower their estrogenicity because of fibroids, fibrocystic breast disease, or endometriosis. Here we have eliminated folic acid and PABA and have increased the amount of choline, inositol, and methionine.

The Next Step

I would like to tell you the system I use for arriving at vitamin prescriptions for each individual, so that you can help yourself. But the system requires experience, and access to the vitamins is through the Atkins Center, not the stores. Therefore, I can only outline what I teach my doctors. If I were teaching one of my young doctors how to do a vitamin program for you, using our building blocks, I would ask him to decide whether there are any special formulas that apply to you. Do you have arthritis, diabetes, allergy? Do you need more energy, or better sleep, or help with your memory or immune system? The first step is to write down all the formulas that apply to you. Then we look for specific deficiencies found on the laboratory reports, especially the trace minerals. We often give extra vitamin C and bioflavonoids. I generally give GLA or EPA nutrients, often both. (If serum cholesterol is high, I favor GLA; if triglycerides are high, I favor EPA.) I usually prescribe antioxidants for everyone.

Most of the building-block formulas have been designed so that the customary adult dose is six capsules or tablets. I often modify this upward or downward according to whether the problem it helps to solve is a major or a minor one. I then write down a tentative vitamin list and add up the number of pills I have prescribed. For patients with complicated medical problems, that total number is often too high — it would prove indigestible. I might then cut the total prescription down by a third, or even a half.

Caveats

Vitamins, like drugs, can cause untoward reactions. But, unlike drug reactions, vitamin reactions rarely take place in the blood stream once the vitamins have been absorbed and assimilated. Here you are protected by the very property that militant antinutritionists seize upon to denigrate nutritional substances — what I call "the expensive urine system." This refers to the fact that the body takes *only what it needs* and excretes the surplus, thus saving you from an overdose but creating a vitamin-rich urinary output. In "the inexpensive drug system," there is no such protection and an overdose can kill.

The adverse effects of vitamins fall into three categories. Almost all of the adverse reactions are gastrointestinal in nature. Too many vitamins sitting in an empty stomach are indigestible enough to cause distress, repeating on you, causing heartburn or some discomfort felt in the pit of your stomach. As they move through the digestive tract, especially if they contain vitamin C or magnesium compounds, especially the oxide, they can cause diarrhea.

The second most common adverse effects are "allergic" reactions, almost always in people with a history of "allergies" to various foods and chemicals. In some people the problem is solved by changing to a hypoallergenic line of vitamins, since the problem is usually in the fillers or binders used in tableting the nutrients, not the nutrient itself. This category of reactions also provides an example of when synthetic may be better than natural, for some people *are* allergic to the food source. Many of these patients are difficult to treat, having traveled from one nutrition doctor to another without achieving success. The roadblock is the Catch-22 situation of not being able to tolerate the very nutrients that we use to overcome this type of sensitivity. What success we have achieved we have done through painstaking use of a gentle homeopathy, or by administering a series of vitamin and mineral injections.

The third group of adverse reactions are true toxicities. An example is the peripheral neuropathy (numbness, tingling in the feet or hands) that comes if doses beyond 1000 milligrams of B_6 are given along with very little other B-complex supplementation. The toxicity of vitamins A and D and the "rebound" effect of suddenly stopping large doses of some vitamins (especially vitamin C) are other good examples. By now, most of these toxicities have been reported upon. Having recognized them, we have built safeguards against them into our building-block system. I do not know of a single example of true vitamin toxicity that has taken place in patients using our system as prescribed.

But you *should* know the toxicity potential of nutritional therapy. For this, let me recommend *my* favorite book (for professionals). It is *Nutritional Influences on Illness* by Melvyn R. Werbach, M.D. The six-page appendix, "Dangers of Supplementation," describes all the nutritional caveats I know about. Contrast this with the thousands of pages in the *Physicians' Desk Reference* devoted to the toxic potential of drugs.

How We Regulate Vitamins

Since we are mainly concerned with gastrointestinal intolerance, we usually ask our patients who are not used to taking vitamins to start with one-third the prescribed dose and, over the first two weeks, gradually build up to full dose. We continually modify our supplement prescription at each subsequent visit, increasing or decreasing formulations as the emphasis shifts. The ability to make these judgments comes with experience, and I can't give general guidelines about this process — it is too specific. I can tell you that we use a "build up, taper down" system, meaning that in the initial stages of therapy we build up the vitamin intake toward maximum effectiveness, and then when we approach an optimal state of health, we strive to cut the vitamin-taking to the necessary minimum.

Does the Diet Ever Change?

In a similar fashion, we start with a strict avoidance diet, which we recognize can be unpleasantly restrictive. The goal is to stay with it long enough to get the maximum clinical benefit from the restrictions. This does not mean until the ideal weight is reached; rather it means when the symptoms due to improper food consumption are under control. Then we start the happier "give-back" phase of dieting. Once my patient's headache or panic attacks or palpitations or other symptoms are under control, I can gradually return some of the foods the patient craves (but never sugar), to see if the symptoms recur. If the patient remains free of symptoms, that food (in the amount given) can stay in the diet; if the symptoms return, at least we are sure the food is a "no-no." We thus gradually work our way back to a diet that represents the best compromise between what we would like to eat and what we can tolerate.

Note that for patients for whom weight loss is also a goal, there is one slight difference. I will not add enough carbohydrate to stop the weight loss, even though the presenting symptoms are controlled.

How We Manage Our Patients

You should by now understand our dietary and nutritional supplement principles, but case management in a complementary center requires much more than that.

About half the patients begin with us already taking some form of medication, sometimes eight or ten different ones. This reflects one of the biggest philosophical differences between orthodox medicine and complementarism. Whereas the apparent objective of orthodoxy is to achieve freedom from illness by use of medications, the clear-cut goal of the new medicine is to achieve wellness *without* medication. *Wellness,* by our definition, means *requiring no medication.*

Our goal, therefore, is to wean the patients from their medications whenever possible. Obviously, there are many instances in which total wellness is no longer possible, and in these cases we may need medications; we may even initiate them. Of course, we can draw upon our nutritional pharmacology, herbal medicine, or homeopathy as safer alternatives to pharmaceuticals.

Unless we perceive that the drug being administered is totally inappropriate or downright dangerous, in which case we stop it immediately, all our drug discontinuances are gradual, visit by visit. We prefer to see these patients at frequent intervals, every week or two, so that the drug withdrawals are done under careful medical supervision.

Selecting a Treatment Protocol

Our patient population, by and large, enters our program with much more serious illness than in the usual internal medical practice. Every visiting doctor who has sat in with us has commented upon that. Our patients, then, need more than prevention; they need treatment.

Our treatment possibilities include nutritional medicine, herbal medicine, acupuncture, chiropractic, homeopathy, bioenergetics, clinical ecology, allergy techniques, biologic (regenerative) medicine, chelation and other infusions, group therapy, neurolinguistic programming, ozone therapy, ultraviolet blood irradiation, an assortment of unclassified techniques, and, of course, *all of orthodox medicine.*

The complementarist is thus provided with an embarrassment of therapeutic riches from which to choose that which he feels may work best. Most of these systems are additive (or complementary); they do not oppose one another. Those that work best standing alone, as do some forms of homeopathy, are less likely to be utilized in our program. I have my own favorite treatment combinations; each of my doctors has a somewhat different emphasis, according to his or her experience. There are many ways to skin a cat; there are many ways to use Complementary Medicine. That is its strength and its elegance.

26

. . .

BUT SUPPOSE YOU WERE
NOT MY PATIENT . . .

Now that I have made you eager to become a complementary
patient (I fervently hope so) and have demonstrated how utterly marvelous it would be to be a patient of ours, I fear I may
have reduced most of you to tears of frustration.

Chances are ninety-nine out of a hundred that we (at the Atkins
Center) won't have the good fortune to be your doctor. Most of you
are geographically too far removed from where we are. And even
when you are not, we may have too long a waiting list or may
charge more than your finances will allow.

Where There's a Will . . .

The point is that I want you to come as close to getting an ideal
health arrangement as possible. Let's see what you can do on your
own. First, let me repeat: *This book was never designed to be a
how-to book; it is a book designed to let the world know that a new
medicine is needed, and that it is ready to become available.* As
this book is written, there are nowhere near enough complementary physicians to supply the medical care required for all those
who should have it. And, as the subject matter of this book indicates, this book is for patients who need doctors, not for do-it-
yourselfers seeking health advice.

So to begin with, let's analyze what you need. To get your health
program going in the right direction, you need to arrange for the
following elements:

- a doctor to oversee and integrate your health care
- a diagnostic facility to evaluate your state of health and your progress
- access to the nutrients and biologicals I recommend as a complementary pharmacology

How Do You Find a Doctor?

First, see if you can find one who *already* has complementary leanings. He may be interested in nutritional medicine, clinical ecology, acupuncture, homeopathy, chelation therapy, or other non-mainstream approaches. Most of these interests are associated with groups of which your doctor-to-be may be a member. (Appendix D contains a list of organizations that give out membership rosters to people who request them.) Remember, a doctor is not obligated to join such a group, so there are some who cannot be located in this way. We call them closet complementarists.

If you locate a doctor in your community through one of these rosters, don't assume you've hit the jackpot. Many doctors are interested in only one aspect of complementary medicine — *only* clinical ecology, or acupuncture, and *not* nutrition, for example. Many specialize in some ailment you don't have. And if you get a nutritionist recommended by the local hospital or medical society, prepare to have a lot of laughs, because you probably already know more about clinical nutrition than he or she does.

The Health Food Store May Be Your Best Bet

Sometimes your best bet is to talk to members of the nutrition underground, which often centers about the staff of your community's most important health food store. Ask: "Which doctors around here practice the best brand of nutritional medicine?" If you get no satisfactory answer, go to the largest nearby city, and then, if necessary, to the nearest metropolis with the same question. I suggest you ask for a nutrition expert rather than some other subdivision of alternative medicine, because nutrition is far and away the most important subspecialty.

One caveat, though. Doctors who are so "into" nutrition that they dispense nutritional supplements in their own office do not figure to be very popular with the health store management, who cannot help feeling a little rejected because of losing such a significant share of their market. But such a doctor may be the very person you are seeking. So be sure to ask the storekeeper whether he may have overlooked a doctor who dispenses.

Now That You Have a Candidate

Your next step is to be sure that the doctor is suitable. You want the doctor to be familiar with the treatment that you now feel, having read this book, would be suitable for you. Ask him or his nurse to outline the general protocol he would follow in treating your condition. If it seems to parallel what I've been saying here, you may want to sign on with him. If not, ask him if he has read or will read this book. After a suitable time, see if you both feel you can work together along these lines. If his ideas seem somewhat different from mine, but he seems to you to know what he is talking about and inspires your confidence, then he may still prove to be the best person you will find. If he is totally unsympathetic with the premise of this book, then it really doesn't sound very promising, does it?

Plan B (and C)

If you still can't locate the right doctor, you may have to work with an orthodox physician who, although open-minded, may not even be aware there is a Complementary Medicine. He may be your own personal physician, one you already like and admire. The next step will be very difficult. Present him with this book, ask him if he is willing to read it, and if and when he does, ask him if he is convinced enough to manage your case while you yourself work with the dietary change and nutritional supplements.

In most cases, if you are taking medications on a daily basis, this will mean your medication requirements will decrease. Both you and your doctor must be aware of that.

Plan C might be to use a combination of an internist whose attitude toward nutritional pharmacology is tolerant, plus a lay nutritionist who does know this field (and this book). Many chiropractors are trained in nutrition and other holistic concepts and they, too, could play this role of second practitioner.

There is even a plan D, and this is risky unless you are very wise. That is, use your present doctor *and* make the necessary nutritional changes on your own, based on your own knowledge and a little more reading. Even here, a *mutual* respect of doctor and patient is required.

Suppose You Don't Need a Doctor?

If you are basically a healthy person and are interested in getting even healthier, and in *preventing* these medical complications I write about, then you can get good guidelines from this book, and you should do very well on your own.

The Diagnostic Aspect

In general, diagnostic testing is provided very nicely by whomever you choose to be your physician. The problem centers around food-intolerance testing, such as the cytotoxic test. Food *allergy* can be tested for in a variety of ways, but too often nonallergic intolerances of real significance are missed. The cytotoxic test would serve this purpose, but it has fallen into disrepute simply because, in my opinion, it is too often neither performed nor interpreted correctly. In the days when blood had only to be collected and mailed in to a few laboratories, the logistics were quite convenient even for residents of remote areas. The problem in cytotoxic testing is that accuracy is lost if the slides are not set up and read within a few hours of the blood drawing. This means, in essence, you have to go to the lab. The lab must be honest enough to know how many tests it can perform on a given day. This means the technician's time must be scheduled.

I believe my help will be needed here. If you write me, enclosing a self-addressed stamped envelope (see page 366), I will send you a list of those cytotoxic laboratories (or those which use a newer technology) whose results I find reliable and reproducible.

What About Supplements?

In the previous chapter, I talked about the building-block system we at the Atkins Center use to prescribe a therapeutic nutritional supplement protocol. You can still come up with a vitamin list without these formulations, which are convenient but not essential.

Make sure you start with a very *broad* basic formula containing at least forty ingredients in doses similar to our Basic Formula. If it requires six capsules a day to get the full dose, so much the better. Ours does.

The basic formula is extremely important, for it prevents most imbalances that might be created when you proceed to the next step, which is to adopt five to ten of the nutritional suggestions that impress you as being most appropriate to your case.

There Is an Art to Vitamin Prescribing

I sincerely hope that you don't *have* to do the prescribing. I hope that, for you, plan A is working and that you have located an experienced, knowledgeable complementary physician.

Nutritional expertise and experience can make the difference between success and failure. The reason may be a single suggestion that the experienced doctor will make — when to use extra folic acid, or magnesium orotate, or anti-yeast protocol, or a thousand other examples.

Suppose Your Doctor Wants to Expand His Horizons

If you wish to receive building-block therapy, you may assume that your doctor does not have access to it. If he is experienced at nutritional prescribing, it should not matter much, because he probably has a very good system of his own. This does not mean that you should feel reticent about discussing some of the nutritional ideas you picked up in this book. (I'm referring to the discussions, not the case histories, whose vitamins may have been appropriate only to those individuals.)

Now, if your doctor is a nutritional neophyte, albeit a willing one, I will personally be more than happy to help him. One way I can do this is to provide him with the nutritional formulations — the actual building blocks we use at the center. Although it is not certain whether we can or should sell our vitamins to individual citizens, it is certain that we can distribute them to other professionals, who in turn can legally prescribe them.

If I haven't handled all the contingencies, there is always plan Z. Write the center (enclosing a self-addressed stamped envelope) and my staff members will try to help you find someone who might help you.

27
• • •

COMMENCEMENT

We've traveled a long way together and I thank you for sharing this journey with me, to the frontiers of the Health Revolution. I'm sure you have noted my deep concern for the future of medicine.

To me it is crystal clear that Complementary Medicine is a better medicine. Remember, I always have the option to practice an excellent state-of-the-art brand of orthodox medicine, but I know when and where I can do better and teach my patients to get better results. Now that Complementary Medicine is itself time-tested, panoramic in scope, and firmly based on scientific evidence, I seldom have to resort to orthodox premises alone.

I cannot believe there could be a fair-minded physician properly exposed to both kinds of medicine who could come to any other conclusion.

The problem is that although we have an abundance of fair-minded physicians, we have a dearth of those who are properly exposed to Complementary Medicine.

The Future Is in Doubt

Although the new medicine is clearly an idea whose time has come, there is an existing power structure pouring billions of dollars into the project of ensuring that it will not. I cannot predict the outcome of this classic struggle. I do know that the new medicine cannot win without help. And there is no one to help but you. We cannot count on help from industry, the profession, or the government. They have declared themselves the enemy of all who would challenge the status quo.

This Is Where You Come In

If you believe the truths I have given you, then I ask for your active participation. And there are things you can do. Let's start with your doctor and doctors you know.

Although most complementary-oriented physicians will read this book, virtually no orthodox physician will. Virtually no orthodox physician will read it even if you give it to him. Nonetheless, I want you to feel it is *your* responsibility to make him aware of the ideas it contains. (Even if you have to spend *your* visit to read *him* some of the pertinent passages.)

An ideologic revolution can take place only in minds that are prepared for it. This may be your revolution, but it is more your doctor's revolution, and his mind is not prepared. Any crack you can produce in his armor may help reopen his once fertile mind and allow for the revolution by gradual evolution I hope we will all achieve.

Watch Our Congress

Keep an eye open for the establishment's attempts to pass legislation that destroys your health freedom. Here you have real clout. It was the outraged public who by its written campaign squelched the odious Pepper bills that would have destroyed Complementary Medicine while it was still an embryo. When, in the future, your conscience calls upon you to act, do so. It's not enough to "let George do it." Both you *and* George must do it.

Keep in Touch, Hear?

Whenever I write a book, I feel it is a communication. I, too, like to be communicated with. I may not be able to answer all your letters, but I would like to read your comments — that I have always done. This time I have a computer, so when you write, your name will be punched in as someone we've made contact with. It will be on our personal mailing list, and I will use it — but only when I feel I have something to benefit you.

Write me, in care of

The Atkins Center for Complementary Medicine
400 East Fifty-sixth Street
New York, New York 10022

Appendix A
The Atkins
(Low-Carbohydrate)
Diet

This is the instruction form patients at the Atkins Center are given when the diet must be low in carbohydrates. There are several blanks that the doctor checks off or fills out according to how strict he feels the diet must be (i.e., what carbohydrate level he chooses for the patient) and to whether several sets of concurrent restrictions must also be invoked.

Carbohydrate Restriction Diet

This is a test* to determine your body's response to taking away virtually all the ready fuel from your diet to see how readily and thoroughly your body utilizes its own stored fat as a source of energy. When you return, your response on the diet, your reading on the ketone analyzer, and your laboratory results will enable us to proceed with the next phase of meal planning. It must be emphasized that the entire test will be negated if you add to the diet so much as a single piece of chewing gum. This is not to be thought of as your permanent diet, but it may provide the basis of your lifetime diet.

This form, as written, describes a diet which does not deal in

---

* Presented as a test to patients who are to be returning to the center after one or two weeks at that level, it also serves as the starting level of a permanent diet for those who find that weight control or one of the other advantages of total carbohydrate restriction is necessary on a long-term basis.

quantities, but does effect certain restrictions. Other restrictions may also be necessary in your case. Abide by them if they are checked off.

_____ NO YEAST OR FERMENTED ITEMS.* This means no cheese, tofu, vinegar, wine, beer, bread (unless unleavened), pasta, etc.

_____ NO CYTOTOXIC FOODS.† If food intolerances are known, through cytotoxic or allergy testing, or from personal experience, they are to be eliminated. Avoid food marked

_____.

_____ NO SALT or _____, LOW TOTAL SODIUM.‡

_____ DIVERSIFIED ROTATION DIET.§ This principle requires that after eating any food in a certain biologic category, you must wait _____ days before having it again.

_____ OTHER.‖ _____

List of Food Permitted

Your diet is to be made up exclusively of foods and beverages from this list. Each item is to be 100% pure and contain no fillers or added ingredients in the sugar or starch families. *If it does not appear specifically on this list, it is not allowed.* You will note this is a qualitative and not a quantitative diet.

ANIMAL FOODS (MEAT, FISH, FOWL, SHELLFISH)

All are allowed, unless sugar, MSG, corn syrup, cornstarch, flour, pickling, nitrites, or other preservatives are used in the preparation.

---

*This set of restrictions is offered to patients in whom an overgrowth of *Candida albicans* is thought to be a clinically significant problem.

†Ideally, we would like to know the results of food-intolerance testing in everyone before devising a semipermanent diet. After studying the results, the clinician must make a judgment as to which of the foods tested most surely need to be restricted. Sometimes he restricts even slightly reactive foods (when there are few reactions, yet severe diet-related symptoms); more often, he restricts only the foods that provoked a severe or moderate reaction.

‡The restriction of salt, or of all sodium, is necessary in some hypertensives and in some fluid-retaining patients.

§A diversified three- or four-day rotational diet is theoretically advisable for everyone because it prevents the development of food (or beverage) addiction; but in practice it is reserved for those for whom food intolerance is a serious problem.

‖Occasionally a no-nightshade, no-dairy-food, no-spicy-food, or other dictum is necessary — for specific reasons.

EGGS

Permitted without restriction.

FATS AND OILS

Despite the furor over "high fat diets," many fats, especially certain oils, are essential to good nutrition. We must include a source of GLA (gamma-linolenic acid) and omega-3 oils (EPA, salmon oil, linseed oil). Olive oil (monounsaturated) is valuable. The best vegetable oils are walnut, soybean, sesame, sunflower, and safflower oils, especially if they are labeled "cold pressed." Butter is far superior to margarine. Mayonnaise is permitted unless you are on yeast restriction. The fat that is part of the meat or fowl you eat is permitted.

For salad dressing use the desired oil plus vinegar or lemon juice and spices. Grated cheese, chopped eggs, or bacon (if allowed) may be added.

Food Allowed in Limited Quantities

Do not exceed the quantities specified in any one day.

CHEESE (HARD, OR SEMISOFT, AGED, YELLOW)

Examples are Swiss, American, cheddar, brie, camembert, blue, mozzarella, gruyere, etc. Goat cheeses are included here. Avoid "diet" cheeses, cheese spreads, or cheese foods such as Velveeta. No gjetost.
You may have up to _____ oz. per day.*

FRESH CHEESES

Cottage, farmer, pot, and ricotta. No diet cheeses. Soybean cheese (tofu) is included in this category.
You may have up to _____ oz. per day.*

*Because of the large number of patients who are milk intolerant, who are reactive to fermented foods, or who react to cheeses on the cytotoxic test, cheese is not permitted for many patients. In uncomplicated weight-control situations, it can usually be given in amounts from 3 to 16 ounces daily. Cottage cheese is preferred when moderation in fat intake is desirable; hard cheese when carbohydrates must be strictly limited.

SALAD VEGETABLES

Leafy greens (lettuce, escarole, romaine, parsley, collards, endive, spinach, etc.), mushrooms, cucumbers, celery, radishes, peppers, bean sprouts.
You may have up to ＿＿ cupsful per day.*

OTHER PERMISSIBLE VEGETABLES

See list below. Some salad items are included in this list and their use is governed by this limitation.

asparagus	kohlrabi	pumpkin
broccoli	mushrooms	turnips
string or wax beans	tomatoes	avocado
cabbage	onions	bamboo shoots
beet greens	spinach	bean sprouts
cauliflower	peppers	water chestnuts
chard	summer squash	snow pea pods
eggplant	zucchini	sauerkraut
kale	okra	

You may have up to ＿＿ cupsful per day.

SPECIAL CATEGORIES †

Olives	up to ＿＿ per day
Avocados	up to ＿＿ per day
Nuts and seeds (no cashews)	up to ＿＿ oz. per day
Lemon/lime juice	up to ＿＿ tsps. per day
Cream (heavy, light, sour)	up to ＿＿ tsps. per day

SWEETENERS AND DESSERTS

Aspartame (Equal, Nutra-Sweet) is the best sweetener. Saccharin and cyclamates (available in Canada and Europe) are/are not permitted.‡ Any combination of two or more sweeteners enhances

---

*Salad intake varies between 2 cups, loosely packed (strict first level of diet), to 6 cups (liberal diet).

†These special categories contain foods that in moderate quantities are suitable for middle levels of the diet.

‡I generally allow the dieter artificial sweeteners in order to ease the transition away from sugar. This does not mean I consider them to be "health foods."

the effect and enables you to use less. Hexitols such as Sorbitol as well as honey, fructose, lactose (milk sugar), maltose (barley malt), and dextrose (corn sugar) are simple sugars and are not allowed.

From time to time ready-made diet desserts appear on the market (diet gelatins, etc.). If you see one, read the label very carefully. Carbohydrate contents should be less than one gram per serving.

BEVERAGES

Consume liberally but do not force fluids beyond your capacity. Avoid caffeine.

The best beverages are water and herbal teas. Spring and mineral waters are preferred to tap water or club soda, but all are allowed. Herbal teas should be free of caffeine, sugar, or barley.

Clear broth (consommé) is permitted if you are not salt restricted.

Decaffeinated coffee is/is not allowed.

Regular coffee or espresso is/is not allowed.*

Tea is allowed up to ＿＿＿ teabags' worth per day. (May brew up to four cups from one teabag.)

Diet soda (caffeine-free) is allowed up to ＿＿＿ cups per day.†

ALCOHOL

Alcohol is not permitted.

Quantities

The diet works best on a "demand feeding" basis, i.e., eat whenever you are hungry, just enough to assuage your hunger and no more. No meal is mandatory; but frequent small feedings are often more effective than 3 square meals. The objective is for the natural appetite reduction of the low-carbohydrate diet to ease you into the consumption of smaller and smaller quantities. Therefore, do not eat everything on your plate "just because it's there."

Note again that the following items are *not* on the diet: bread,

---

*In most cases, I do not allow the use of caffeine. When breaking the coffee habit, I often allow regular tea.
†I generally allow the dieter artificial sweeteners in order to ease the transition away from sugar. This does not mean I consider them to be "health foods."

flour-containing items, fruits, juices, honey, milk or skimmed milk, yogurt, canned soups, dairy substitutes, catsup, sweet condiments, and relishes.

Avoid these common mistakes: Using "diet" products (candy, fruit, bread, ice cream, etc.), food containing sugar (coleslaw), liquid medications, cough syrup, cough drops, lozenges, Ex-Lax, Aspergum.

Symptoms on the Diet

We expect you to feel physically improved on the diet — that is the reason we have prescribed it. Some people, however, experience symptoms which we will note here.

Symptoms occurring on the first two days of the diet probably represent either an untoward reaction to one (or more) of the new vitamins or are really withdrawal symptoms representing the sudden removal of a food or beverage you were actually addicted to. Symptoms beginning the second or third day (fatigue, weakness, irritability, etc.) represent the metabolic changeover from carbohydrate to your stored body fat as a primary fuel. In all cases if symptoms are tolerable, continue the diet to see if they diminish by the fourth day. If they do not, omit the vitamins and/or add some starch (bread or whole grain) to the diet for a few days and then return to the diet.

When weight loss is too rapid, there may be weakness representing salt depletion. In this case you should be able to correct matters by taking in salty broth and potassium-rich foods (parsley and sunflower seeds).

The most frequent untoward reaction is constipation. It is appropriate to add unprocessed miller's bran and herbal laxatives if your bowel movement begins to slow down. Nausea and stomach distress, however, would more likely be due to the vitamins than to the diet. If this happens, omit the vitamins for a few days and resume at approximately half the dosage.

Exercise

Maximum achievable physical conditioning is a must. This must include (a) aerobic exercise for heart conditioning, (b) limbering-stretching and strength exercises for all muscle groups, and (c) recreational exercise for *your enjoyment*.

Start at the level you are now at, and gradually and steadily build up in all these categories.

[The rest of the instructions are the personalized support program for each individual patient.]

• • •

Appendix B
The Meat and Millet
(Insulin Regulation)
Diet

This is the instruction form patients are given when their weight is at or below its ideal level and a strict low-carbohydrate diet is therefore not advisable.

Insulin Regulation Diet

There are several diets that patients of the Atkins Center may follow according to their dietary needs. The Insulin Regulation Diet is one such diet. It is based on the recognition that our single most important dietary need is to regulate and stabilize our blood sugar. This is achieved by eliminating sugar, glucose-containing foods, and refined carbohydrates. You will accomplish this if you follow these instructions to the letter between now and your next visit. At that point you will be re-evaluated, through an analysis of your verbal and laboratory responses, and your diet will be modified if need be, so that an individual diet prescription can begin to emerge.

This form, as written, describes a diet which does not deal in quantities, but does effect certain restrictions. Other restrictions may also be necessary in your case. Abide by them if they are checked off.

———— NO YEAST OR FERMENTED ITEMS.* This means no cheese, tofu, vinegar, wine, beer, bread (unless unleavened), pasta, etc.

*This set of restrictions is offered to patients in whom an overgrowth of *Candida albicans* is thought to be a clinically significant problem.

_____ NO CYTOTOXIC FOODS.* If food intolerances are known, through cytotoxic or allergy testing, or from personal experience, they are to be eliminated. Avoid food marked

_____.

_____ NO SALT or _____, LOW TOTAL SODIUM.†

_____ DIVERSIFIED ROTATION DIET.‡ This principle requires that after eating any food in a certain biologic category, you must wait _____ days before having it again.

_____ OTHER § _____

List of Foods Permitted

Your entire diet is to be made from choices within the categories below. If these items are part of a prepared food which also contains ingredients that are *not* permitted, then none of that food is permitted.

ANIMAL FOODS (MEAT, FISH, FOWL, SHELLFISH)

All are allowed, unless sugar, MSG, corn syrup, cornstarch, flour, pickling, nitrites, or other preservatives are used in the preparation.

EGGS

Permitted without restriction.

NUTS, SEEDS, SOYBEANS

All types, including nut butters (without sugar or glucose), soy flour, textured soy protein. (Fermented soy products, i.e., tofu and miso, are not allowed on the non-yeast diet.)

---

*Ideally, we would like to know the results of food-intolerance testing in everyone before devising a semipermanent diet. After studying the results, the clinician must make a judgment as to which of the foods tested most surely need to be restricted. Sometimes he restricts even slightly reactive foods (when there are few reactions, yet severe diet-related symptoms); more often, he restricts only the foods that provoked a severe or moderate reaction.

†The restriction of salt, or of all sodium, is necessary in some hypertensives and in some fluid-retaining patients.

‡A diversified three- or four-day rotational diet is theoretically advisable for everyone because it prevents the development of food (or beverage) addiction; but in practice it is reserved for those for whom food intolerance is a serious problem.

§Occasionally a no-nightshade, no-dairy-food, no-spicy-food, or other dictum is necessary — for specific reasons.

DAIRY PRODUCTS

Milk: Contains lactose, a simple sugar. Can be a problem to the lactose-intolerant. (Include buttermilk, unflavored yogurt in this category.) You may have _____.*

Cheeses: All cheese, from aged, hard varieties to cottage cheese or ricotta, are low in lactose (carbohydrate), but all are fermented by some form of mold or culture. You may have _____.†

Cream and butter are/are not OK.‡

Never use nondairy lighteners or margarine.

FATS AND OILS

Despite the furor over "high fat diets," many fats, especially certain oils, are essential to good nutrition. We must include a source of GLA (gamma-linolenic acid) and omega-3 oils (EPA, salmon oil, linseed oil). Olive oil (monounsaturated) is valuable. The best vegetable oils are walnut, soybean, sesame, sunflower, and safflower oils, especially if they are labeled "cold pressed." Butter is far superior to margarine. Mayonnaise is permitted unless you are on yeast restriction. The fat that is part of the meat or fowl you eat is permitted.

The Carbohydrates in Your Diet

The basic principle of this diet is to eliminate sugars (simple carbohydrates) and replace them with starches (complex carbohydrates). To avoid undesired weight loss, you must replace sugar carbohydrates with vegetables and grains.

VEGETABLES AND GRAINS (COMPLEX CARBOHYDRATES)

All vegetables, steamed and cooked, can be taken freely. Grains are allowed as whole grains or cereals. White flour is a refined carbohydrate and must be avoided. Bread and crackers are made with yeast and are/are not allowed.§ Matzo or sourdough bread are examples of "no yeast." Rice cakes are without wheat or yeast.

---

* Most often, no milk is allowed. In growing children, up to 16 ounces is often allowed. Milk is a source of lactose, one of the simple sugars.

† Cheese is restricted when a no-yeast diet is necessary.

‡ Cream and butter are permitted unless there is a severe dairy intolerance.

§ Decision is based on presence of yeast or wheat intolerance.

Some vegetables and grains with high carbohydrate content include brown rice, kasha, oats, corn, cracked wheat, millet, peas, lentils, beans, yams, parsnips, acorn squash, plantain, and cashews. These are/are not OK.*

FRUIT

A most important point is that fruit carbohydrate is generally a simple sugar, consisting of glucose and fructose, the same as white sugar. According to our appraisal of your need for glucose restriction, your fruit intake should be limited to _____.†
Avoid fruit juice. However, lemon, lime, and vegetable juices, avocados, and olives are allowed.

Other Foods and Beverages

CONDIMENTS

Condiments are generally allowed, but there are exceptions. Try to use herbal seasonings (oregano, thyme, cinnamon, etc.). Most prepared condiments will prove incorrect, containing sugar or corn syrup, or for some, salt or fermentation. Pepper is a very common cause of food allergy. Please, no catsup or other sweet condiment.

SWEETS AND DESSERTS

Since this is the primary restriction on the diet, we cannot offer much more here except this advice: "Don't leave room for dessert." For those who have a sweet tooth, the most sensible choice is to use artificial sweeteners, all of which have been implicated as "problem foods."

I generally recommend combinations of all available noncarbohydrate sweeteners: aspartame (Equal, Nutra-Sweet), saccharin and cyclamates (available in Canada and Europe).‡

Notice that hexitols (Sorbitol), honey, fructose, lactose (milk sugar),

---

*Decision is based on whether carbohydrates need *some* restriction, as in slightly overweight subjects.

†This is the difficult decision. When blood sugar control is paramount, no fruit is allowed. If the blood glucose dynamics are relatively normal, then I may allow up to a half piece per meal.

‡I generally allow the dieter artificial sweeteners in order to ease the transition away from sugar. This does not mean I consider them to be "health foods."

maltose (barley malt), and dextrose (corn sugar) are simple sugars and are not allowed.

BEVERAGES

Consume liberally but do not force fluids beyond your capacity. Avoid caffeine.

The best beverages are water and herbal teas. Spring and mineral waters are preferred to tap water or club soda, but all are allowed. Herbal teas should be free of caffeine, sugar, or barley.

Clear broth (consommé) is permitted if you are not salt restricted.

Decaffeinated coffee is/is not allowed.

Regular coffee or espresso is/is not allowed.*

Tea is allowed up to ____ teabags' worth per day. (May brew up to four cups from one teabag.)

Diet soda (caffeine-free) is allowed up to ____ cups per day.†

ALCOHOL

Alcohol is not permitted.

Quantities

The general rule is to eat the amount that makes you comfortable, whenever you feel like eating. Often, frequent small snacks accomplish this better. A sizable breakfast that contains protein is encouraged.

If you wish to lose weight, you should restrict your carbohydrates and cut your quantities to the level where hunger is assuaged but no more. If you still remain overweight, you should be placed on another diet: the Atkins Center Low-Carbohydrate Diet.

Symptoms on the Diet

Most people feel better from the very beginning. Some, however, will notice worsening immediately that almost always represents withdrawal from addiction, be it to caffeine, sugar, juices,

---

*In most cases, I do not allow the use of caffeine. When breaking the coffee habit, I often allow regular tea.

† I generally allow the dieter artificial sweeteners in order to ease the transition away from sugar. This does not mean I consider them to be "health foods."

milk, or some specific allergy food that has been removed. This can prove fortunate, for it means that after a few days, when the withdrawal is completed, you will feel better than before.

For some, taking a large quantity of vitamins and minerals in effective doses may produce symptoms of a gastrointestinal nature. If this happens, go back to your previous vitamin level and add the new ones, a few at a time, until you build up to the prescribed level.

If any discontinuance of medications has taken place, this could cause the return of symptoms for which they were originally prescribed. If this is suspected, you must call one of our staff physicians.

One common problem is a change in bowel habits, usually constipation. Unprocessed miller's bran, herbal laxatives, or large doses of vitamin C (5 to 20 grams a day) may be helpful in these cases.

Exercise

Maximum achievable physical conditioning is a must. This must include (a) aerobic exercise for heart conditioning, (b) limbering-stretching and strength exercises for all muscle groups, and (c) recreational exercise for *your enjoyment*.

Start at the level you are now at, and gradually and steadily build up in all these categories.

■ ■ ■

Appendix C
Prescriptive Formulas

I sometimes feel rather peeved with doctor-authors who won't provide their readers with a full disclosure of the secrets behind their success. I see no point in not giving the reader the formulas we use as nutritional backup in dealing with various conditions. Of course, the further secret that I can't give you is knowing which ones to use on whom and how much to take.

The two Basic formulas provide sound nutrition for almost everyone, and 3 to 6 tablets a day is what I generally prescribe. For the other formulas that is also the general dosage level, although in my clinical practice I sometimes prescribe more tablets as the clinical urgencies require. With cancer patients, for instance, I sometimes prescribe up to 12 Antioxidant Formula capsules a day. However, as I said in the Preface, this is *not* an invitation to be your own doctor. You should have a physician of your own who understands nutrition and who will help you choose the best levels for you.

I'd also like to point out that none of these formulas is the total treatment protocol for the condition it relates to. Each formula is usually just one of the elements in our building-block system of prescribing. A patient with, for example, arthritis is generally receiving not just the Basic Formula and the Anti-arthritic Formula but also a number of supplemental nutrients, varying with the particular type and severity of his arthritis and relating as well to any other conditions he may be suffering from. This highly individualized approach contributes strongly to our success.

These formulas are updated every year or two as new nutritional refinements are worked out, so if you should see a label from the Atkins Center with, let us say, a different Antifatigue Formula, that will be the reason.

Basic Formula (Yeast-Free*)

Each tablet contains:

Vitamin A (beta carotene)	500 IU ⎫
Vitamin A (acetate)	500 IU ⎭
Vitamin D_2	30 IU
Thiamine (HCl) (B_1)	10 mg
Riboflavin (B_2)	8 mg
Ascorbate acid (from calcium ascorbate)	160 mg
Niacin (B_3)	5 mg ⎫
Niacinamide (B_3)	10 mg ⎭
Pyridoxine	10 mg
Pyridoxal-5 phosphate	2 mg
Biotin	40 mcg
Folic acid	400 mcg
Vitamin B_{12} (cyanocobalamin)	60 mcg
Vitamin E (dl-alpha tocopheryl acetate)	30 IU
Copper (copper sulfate)	300 mcg
Magnesium (from magnesium oxide)	5 mg
Calcium (from calcium ascorbate)	10 mg
Choline (bitartrate)	80 mg
Inositol	50 mg
PABA	150 mg
Manganese (amino acid chelate)	4 mg
Zinc (amino acid chelate)	8 mg
Citrus bioflavonoids	66.6 mg
Chromium (amino acid chelate)	30 mcg
Selenium (sodium selenite)	30 mcg
L-cysteine	25 mg
Molybdenum (amino acid chelate)	20 mcg
Vanadium pentoxide	20 mcg
Octacosanol	25 mcg

*All our formulas are yeast-free, because of the large number of patients with yeast sensitivities or candidiasis.

Basic Formula (Low-Estrogen*)

Each tablet contains:

Vitamin A (beta carotene)	500 IU ⎫
Vitamin A (acetate)	500 IU ⎬
Vitamin D_2	30 IU
Thiamine (HCl) (B_1)	10 mg
Riboflavin (B_2)	8 mg
Ascorbate Acid (from calcium ascorbate)	150 mg
Niacin (B_3)	5 mg ⎫
Niacinamide (B_3)	10 mg ⎬
Pyridoxine (B_6)	10 mg
Pyridoxal-5 phosphate (B_6)	2 mg
Biotin	40 mcg
Vitamin B_{12} (cyanocobalamin)	60 mcg
Vitamin E (dl-alpha tocopheryl acetate)	30 IU
Copper (copper sulfate)	300 mcg
Methionine	166 mg
Magnesium (from magnesium oxide)	105 mg
Calcium (from calcium ascorbate)	10 mg
Choline (bitartrate)	166 mg
Inositol	100 mg
Manganese (amino acid chelate)	4 mg
Zinc (amino acid chelate)	8 mg
Citrus bioflavonoids	66.6 mg
Chromium (amino acid chelate)	30 mcg
Selenium (sodium selenite)	30 mcg
L-cysteine	25 mg
Molybdenum (amino acid chelate)	20 mcg
Vanadium pentoxide	20 mcg
Octacosanol	25 mcg

*The Low-Estrogen Basic Formula contains no folic acid or PABA, which stimulate the production of estrogen, and is designed for women who should be on an estrogen-decreasing protocol (see the table on page 166).

Sleep Formula

Each tablet contains:

L-tryptophan	350 mg
Inositol	250 mg
Niacinamide	100 mg
Calcium pantothenate	100 mg
Calcium (from 150 mg calcium carbonate)	60 mg
Magnesium (from 125 mg magnesium carbonate)	37.5 mg

Acute Infection Formula

Each tablet contains:

Beta carotene	5000 IU
Vitamin A	3333 IU
Quercetin	80 mg
Zinc (gluconate)	25 mg
Ascorbic acid	500 mg
Calcium pantothenate	80 mg
Citrus bioflavonoids	80 mg
Selenium	30 mcg
Magnesium (ascorbate)	15 mg
Garlic	160 mg
Folic acid	400 mcg
N, N-dimethylglycine HCl	20 mg
Pyridoxine HCl	4 mg
Riboflavin	2 mg
Copper (chelate)	1 mg
Niacinamide	15 mg

Antihypertensive Formula

Each tablet contains:

Magnesium orotate	300 mg
Magnesium oxide	200 mg
Potassium orotate	125 mg
L-taurine	200 mg
Pyridoxine HCl	75 mg
Inositol	100 mg
Garlic (with allicin)	200 mg

Cardiovascular Formula

Each tablet contains:

Pyridoxine HCl	25 mg
Niacinamide	25 mg
Vitamin E (dl-alpha tocopheryl acetate)	75 IU
Copper (copper sulfate)	1.5 mg
Magnesium (orotate)	200 mg
L-taurine	200 mg
L-carnitine	100 mg
Garlic (allicin-free)	200 mg
Bromelain	100 mg
Selenium (sodium selenite)	25 mcg
Chromium (amino acid chelate)	25 mcg
Coenzyme Q_{10}	5 mg

Anti-arthritic Formula

Each tablet contains:

Niacinamide	250 mg
Calcium ascorbate	150 mg
Calcium pantothenate	150 mg
Zinc (sulfate)	15 mg
Manganese (sulfate)	15 mg
Copper (sulfate)	4 mg
Selenium	25 mcg
Pyridoxine HCl	50 mg
Vitamin E (dl-alpha tocopheryl acetate)	60 IU

Antifatigue Formula

Each tablet contains:

Thiamine HCl	75 mg
Pyridoxine HCl	30 mg
Vitamin B_{12} (cyanocobalamin)	75 mcg
Folic acid	400 mcg
PABA	300 mg
Choline (bitartrate)	150 mg
L-methionine	150 mg
N, N-dimethyglycine	50 mg
L-phenylalanine	150 mg
Octacosanol	1.25 mg

Antidepressant Formula

Each tablet contains:

Vitamin B_6	150 mg
Niacinamide	100 mg
Niacin	25 mg
Ascorbic acid	300 mg
Zinc (chelate)	15 mg
Manganese (chelate)	5 mg
Folic acid	400 mcg
Vitamin B_{12}	100 mcg
Choline (bitartrate)	100 mg
L-tryptophan	300 mg

Painkiller Formula

Each tablet contains:

DL phenylalanine	300 mg
L-tryptophan	300 mg
DL methionine	125 mg
L-serine	35 mg
Adenoisine monophosphate	1 mg
Gamma-amino butyric acid	25 mg
Thiamine HCl	15 mg
Pyridoxine HCl	10 mg
Ascorbic acid	50 mg
Zinc (zinc sulfate)	5 mg
Manganese (manganese sulfate)	5 mg
Copper (copper sulfate)	1 mg

Osteoporosis Formula

Each tablet contains:

Calcium carbonate	150 mg
Calcium orotate	200 mg
Calcium ascorbate	150 mg
Total calcium	90 mg
Magnesium carbonate	150 mg
Magnesium orotate	200 mg
Total magnesium	65 mg
Vitamin D_2	75 IU
Vitamin A (beta carotene)	400 IU
Vitamin A (as palmitate)	400 IU
Folic acid	800 mcg
Silicon (as silica)	100 mg
Zinc orotate	15 mg
Chrondroitin sulfate A	200 mg

Heart Rhythm Formula

Each tablet contains:

Magnesium orotate	300 mg
Potassium orotate	150 mg
Garlic (with allicin)	200 mg
Inositol	150 mg
Choline (bitartrate)	150 mg
L-taurine	100 mg
Manganese (from manganese sulfate)	20 mg
Octacosanol	1 mg
Hawthorne extract powder	100 mg

Antioxidant Formula

Each capsule contains:

Vitamin E succinate (natural)	100 IU
Glutathione	25 mg
N, N-Dimethylglycine	25 mg
Pantothenic acid (d-calcium pantothenate)	25 mg
Magnesium ascorbate	100 mg
L-cysteine	200 mg
Zinc (zinc gluconate)	7.5 mg
Pyridoxal-5 phosphate	2 mg
Beta carotene (vitamin A equivalent)	7500 IU
Selenium (sodium selenite)	60 mcg
Choline bitartrate	100 mg
Citrus bioflavonoids	200 mg
Manganese (chelate)	2 mg

Lipid Formula

Each tablet contains:

Ascorbic acid	400 mg
Timed niacin	250 mg
Pectin	200 mg
Guar gum	200 mg
Pantethine	45 mg
Niacinamide	25 mg
Pyridoxine HCl	5 mg
Copper (chelate)	1 mg
Folic acid	400 mcg
GTF chromium	40 mcg

DM (Diabetes Mellitus) Formula

Each capsule contains:

Ascorbic acid	300 mg
Inositol	150 mg
D-alpha tocopherol	60 IU
L-carnitine	50 mg
Niacinamide	50 mg
Magnesium (chelate)	15 mg
Zinc (chelate)	10 mg
Manganese (chelate)	5 mg
CoQ_{10}	5 mg
Pyridoxal-5 phosphate	2 mg
GTF chromium	50 mcg

Allergy Formula

Each tablet contains:

Pantethine	60 mg
Calcium pantothenate	110 mg
Quercetin	140 mg
Vitamin C	500 mg
Catechin	60 mg
Citrus bioflavonoids	100 mg
Niacinamide	20 mg

• • •

Appendix D
Organizations

The following is a list of organizations involved in various forms of Complementary Medicine that will give out membership rolls to members of the public who write to them. They may put you on the track of a complementary physician in your area.

Academy of Orthomolecular
  Psychiatry
1691 Northern Boulevard
Manhasset, New York 11030

American Academy of Environmen-
  tal Medicine
Box 16106
Denver, Colorado 80216

American College of Advancement
  in Medicine
23121 Verdugo Drive
Suite 204
Laguna Hills, California 92653

American Holistic Medical
  Association
6932 Little River Turnpike
Annandale, Virginia 22003

International Academy of Holistic
  Health and Medicine
218 Avenue B
Redondo Beach, California 90277

International Academy of Preventive
  Medicine
Box 25276
Shawnee Mission, Kansas 66225

International College of Applied
  Nutrition
Box 386
La Habra, California 90631

Northwest Academy of Preventive
  Medicine
15615 Bellevue-Redmond Road
Suite E
Bellevue, Washington 98008

Orthomolecular Medical Society
6551 West Century Boulevard
Suite 114
Los Angeles, California 90045

References

Chapter 1. Medicine's Dual Traditions

1. Hahnemann, Samuel. *The Organon of Medicine*, translated with Preface by William Boericke (Philadelphia: Boericke and Tafel, 1922).
2. Rush, Benjamin. *Sixteen Introduction Lectures to Courses of Lectures upon the Institutes and Practice of Medicine, Delivered in the University of Pennsylvania* (Philadelphia: Bradford and Inskeep, 1811), p. 165.
3. Coulter, Harris L. *Divided Legacy. A History of the Schism in Medical Thought*, vol. III (Washington, D.C.: McGrath, 1973), p. 90.
4. Ibid., p. 63.
5. *Proceedings of the Connecticut Medical Society for 1850*. Bound pamphlets printed in Norwich and Hartford, vol. 124, p. 53.
6. Coulter, op. cit., p. 404.
7. Ibid., pp. 298–302.
8. Cited in Diesendorf, M. *The Magic Bullet* (Canberra: Society for Social Responsibility in Science, 1976), p. 2.

Chapter 6. Diabetes: The Basic Epidemic

1. Stout, R. "Diabetes and Arteriosclerosis: The Role of Insulin," *Diabetologie* 16 (1979), p. 14.
2. Cleave, T. L. *The Saccharin Disease: Conditions Caused by the Taking of Refined Carbohydrates, Such as Sugar and White Flour* (New Canaan, Connecticut: Keats, 1978).
3. Katzen, H. M., and Mahler, R. J., eds. *Diabetes, Obesity and Vascular Disease*, 2 vols. (New York: Halsted Press, 1978).
4. Reiser, S., and Szepesi, B., "SCOGS Report on the Health Aspect of

Sucrose Consumption," Letter to the Editor, *American Journal of Clinical Nutrition* 31 (1978), pp. 9–11.

5. Eisenbarth, G. S. "Type I Diabetes Mellitus: A Chronic Autoimmunic Disease," *New England Journal of Medicine* 314 (1986), pp. 1360–68.

6. University Group Diabetes Program. "A Study of the Effects of Hypoglycemia Agents on Vascular Complications in Patients with Adult-Onset Diabetes," *Diabetes* 19, suppl. 2 (1970), pp. 747–832.

7. Mertz, W., and Schwarz, K. "Chromium (III) and the Glucose Tolerance Factor," *Archives of Biochemistry and Biophysics* 85 (1959), pp. 292–95.

8. Houtsmiller, A. J., et al. "Favorable Influences of Linoleic Acid on the Progression of Diabetic Micro- and Macroangiopathy in Adult-Onset Diabetes Mellitus," *Progress in Lipid Research* 20 (1981), pp. 377–86.

9. Passariello, N., et al. "Effects of Pyridoxine Alpha-Ketoglutarate on Blood Glucose and Lactate in Type I and Type II Diabetics," *International Journal of Clinical Pharmacology and Therapeutic Toxicology* 21 (1983), pp. 252–56.

10. Shigeta, Y., et al. "Effect of Coenzyme Q_7 Treatment on Blood Sugar and Ketone Bodies of Diabetics," *Journal of Vitaminology* 12 (1966), p. 293.

11. Coggeshall, J. C., et al. "Biotin Status and Plasma Glucose in Diabetics," *Annals of the New York Academy of Science* 447 (1985), pp. 389–92.

Chapter 7. Hypoglycemia: Everybody Has Some

1. Joint statement by the American Diabetes Association, the Endocrine Society, and the American Medical Association. "Special Report: Statement on Hypoglycemia," *Diabetes* 22 (1973), p. 137.

2. In the absence of glucose, the brain can utilize ketone bodies, the fuel derived from fat metabolism. However, this mechanism takes hours to mobilize in some individuals. These are the ones subject to low-glucose symptoms.

3. Sanders, L. R., et al. "Refined Carbohydrate as a Contributing Factor in Reactive Hypoglycemia," *Southern Medical Journal* 75 (1982), p. 1072.

4. Aiuti, F., and Paganelli, R. "Food Allergy and Gastrointestinal Diseases," *Annals of Allergy* 5 (1983), pp. 275–80.

Chapter 8. Candida Albicans: *The Complementarist's Diagnosis*

1. Truss, C. O. *The Missing Diagnosis* (Birmingham: C. O. Truss, 1983).
2. Crook, W. G. *The Yeast Connection* (Jackson, Tennessee: Professional Books, 1985).
3. Dubos, R. J., and Schaedler, R. W. "Effective Nutrition on the Resistance of Mice to Endotoxin and on the Bactericidal Power of Their Tissues," *Journal of Experimental Medicine* 110 (1959), pp. 935–50.
4. Odds, F. C. *Candida and Candidiasis* (Baltimore: University Park Press, 1979), p. 142.
5. Horas, Carol V. *Vaginal Health* (Tohey Publishing Company, 1975).
6. Berger, Stuart. "Doctor's Orders," *New York Post*, November 1984.
7. Blonz, Edward. Commentary, *Journal of the American Medical Association* 256: 22 (December 12, 1986), pp. 3138–39.
8. Horas, op. cit., p. 174.
9. Eggleston, D. W. "Effect of Dental Amalgam and Nickel Alloys on T-Lymphocytes: Preliminary Report," *Journal of Prosthetic Dentistry* 51:5 (May 1984), pp. 617–23.

Chapter 9. Mercury Amalgam Toxicity: What Have Our Dentists Wrought?

1. Fasciara, G. *Are Your Dental Fillings Hurting You?* (Springfield, Massachusetts: Health Challenge Press, 1986).
2. Fredericks, Carlton. "Mercury: The Poison That Migrates from Your Molars," *Let's Live* (July 1984).
3. Huggins, H., and Pinto, O. "Mercury Poisoning in America," *Journal of the International Academy of Preventive Medicine* III: 2 (December 1976).
4. Pike, R., and Brown, M. *Nutrition: An Integrated Approach* (New York: John Wiley & Sons, 1984).
5. "Mercury Amalgams: An Environmental Health Problem?" *Complementary Medicine Magazine* 1:2 (November/December 1985).
6. Ibid.
7. Eggleston, D. W. "Effect of Dental Amalgam and Nickel Alloys on T-Lymphocytes: Preliminary Report," *Journal of Prosthetic Dentistry* 51:5 (May 1984), pp. 617–23.
8. "Mercury Amalgams."
9. Svare, C. W., et al. "The Effect of Dental Amalgams on Mercury Levels in Expired Air," *Journal of Dental Research* 60:9 (September 1981), pp. 1668–71.

10. Nakamura, N., and Kawahara, H. "Cellular Responses to the Dispersion of Amalgams in Vitro," *Journal of Dental Research* 58:8 (August 1979), p. 1790.
11. Abbotts, J. *Disposable Consumer Items: The Overlooked Mercury Problem* (Washington, D.C.: Center for Study of Responsive Law, 1981).
12. "Mercury Amalgams."
13. See *Dentist* 64:2 (March/April 1986).

Chapter 10. Headache: Prevention Is the Cure

1. Grant, E. C. "Food Allergies and Migraine," *Lancet* (May 5, 1979), pp. 966–69.
2. Davben, R. D. "Headache Syndromes," *Modern Medicine* 54 (August 1986), p. 70.
3. Egger, J., et al. "Is Migraine Food Allergy?: A Double-Blind Controlled Trial of Oligoantigenic Diet Treatment," *Lancet* (October 29, 1984), pp. 719–21.
4. AFP News Brief 35: 2 (February 1987), p. 326.
5. Johnson, E. S., et al. "Efficacy of Feverfew as a Prophylactic Treatment of Migraine," *British Medical Journal* 291 (1985), pp. 569–73.

Chapter 11. Female Problems: The Nutritional Approach

1. Lauersen, N., and Stukane, F. *Premenstrual Syndrome and You* (New York: Simon & Schuster, 1983).
2. Information supplied by Nora Coffey, president of the HERS Foundation.
3. Napoli, M., ed. "Report from the Women and Cancer Conference," *Health Facts* X:79 (December 1985).
4. Cutler, G. B., Jr., et al. "Therapeutic Applications of Lutenizing-Hormone-Releasing Hormone and Its Analogs," *Annals of Internal Medicine*, 102:5 (May 1985), pp. 643–57. See also Dizerega, C., et al. "Endometriosis: Role of Ovarian Steroids in Initiation, Maintenance and Suppression," *Fertility and Sterility* 33 (June 1980), p. 6.
5. Fredericks, Carlton. *Breast Cancer: A Nutritional Approach* (New York: Grosset & Dunlap, 1977).
6. Butterworth, C. E., et al. "Improvement in Cervical Dysplasia Associated with Folic Acid Therapy in Users of Oral Contraceptives," *American Journal of Clinical Nutrition* 35 (1982), pp. 73–82.
7. Osteoporosis-Consensus Conference, *Journal of the American Medical Association* 252 (August 10, 1984), p. 6.
8. Nordin, B. E., et al. "A Prospective Trial of the Effect of Vitamin D

Supplementation on Metacarpal Bone Loss in Elderly Women," *American Journal of Clinical Nutrition* 43:3 (1985), pp. 470–74.

9. Budoff, Penny Wise. *No More Menstrual Cramps & Other Good News* (New York: Putnam, 1980), p. 249.

10. "Premenstrual Syndrome Keeps Doctors Guessing," *New York Times*, January 1986.

11. Lauersen, op. cit.

12. Brush, M. G. "Efamol (Evening Primrose Oil) in the Rx of the PM Syndrome," in Horrobin, D., ed. *Clinical Uses of Essential Fatty Acids* (Montreal: Eden Press, 1982), pp. 155–61.

13. Horrobin, D. F., in Bland, J., ed. *1984–85 Yearbook of Nutritional Medicine* (New Canaan, Connecticut: Keats, 1986), pp. 23–25. See also Horrobin, D. F. "The Role of Essential Fatty Acids and Prostaglandins in the PM Syndrome," *Journal of Reproductive Medicine* 28 (1983), pp. 465–81.

14. Goei, G. S., et al. "Dietary Patterns of Patients with Premenstrual Tension," *Journal of Applied Nutrition* 34 (1982), p. 1.

15. Abraham, G. "Premenstrual Tension," in *Current Problems in Obstetrics and Gynecology* (Chicago: Yearbook Medical Publishers, 1981).

16. Bland, J. *1986: A Year in Nutritional Medicine* (New Canaan, Connecticut: Keats, 1986).

17. Lauersen, op, cit.

18. Abraham, op. cit.

Chapter 13. Coronary Heart Disease: The Death of Most of Us

1. CASS Principal Investigators and Their Associates. "The Coronary Artery Surgery Study (CASS): A Randomized Trial of Coronary Artery Bypass Surgery," *Journal of the American College of Cardiology* 3 (1984), pp. 114–28.

Chapter 14. Chelation: A Wonder Regimen for Coronary Disease

1. Richard Casdorph, M.D., did demonstrate a series of patients tested and retested by the RNCA, all of whom showed improvements in resting ejection fraction after chelation. However, in most cases this improvement was slight, and no exercise testing was reported.

2. Crohn, L. Lecture on tape, with the American College of Advancement in Medicine.

3. For a concise and enlightened discussion of Dr. Clarke's effort, see *Chelation EDTA*, by Morton Walker and Garry Gordon (New York: M. Evans, 1982), pp. 72–74.

4. Kitchell, J. R., et al. "The Treatment of Coronary Artery Disease with Disodium EDTA. A Reappraisal," *American Journal of Cardiology* 11 (1963), pp. 501–6.
5. Present evidence from autopsies indicates that death in these cases was not directly due to chelation but to pre-existing conditions that had not been examined for before administering the agent.
6. Cranton, E. *Bypassing Bypass* (New York: Stein & Day, 1984), p. 85.

Chapter 15. Cholesterol Revisited

1. *Practical Cardiology*, 6:6 (1980), p. 157.
2. Frick, M. H., et al. "Helsinki Heart Study. Primary Prevention Trial with Gemfibrozil in Middle-aged Men with Dyslipedemia: Safety of Treatment Changes in Risk Factors and Incidents of Coronary Heart Disease," *New England Journal of Medicine* 317 (1987), pp. 1237–45. See also Werhmacher, W. H. "Comments on the Helsinki Heart Study," *IM* 9:3 (1988), pp. 83–88.
3. Lipid Research Clinics Program. "The Lipid Research Clinics Coronary Primary Prevention Results," *Journal of the American Medical Association* 251 (1984), pp. 351–64.
4. Cranton, E. *Bypassing Bypass* (New York: Stein & Day, 1984).
5. Demopoulos, H. B., et al. *Journal of the American College of Toxicology* (1983), pp. 173–84.
6. Taylor, C. Bruce. "Spontaneously Occurring Angiotoxic Derivations of Cholesterol," *American Journal of Clinical Nutrition* 32 (January 1979), pp. 40–57.
7. Cook, Robert P. *Cholesterol: Chemistry, Biochemistry and Pathology* (New York: Academic Press, 1958). Cook found that when he gave 150 grams of egg yolk powder (approximately 25 percent cholesterol and 15.2 percent lecithin) in 400 milligrams of milk two times a day for forty-eight straight days to men, there was an increase in cholesterol count. However, the rise was transient and the count soon returned to pre-existing levels when these individuals were taken off this unusually high cholesterol diet.
8. Passwater, R. *Super Nutrition for Healthy Hearts* (New York: Deal Press, 1977). See also Flynn, M. A., et al. "Effects of Dietary Egg on Human Serum Cholesterol and Triglycerides," *American Journal of Clinical Nutrition* 32 (May 1979), pp. 1051–57. Also: Krombout, D., et al. "The Inverse Relation Between Fish Consumption and 20 Year Mortality from Coronary Heart Disease," *New England Journal of Medicine* 312 (1985), pp. 1205–9.

9. Raymond, C. A. "Dietary Cholesterol Still a Lively Discussion Topic," *Journal of the American Medical Association* 259 (1988), pp. 1435–36.

10. Grundy, S. M., et al. "Influence of Nicotinic Acid on Metabolism of Cholesterol and Triglycerides in Man," *Lipid Research* 22 (1981), pp. 24–36.

11. Saynor, R. "Effects of Omega-3 Fatty Acids on Serum Lipids," *Lancet* 2 (1984), pp. 696–97. See also Harris, W. S., et al. "Dietary Omega-3 Fatty Acids Prevent Carbohydrate Induced Hypertriglyceridemia," *Metabolism* 33 (1984), pp. 1016–19.

12. Krombout, op. cit.

13. Dobson, H. M., et al. "The Effect of Ascorbic Acid on the Seasonal Variations in Serum Cholesterol Levels," *Scottish Medical Journal* 29 (1984), pp. 176–82.

14. Arsenio, L., et al. "Effectiveness of Long-term Treatment with Pantethine in Patients with Dyslipidemia," *Clinical Therapeutics* 8 (1986), pp. 537–45.

15. Abdel-Aziz, M. T., et al. "Effect of Carnitine on Blood Lipid Pattern in Diabetic Patients," *Nutritional Reports International* 29 (1984), p. 1071.

16. Railes, R., and Albrink, M. J. "Effect of Chromium Chloride Supplementation on Glucose Tolerance and Serum Lipids Including High Density Lipoprotein of Adult Men," *American Journal of Clinical Nutrition* 34 (1981), pp. 2670–78.

17. Simons, L. A., et al. "Long-term Treatment of Hypercholesterolaemia with a New Palatable Formulation of Guar Gum," *Atherosclerosis* 45:1 (1982), pp. 101–8.

18. Kay, R. M., and Truswell, A. S. "Effect of Citrus Pectin on Blood Lipids and Fecal Steroid Excretion," *American Journal of Clinical Nutrition* 30:2 (1977), pp. 171–75.

19. Kuusisto, R., et al. "Effect of Activated Charcoal on Hypercholesterolaemia," *Lancet* 2 (1986), pp. 366–67.

20. Ernst, E., et al. "Garlic and Blood Lipids," *British Medical Journal* 291 (1985), p. 139. See also Bordia, A. "Effect of Garlic on Blood Lipids in Patients with Coronary Heart Disease," *American Journal of Clinical Nutrition* 34 (1981), pp. 2100–3.

21. Nakazawa, K., and Murata, K. "The Therapeutic Effect of Chondroitin Polysulphate in Elderly Atherosclerotic Patients," *Journal of International Medical Research* 6:3 (1978), pp. 217–25.

22. Mattson, F. H., et al. "Optimizing the Effect of Plant Sterols on Cholesterol Absorption in Man," *American Journal of Clinical Nutrition* 35 (1982), pp. 697–700.

Chapter 17. Heart Rhythm Disturbances: The Drugless Approach

1. Rasmussen, H. S., et al. "Intravenous Magnesium in Acute Infarction," *Lancet* 1 (February 1986), pp. 234–36.
2. Lesser, F. "The Costs of Treating High Blood Pressure?" *Science*, 1985.
3. Cantarow and Trumper, *Clinical Biochemistry* (Philadelphia: W. B. Saunders, 1975).
4. Harrison, T. "Glucose Deficiency as a Factor in Production of Symptoms Referable to Cardiovascular System," *American Heart Journal* 26 (August 1943), pp. 147–63.
5. Dobmeyer, D. J., et al. "The Arrhythmogenic Effects of Caffeine in Human Beings," *New England Journal of Medicine* 308:14 (1983), pp. 814–16.
6. Boudoulas, H., et al. "Metabolic Studies in Mitral Valve Prolapse Syndrome," *Circulation* 61 (1980), p. 1200.
7. Reinhart, R., et al. "Hypermagnesium in Patients Entering the ICU," *Critical Care Medicine* 13:6 (1985), p. 506.
8. Frances, Y., et al. "Long-term Follow-up of Mitral Valve Prolapse and Latent Tetany. Preliminary Data," *Magnesium* 5 (1986), pp. 175–81. See also Fernandes, J. S., et al. "Therapeutic Effect of a Magnesium Salt in Patients Suffering from Mitral Valvular Prolapse and Latent Tetany," *Magnesium* (1985), p. 283.
9. Sangiori, G. B., et al. "Serum Potassium Levels, Red-Blood Cell Potassium and Alterations of the Repolarization Phase of Electrocardiography in Old Subjects," *Age and Aging* 13 (1984), p. 309. See also Dychner, T., and Wester, P. D. "Magnesium and Potassium in Serum and Muscle in Relation to Disturbance of Cardiac Rhythm," in Cantin, M., and Seelig, M., eds. *Magnesium in Health and Disease* (New York: Spectrum, 1980), pp. 551–57.
10. DiPalma, J. R., et al. "Cardiovascular and Antiarrhythmic Effects of Carnitine," *Archives Internationales de Pharmacodynamie et de Therapie* 217 (1975), pp. 246–50.
11. Fugiaka, T., et al. "Clinical Study of Cardiac Arrhythmias Using a 24-Hour Continuous Electro Cardiographic Recorder (5th Report): Antiarrhythmic Action of Coenzyme Q_{10} in Diabetics," *Tohoku Journal of Experimental Medicine* (1983), pp. 453–63.
12. Chazov, E. L., et al. "Taurine and Electrical Activity of the Heart," *Circulation Research* 34–5, suppl. III (1974), pp. 11–21.
13. Nygaard, et al. "Adverse Reactions to Antiarrhythmic Drugs During Therapy for Ventricular Arrhythmias," *Journal of the American Medical Association* 256 (July 4, 1986), pp. 55–57.

Chapter 18. Hypertension: The Great Pharmaceutical Rip-off

1. Grobbee, D. E., and Hofman, A. "Does Sodium Restriction Lower the Blood Pressure?" *British Medical Journal* 293 (1986), pp. 27–29. See also McCarron, D. A., et al. "Blood Pressure and Nutrient Intake in the U.S.," *Science* 224 (1984), pp. 1392–98.

2. Cohen, N., et al. "Obesity and Hypertension. Demonstration of a 'Floor Effect,' " *American Journal of Medicine* 80 (1986), pp. 177–81.

3. Aherns, R. A., et al. "Moderate Pressure Ingestion and Blood Pressure in the Rat," *Journal of Nutrition* 110 (1980), pp. 725–31.

4. "Final Report of the Subcommittee on Nonpharmacological Therapy of the 1984 Joint National Committee on Detection, Evaluation, and Treatment of High Blood Pressure," *Hypertension* 8:5 (1986), pp. 444–67.

5. Lucas, C. P., et al. "Insulin and Blood Pressure in Obesity," *Hypertension* 7 (1985), pp. 702–706. See also Singer, P., et al. "Postprandial Hyperinsulinemia in Patients with Mild Essential Hypertension," *Hypertension* 7 (1985), pp. 182–86. Also: Modan, M., et al. "Hyperinsulinemia: A Link Between Hypertension, Obesity and Glucose Tolerance," *Journal of Clinical Investigations* 75 (1985), pp. 809–17. Also: Manicardi, V., et al. "Evidence for an Association of High Blood Pressure and Hyperinsulinemia in Obese Man," *Journal of Clinical Endocrinological Metabolism* 62 (1986), pp. 1302–4.

6. Reaven, G. M., et al. "Hyperglycemia, Hyperinsulinemia, and Insulin Resistance in Patients with Hypertension," *Clinical Research* 35 (1987), p. 605A. See also Olefsky, J. M., and Farquhar, J. W. "Reappraisal of the Role of Insulin in Hypertriglyceridemia," *American Journal of Medicine* 57 (1974), pp. 551–60.

7. Norris, P. G., et al. "Effect of Dietary Supplementation with Fish Oil on Systolic Blood Pressure in Mild Essential Hypertension," *British Medical Journal* 293 (1986), p. 104. See also Singer, P., et al. "Lipid and Blood-Pressure Lowering Effect of Mackerel Diet in Man," *Atherosclerosis* 49:1 (1983), pp. 99–108.

8. Soma, M., et al. "The Effects of Hydrogenated Coconut Oil, Safflower Oil, and Evening Primrose Oil on Development of Hypertension and Sodium Handling in Spontaneously Hypertensive Rats," *Canadian Journal of Physiology and Pharmacology* 63 (1985), pp. 325–30.

9. Azuma, J., et al. "Therapeutic Effect of Taurine in Congestive Heart Failure: A Double-Blind Crossover Trial," *Clinical Cardiology* 8 (1985), pp. 276–82.

10. Resnick, L. M., Laragh, J. H., et al. "Intracellular Free Magnesium

in Erythrocytes of Essential Hypertension," *Proceedings of the National Academy of Science* 81 (1984), pp. 6511–15.

11. Resnick, L. M., et al. Endocrine Society Meeting, June 8, 1983, abstract 385; Cohen, L. "Magnesium and Hypertension," *Magnesium Bulletin* 8 (1986), pp. 93–94.

12. Dyckner, T., and Wester, O. "Effect of Magnesium on Blood Pressure," *British Medical Journal* 286 (1983), pp. 1847–49.

13. Grobbee, D. E., and Hofman, A. "Effects of Calcium Supplementation," *Lancet* 2 (1986), pp. 703–7. See also McCarron, D. A., and Morris, C. D. "Blood Pressure Response to Oral Calcium in Persons with Mild to Moderate Hypertension. A Randomized, Double-Blind, Placebo-Controlled Crossover Trial," *Annals of Internal Medicine* 103 (1985), pp. 825–31. Also: McCarron, D. A. "Is Calcium More Important Than Sodium in the Pathogenesis of Essential Hypertension?" *Hypertension* 7:4 (1985), p. 60727.

14. Yamagani, T., et al. "Bioenergetics in Clinical Medicine," *Research Communications in Chemical Pathology and Pharmacology* 14 (1976), p. 721.

15. *The Townsend Letter* 44 (January 1987), p. 411.

Chapter 20. Multiple Sclerosis: It Can Be Halted

1. Craelius, W. "Comparative Epidemiology of Multiple Sclerosis and Dental Caries," *Journal of Epidemiology and Community Health* 32 (1972), pp. 155–65.

2. Ingalls, T. H. "Triggers for Multiple Sclerosis," Letter to the Editor, *Lancet* 2 (1986), p. 160.

3. Nightingale, S. L. "From the Food and Drug Administration," *Journal of the American Medical Association* 256 (1986), p. 3075.

4. French, J. M. "MaxEPA in Multiple Sclerosis," *British Journal of Clinical Practice Symp.* suppl. 31 (1984), pp. 117–21. See also Cherayil, G. D. "Sialic Acid and Fatty Acid Concentrations in Lymphocytes, Red Blood Cells and Plasma from Patients with Multiple Sclerosis," *Journal of Neurological Science* 63 (1984), pp. 1–10.

5. Horrobin, D. "Multiple Sclerosis: The Rational Basis for Treatment with Colchicine and Evening Primrose Oil," *Medical Hypotheses* 5 (1979), pp. 365–78. See also Simpson, L. O., et al. "Dietary Supplementation with Efamol and Multiple Sclerosis," *New Zealand Medical Journal* 98 (1985), pp. 1053–54.

Chapter 21. Irritable Bowel Syndrome and the Many Ways to Heal It

1. Dotewall, G., et al. "Symptoms in Irritable Bowel Syndrome," *Scandinavian Journal of Gastroenterology* 79 (1982), pp. 16–19.
2. Strober, W., and James, S. P. "The Immunologic Basis of IBD," *Journal of Clinical Immunology* 6 (1986), pp. 415–32.
3. Gillespie, I., and Thomson, T. J. *Gastroenterology: An Integrated Course*, 3rd ed. (New York: Churchill Livingston Publications, 1983), p. 233.
4. Stefananini, G. F., et al. "Efficacy of Oral Disodium Cromoglycate in Patients with Irritable Bowel Syndrome and Positive Skin Prick Tests to Foods," Letter to the Editor, *Lancet* 1 (1986), pp. 207–8. See also Finn, R., et al. "Expanding Horizons of Allergy and the Total Allergy Syndrome," *Clinical Ecology* 3:3 (1985), pp. 129–31. Also: Smith, M. A., et al. "Food Intolerance, Atopy and Irritable Bowel Syndrome," *Lancet* 2 (November 9, 1985), p. 1064. Also: Alun Jones, V., and Hunter, J. Q. "Food Intolerance in Irritable Bowel Syndrome," *Clinical Ecology* 3:1 (1985), pp. 35–38. Also: Petitpierre, M., et al. "Irritable Bowel Syndrome and Hypersensitivity to Food," *Annals of Allergy* 54 (1985), pp. 538–40. Also: Jenkins, H. P., et al. "Food Intolerance: A Major Cause of Infantile Colitis," *Archives of Disease in Childhood* 59:4 (1984), pp. 326–29. Also: Alun Jones, V. A., et al. "Food Intolerance: A Major Factor in the Pathogenesis of Irritable Bowel Syndrome," *Lancet* 2 (1982), pp. 1115–17. Also: Siegel, J. "Inflammatory Bowel Disease: Another Possible Facet of the Allergic Diathesis," *Annals of Allergy* 47 (1981), pp. 92–94.
5. Hodges, P., et al. "Vitamin and Iron Intake in Patients with Crohn's Disease," *Journal of the American Dietetic Association* 84:1 (1984), pp. 52–58.
6. Baum, C. L., et al. "Antifolate Actions of Sulfasalazine on Intact Lymphocytes," *Journal of Laboratory and Clinical Medicine* 97:6 (1981), pp. 779–84. See also Halstead, C. H., et al. "Sulfasalazine Inhibits the Absorption of Folates in Ulcerative Colitis," *New England Journal of Medicine* 305:25 (1981), p. 1513.
7. Grimes, D. S. "Refined Carbohydrate, Smooth Muscle Spasm and Disease of the Colon," *Lancet* 1 (1976), pp. 395–97.
8. Penny, W. J., et al. "Relationship Between Trace Elements, Sugar Consumption, and Taste in Crohn's Disease," *Gut* 24:4 (1983), pp. 288–92. See also Mayberry, J. F., et al. "Diet in Crohn's Disease," *Digestive Diseases and Sciences* 26:5 (1981), pp. 444–48.

9. Brandes, J. W., and Lorenz-Meyer, H. "Sugar Free Diet: A New Perspective in the Treatment of Crohn's Disease: Randomized, Control Study," *Zeitschrift fur Gastroenterologie* 19:1 (1981), pp. 1–12.
10. Ellestad-Sayed, J. J., et al. "Pantothenic Acid, Coenzyme A, and Human Chronic Ulcerative and Granulomatous Colitis," *American Journal of Clinical Nutrition* 29 (1976), pp. 1333–38.
11. Carruthers, L. B. "Chronic Diarrhea Treated with Folic Acid," *Lancet* 1 (1946), p. 849.
12. Elsborg, L., and Larsen, L. "Folate Deficiency in Chronic Inflammatory Bowel Disease," *Scandinavian Journal of Gastroenterology* 14 (1979), pp. 1019–24.
13. Page, P. C., and Bercovitz, Z. "The Absorption of Vitamin A in Chronic Ulcerative Colitis," *American Journal of Digestive Disorders* 10 (1983), pp. 174–77.
14. Schoelmerich, J., et al. "Zinc and Vitamin A Deficiency in Patients with Crohn's Disease Is Correlated with Activity but Not with Localization or Extent of the Disease," *Hepatogastroenterology* 32:1 (1985), pp. 34–38.
15. Kruis, W., et al. "Zinc Deficiency as a Problem in Patients with Crohn's Disease and Fistula Formation," *Hepatogastroenterology* 32:3 (1985), pp. 133–34. See also Solomons, N. W., et al. "Zinc Deficiency in Crohn's Disease," *Digestion* 16 (1977), p. 87.
16. Russell, R. I. "Magnesium Requirements in Patients with Chronic Inflammatory Disease Receiving Intravenous Nutrition," *Journal of the American College of Nutrition* 4:5 (1985), pp. 553–58.
17. Rosenberg, I. H., et al. "Nutritional Aspects of Inflammatory Bowel Disease," *Annual Review of Nutrition* 5 (1985), pp. 463–84.
18. Penny, op. cit.

Chapter 22. Arthritis: The Great Proving Ground

1. Arthritis Foundation. "Arthritis, Unproven Remedies," published by Public Education Department, #4240-7-81.
2. Arthritis Foundation. "Arthritis, Basic Facts and Answers to Your Questions," published by Public Education Department, #4001-6-83.
3. Skoldstam, L., et al. "Effects of Fasting and Lactovegetarian Diet on Rheumatoid Arthritis," *Scandinavian Journal of Rheumatology* 8 (1979), pp. 249–55.
4. Hicklin, J. A., et al. "The Effect of Diet in Rheumatoid Arthritis," *Clinical Allergy* 10 (1980), p. 463.
5. Darlington, L. G., et al. "Placebo-Controlled, Blind Study of Dietary

Manipulation Therapy in Rheumatoid Arthritis," *Lancet* (February 1, 1986), pp. 236–38. See also Kroker, G. F., et al. "Fasting and Rheumatoid Arthritis: A Multicenter Study," *Clinical Ecology* 2 (1984), pp. 137–44. Also: Uden, A. M., et al. "Neutrophil Functions and Clinical Performance After Total Fasting in Patients with Rheumatoid Arthritis," *Annals of the Rheumatic Diseases* 42:1 (1983), pp. 45–51. Also: Sundquist, T., et al. "Influence of Fasting on Intestinal Permeability and Disease Activity in Patients with Rheumatoid Arthritis," *Scandinavian Journal of Rheumatology* 11:1 (1982), pp. 33–38.

6. Bjarnason, I., et al. "Intestinal Permeability and Inflammation in Rheumatoid Arthritis: Effects of Non-Steroidal Anti-Inflammatory Drugs," *Lancet* 2 (November 24, 1984), pp. 1171–74.

7. General Practitioners Research Group. "Calcium Pantothenate in Arthritic Conditions," *Practitioner* 224 (1980), pp. 208–11.

8. Mullen, A., and Wilson, C. W. M. "The Metabolism of Ascorbic Acid in Rheumatoid Arthritis," *Proceedings of the Nutrition Society* 35 (1976), pp. 8A–9A. See also Roberts, P., et al. "Vitamin C and Inflammation," *Medical Biology* 62 (1984), p. 88. Also: Bland, J. H., and Cooper, S. M., "Osteoarthritis: A Review of the Cell Biology Involved and Evidence for Reversibility. Management Rationally Related to Known Genesis and Pathophysiology," *Seminars in Arthritis and Rheumatism* 14:2 (1984), pp. 106–33. Also: Schwartz, E. R. "The Modulation of Osteoarthritic Development by Vitamins C and E," *International Journal for Vitamin and Nutrition Research* suppl. 26 (1984), pp. 141–46. Also: Ptind, S. P. A., et al. "Effect of Purified Growth Factors on Rabbit Articular Chondrocyte in Monolayer Culture. Sulfated Proteoglycan Synthesis," *Arthritis and Rheumatism* 25 (1982), pp. 1228–38.

9. Brown, D. H., et al. "Serum Copper and Its Relationship to Clinical Symptoms in Rheumatoid Arthritis," *Annals of the Rheumatic Diseases* 38:2 (1979), pp. 174–76. See also Hangarter, W. "Copper Salicylate in Rheumatoid Arthritis and Rheumatism-like Degenerative Disease," *Medizinische Welt* 31 (1980), p. 1625.

10. Kremer, J. M., et al. "Effect of Manipulation of Dietary Fatty Acids on Clinical Manifestations of Rheumatoid Arthritis," *Lancet* 1 (1985), pp. 184–87. See also Sperling, R. I., reported in *Medical World News*, July 14, 1986. Also: Horrobin, D. F. "The Importance of Gamma Linolenic Acid and Prostaglandin E_1 in Human Nutrition and Medicine," *Journal of Holistic Medicine* 3 (1981), pp. 118–39.

11. Hansen, T. M., et al. "Treatment of Rheumatoid Arthritis with Prostaglandin E_1 Precursors Cislinoleic Acid and Gamma Linolenic

Acid," *Scandinavian Journal of Rheumatology* 12 (1983), p. 85.

12. Goebel, K. M., et al. "Intrasynovial Orgotein Therapy in Rheumatoid Arthritis," *Lancet* 1 (1981), pp. 1015–17.

13. Gerber, D. A., et al. "Specificity of a Low Free Serum Histidine Concentration for Rheumatoid Arthritis," *Journal of Chronic Diseases* 30 (1977), p. 115.

Chapter 23. Cancer Therapy: Orthodoxy's Most Willful Negligence

1. Revici, E. *Research in Physiopathology as Basis of Guided Chemotherapy* (New York: Van Nostrand, 1961). See also Keith Brown, R. *AIDS, Cancer, and the Medical Establishment* (New York: Robert Speller, 1986).

2. Wolf, M., and Ransberger, K. *Enzyme Therapy* (New York: Vantage Press, 1972).

3. Kelley, W. D. *An Ecological Approach to the Successful Treatment of Malignancy* (New York: The Kelley Foundation, 1969).

4. Bristol, J. B. "Sugar, Fat, and the Risk of Colorectal Cancer," *British Medical Journal* 291 (1985), p. 1457. See also Seely, S., and Horrobin, D. F. "Diet and Breast Cancer: The Possible Connection with Sugar Consumption," *Medical Hypotheses* 11:3 (1983), pp. 319–27. Also: Carroll, K. K. "Dietary Factors in Hormone-Dependent Cancers," in Winick, M., ed., *Current Concepts in Nutrition*, vol. 6, *Nutrition and Cancer* (New York: John Wiley, 1977), pp. 25–40.

5. Menkes, M. S., et al. "Serum Beta-Carotene, Vitamins A and E, Selenium and the Risk of Lung Cancer," *New England Journal of Medicine* 315 (1986), p. 1250.

6. Graham, S., et al. "Dietary Factors in the Epidemiology of Cancer of the Larynx," *American Journal of Epidemiology* 113:6 (1981), pp. 675–80.

7. Blondell, J. M. "The Anticarcinogenic Effect of Magnesium," *Medical Hypotheses* 6 (1980), pp. 863–71.

8. Bailey, Herbert. *Krebiozen — Key to Cancer* (New York: Hermitage House, 1955).

9. Nieper, Hans, *Cancer Control Journal* 2:5 (1974).

10. Bailar, J. C., 3rd, and Smith, E. M. "Progress Against Cancer," *New England Journal of Medicine* 314 (1986), pp. 1226–32.

Chapter 24. The Cutting Edge of Complementary Nutrition

1. Pike, R. L., and Brown, M. L. *Nutrition: An Integrated Approach* (New York: Macmillan, 1986).

2. Horrobin, D. F. "The Role of Essential Fatty Acids and Prostaglandins in the Premenstrual Syndrome," *Journal of Reproductive Medicine* 23 (1983), pp. 465–68. See also Ockerman, P. A., et al. "Evening Primrose Oil as a Treatment of the Premenstrual Syndrome," *Recent Advances in Clinical Nutrition* 2 (1986), pp. 404–5.

3. Wright, S. "Atopic Dermatitis and Essential Fatty Acids," *Acta Dermato-Venereologica* (Stockholm) suppl. 114 (1985), pp. 143–45.

4. Manthorpe, R., et al. "Primary Sjogren's Syndrome Treated with Efanol/Efavit. A Double-Blind Cross-Over Investigation," *Rheumatology International* 4 (1984), pp. 165–67.

5. Manko, M. S., et al. "Reduced Levels of Prostaglandin Precursors in the Blood of Atopic Patients," *Prostaglandin Leukotrienes and Medicine* 9:6 (1982), pp. 615–28. See also Stenius-Aarniala, B., et al. *Annals of Allergy* 55:2 (1985), pp. 490–94.

6. Chaintrevil, J., et al. "Effects of Dietary Gamma-Linolenate Supplementation," *Human Nutrition. Clinical Nutrition* 38 (1984), pp. 121–30. See also Soma, M., et al. "The Effects of Hydrogenated Coconut Oil, Safflower Oil, and Evening Primrose Oil on Development of Hypertension and Sodium Handling in Spontaneously Hypertensive Rats," *Canadian Journal of Physiology and Pharmacology* 63 (1985), pp. 325–30.

7. Glen, E., et al. "Possible Pharmacological Approaches," in Edwards, C., and Littleton, J., eds., *Pharmacological Treatments for Alcoholism* (London, 1984), pp. 331–40.

8. Pye, J. K., et al. "Clinical Experience of Drug Treatments for Mastalgia," *Lancet* 2 (1985), pp. 373–77.

9. Belch, J. J. F., et al. "Evening Primrose Oil (Efanol) in the Treatment of Raynaud's Phenomenon: A Double-Blind Study," *Thrombosis and Haemostasis* 54 (1985), pp. 490–94.

10. Jamal, G. A., et al. "Gamma-Linolenic Acid in Diabetic Neuropathy," *Lancet* 1 (1986), p. 1098.

11. Ansell, D., et al. "The Effect of Efaniol and Efaniol Marine on Patients with Rheumatoid Arthritis," Florence, Italy, 6th International Congress on Prostaglandins, June 3, 1986.

12. Field, E. J., and Joyce, G. "Multiple Sclerosis: Effect of Gamma-Linolenate Administration," *European Neurology* 22 (1983), pp. 75–83.

13. Zurier, R. B., et al. "Prostaglandin E$_1$ Treatment of NZB/W Mice, I," *Arthritis and Rheumatism* (1977), pp. 723–28.

14. Strong, A. M. M., et al. "The Effect of Oral Linoleic Acid and Gamma-Linoleic Acid," *British Journal of Clinical Practice* (November/December 1985), p. 444.

15. Colquhoun, V., and Bunday, S. "A Lack of Essential Fatty Acids as a Possible Cause for Hyperactivity in Children," *Medical Hypotheses* 7 (1981), pp. 681–86. See also Critchley, E. M. R. "Evening Primrose Oil in Parkinsonian and Other Tremors," in Horrobin, D. F., ed., *Clinical Uses of Essential Fatty Acids* (Montreal, 1982), pp. 205–8.

16. van der Merwe, C. F. "The Reversibility of Cancer," *South African Medical Journal* 65 (1984), p. 712.

17. Kremer, J. M., et al. "Effects of Manipulation of Dietary Fatty Acid on Clinical Manifestations of Rheumatoid Arthritis," *Lancet* 1 (1985), pp. 184–87. See also Sperling, R. I.: Reported in *Medical World News*, July 14, 1986.

18. Lee, T. H., and Arin, J. P. "Prospects for Modifying the Allergic Response by Fish Oil Diets," *Clinical Allergy* 16:2 (1986), pp. 89–100.

19. French, J. M. "MaxEPA in Multiple Sclerosis," *British Journal of Clinical Practice* symp. suppl. 31 (1984), pp. 117–21.

20. Nestel, P. *American Journal of Clinical Nutrition* 43 (1986), pp. 752–57. See also Phillipson, B. E., et al. "Reduction of Plasma Lipids, Lipoproteins, and Apoproteins by Dietary Fish Oils in Patients with Hypertriglyceridemia," *New England Journal of Medicine* 312 (1985), pp. 1210–16.

21. Nieper, Hans. "Capillarographic Criteria on the Effect of Magnesium Orotate EPL Substances and Clofibrate on the Elasticity of Blood Vessels," *Agressologie* 15:1 (1974), pp. 73–77.

22. Gaby, A. R. "Aspartic Acid Salts and Fatigue," *Current Nutritional Therapeutics*, November 1982.

23. Azuma, J., et al. "Beneficial Effect of Taurine on Congestive Heart Failure," *Research Communications in Chemical Pathology and Pharmacology* 435 (1984), p. 261.

24. Chazov, E. L., et al. "Taurine and Electrical Activity of the Heart," *Circulation Research* 35:5, suppl. III (1974), pp. 11–21.

25. Mantovani, J., et al. "Effects of Taurine on Seizures and Growth Hormone Release in Epileptic Patients," *Archives of Neurology* 35 (1979), p. 672.

26. Tripp, M. E., et al. "Systemic Carnitine Deficiency Presenting as Familial Endocardial Fibroelastosis: A Treatable Cardiomyopathy," *New England Journal of Medicine* 305 (1982), p. 385.

27. DiPalma, J. R., et al. "Cardiovascular and Antiarrhythmic Effects of Carnitine," *Archives Internationales de Pharmacodynamie et de Therapie* 217 (1975), pp. 246–50.

28. Cherchi, A., et al. "Effects of L-Carnitine on Exercise Tolerance in

Chronic, Stable Angina," *International Journal of Clinical Pharmacology, Therapy, and Toxicology* 23:10 (1985), pp. 569–72. See also Ferrari, R., et al. "The Metabolical Effects of L-Carnitine in Angina Pectoris," *International Journal of Cardiology* 5 (1984), p. 213. Also: Kosolcharoen, P., et al. "Improved Exercise Tolerance After Administration of Carnitine," *Current Therapeutic Research* (November 1981), pp. 753–64.

29. Abdel-Aziz, M. T., et al. "Effect of Carnitine on Blood Lipid Pattern in Diabetic Patients," *Nutritional Reports International* 29 (1984), p. 1071. See also Bougneres, P. F., et al. *Lancet* (June 1979), pp. 1401–2.

30. Nieper, Hans. *Revolution in Technology, Medicine & Society* (MIT Verlag, 1985), p. 235.

31. Ibid., p. 249.

32. Bliznakov, E. G., and Hunt, G. *The Miracle Nutrient Coenzyme Q10* (New York: Bantam Books, 1986).

33. Folkers, K., ed. *Biomedical and Clinical Aspects of Coenzyme Q* (Amsterdam: Elsevier Science Publishers, 1984), pp. 252–62.

34. Kamikawa, T., et al. "Effects of Coenzyme Q10 on Exercise Tolerance in Chronic Stable Angina Pectoris," *American Journal of Cardiology* 56 (1985), p. 247. See also Folkers, op. cit., p. 247.

35. Kishi, T., et al. "Bioenergetics in Clinical Medicine," *Journal of Medicine* 7 (1976), p. 307.

36. Shigeta, Y., et al. "Effect of Coenzyme Q7 Treatment," *Journal of Vitaminology* 12 (1966), p. 293.

37. Mortensen, S. A., et al. "Long-Term Coenzyme Q10 Therapy," *Drugs Exp. Clin. Res.* 11:8 (1985), pp. 581–93.

38. Fugioka, T., et al. "Antiarrhythmic Action of Coenzyme Q10 in Diabetics," *Tohoku Journal of Experimental Medicine* 141: suppl. (1983), pp. 453–63.

39. Folkers, K., et al. "Effective Therapy of Cardiomyopathy with Coenzyme Q10," *Proceedings of the National Academy of Science* 82 (1985), p. 901. See also Judy, W. V., et al., in International Symposium on Coenzyme Q, *Biomedical and Clinical Aspects of Coenzyme Q* 4 (1984), pp. 353–67. Also: Langsjoen, P. H., et al. "Response of Patients in Classes III and IV of Cardiomyopathy to Therapy in a Blind and Crossover Trial with Coenzyme Q10," *Proceedings of the National Academy of Science* 82 (1985), pp. 4240.

40. Middleton, E., Jr., and Drzewiecki, G. "Flavonoid Inhibition of Human Basophil Histamine Release Stimulated by Various Agents," *Biochemical Pharmacology* 33:21 (1984), p. 3333.

41. Prerovsky, et al. *Angiologica* 9:408–14. See also Perce, F., et al.

"Mucosal Mast Cells. Effect of Quercetin and Other Flavonoids on Antigen Induced Histamine Secretion from Rate Intestinal Mast Cells," *Journal of Allergy and Clinical Immunology* 73 (1984), pp. 819–23. Also: Middleton, E., and Drzewiecki, G. "Naturally Occurring Flavonoids and Human Basophil Histamine Release," *International Archives of Allergy and Applied Immunology* 77 (1985), pp. 155–57. Also: Wendt, P., et al. "The Use of Flavonoids as Inhibitors of Histadine Decarboxylase in Gastric Disease, Experimental and Clinical Studies," *Naunyn-Schmiedeberg's Archives of Pharmacology* 313: suppl. 238 (1980), p. 238.

42. Truss, C. O. "Metabolic Abnormalities in Patients with Chronic Candidiasis: The Acetaldehyde Hypothesis," *Journal of Orthomolecular Psychiatry* 13 (1983), p. 66. See also Watanabe, A., et al. "Lowering of Blood Acetaldehyde but Not Ethanol Concentrations by Pantethine Following Alcohol Ingestion: Different Effects in Flushing and Non-flushing Subjects," *Alcoholism — Clinical and Experimental Research* 9 (1985), p. 272.

43. Cattin, L., et al. "Treatment of Hypercholesterolemina with Pantethine and Fenofibrate: An Open Randomized Study on Forty-three Subjects," *Current Therapeutic Research* 38:3 (1985), pp. 386–95. See also "Pantethine Treatment of Hyperlipidemia," *Clinical Therapeutics* 8 (1986), p. 537. Also: Galeone, F., et al. "The Lipid Lowering Effect of Pantethine in Hyperlipidemic Patients: A Clinical Investigation," *Current Therapeutic Research* 34 (1983), pp. 383–90. Also: Maioli, M., et al. "Effect of Pantethine on the Subfractions of HDL in Dislipemic Patients," *Current Therapeutic Research* 35 (1984), p. 307. Also: Angelico, M., et al. "Improvement in Serum Lipid Profile in Hyper-Lipoproteinaemic Patients After Treatment with Pantethine: A Crossover, Double-Blind Trial Versus Placebo," *Current Therapeutic Research* 33 (1983), p. 1091.

44. Prisco, D., et al. "Effect of Pantethine Treatment on Platelet Aggregation and Thromboxane A_2 Production," *Current Therapeutic Rech* 35 (1984), p. 700.

45. Cureton, T. *The Physiologic Effects of Wheat Germ Oil on Humans in Exercise* (Charles C. Thomas, 1972).

46. Snider, S. R. "Octacosanol in Parkinsonism," *Annals of Neurology* 16 (1984), p. 723.

INDEX